Imaging Coronary Arteries

David A. Dowe
Massimo Fioranelli
Paolo Pavone

Editors

Imaging Coronary Arteries

Second edition

In collaboration with
Roberto Leo

With a collection
of clinical cases

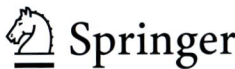

Editors
David A. Dowe
Coronary CTA Program Director
Atlantic Medical Imaging
Galloway, NJ, USA

Massimo Fioranelli
Head of Heart Center
Casa di Cura Mater Dei
Rome, Italy
Scientific Director of the
Centro Studi in Scienze della Vita
"Guglielmo Marconi" University
Rome, Italy

Paolo Pavone
Radiology Department
Casa di Cura Mater Dei
Rome, Italy

ISBN 978-88-470-2681-0   e-ISBN 978-88-470-2682-7 (eBook)
DOI 10.1007/978-88-470-2682-7
Springer Milan Heidelberg New York Dordrecht London

Library of Congress Control Number: 2012951304

© Springer-Verlag Italia 2013
This work is subject to copyright. All rights are reserved by the Publisher, whether the whole or part of the material is concerned, specifically the rights of translation, reprinting, reuse of illustrations, recitation, broadcasting, reproduction on microfilms or in any other physical way, and transmission or information storage and retrieval, electronic adaptation, computer software, or by similar or dissimilar methodology now known or hereafter developed. Exempted from this legal reservation are brief excerpts in connection with reviews or scholarly analysis or material supplied specifically for the purpose of being entered and executed on a computer system, for exclusive use by the purchaser of the work. Duplication of this publication or parts thereof is permitted only under the provisions of the Copyright Law of the Publisher's location, in its current version, and permission for use must always be obtained from Springer. Permissions for use may be obtained through RightsLink at the Copyright Clearance Center. Violations are liable to prosecution under the respective Copyright Law.

The use of general descriptive names, registered names, trademarks, service marks, etc. in this publication does not imply, even in the absence of a specific statement, that such names are exempt from the relevant protective laws and regulations and therefore free for general use.

While the advice and information in this book are believed to be true and accurate at the date of publication, neither the authors nor the editors nor the publisher can accept any legal responsibility for any errors or omissions that may be made. The publisher makes no warranty, express or implied, with respect to the material contained herein.

Cover design: Ikona S.r.l., Milan, Italy
Typesetting: C & G di Cerri e Galassi, Cremona, Italy
Printing and binding: Grafiche Porpora, Segrate (MI), Italy
Printed in Italy

Springer-Verlag Italia S.r.l., Via Decembrio 28, 20137 Milan

Springer is a part of Springer Science+Business Media (www.springer.com)

Preface to the Second Edition

Coronary artery disease (CAD) is one of the leading causes of death in developed countries, yet for many years the prediction of clinical events has been reliant upon methods with substantial drawbacks. Non-invasive, indirect examinations such as Framingham risk factors, thorough clinical examination, EKG and the treadmill test yield valid information but certainly do not provide a safe and complete assessment of the presence of CAD. Even nuclear medicine techniques provide only indirect information on the presence of disease and are not always specific. On the other hand, direct imaging of the coronary arteries using selective coronary angiography, possible since the 1960s, is an invasive procedure that is not well tolerated by patients; this remains true despite progress in catheter and guidewire design and the development of stenting procedures that allow diagnosis and therapy within the same clinical setting.

Coronary CT angiography has been proposed relatively recently as an alternative to selective coronary angiography. Progress in equipment design has transformed what was originally a research tool into a reliable, clinically accepted procedure that is easy to perform. The widely debated issue of X-ray dose has now been partially solved as we have moved from an absolutely unacceptable dose of 25-30 mSv to a routine dose of 3-5 mSv or even 1 mSv. Furthermore, a reduction in the acquisition time has permitted the contrast medium dose to be consistently lowered from 120-150 ml to 40-50 ml. Acceptance of coronary CT angiography continues to grow, although there is still no consensus on its role as a non-invasive diagnostic test in intermediate risk patients.

Looking beyond coronary CT angiography, magnetic resonance angiography (MRA) of the coronary arteries has been the subject of considerable clinical research but has not yet entered general clinical practice despite advances on various fronts. A further significant advance is the use of techniques that allow imaging of the coronary arterial walls during selective coronary angiography (intravascular ultrasound, IVUS, and optical coherence tomography, OCT); this approach is improving our understanding of CAD and providing better evidence of the type of vascular wall involvement.

This new edition of Imaging Coronary Arteries fully reflects the latest advances in coronary CT angiography and includes extensively revised or entirely new chapters on IVUS, catheter angiography and OCT as well as discussion of the role of nuclear imaging and MRA. A further very significant new feature is the inclusion of 74 clinical cases that will serve to illustrate the wide range of clinical cases encountered in daily practice and to demonstrate the utmost importance of correlation of clinical and imaging findings.

The editors would like to express their gratitude to all who have been involved in the preparation of this edition, which will without doubt be of great interest to radiologists, cardiologists, CT technologists and others. Special thanks are due to Dr. Marco Rengo, Dr. Carlo Nicola De Cecco, Dr. Davide Bellini, Dr. Damiano Caruso and Dr. Marco Maria Maceroni for their support in the preparation of the updated chapters 2, 3, 4, 8 and 9.

November 2012

David A. Dowe
Massimo Fioranelli
Paolo Pavone

Preface to the First Edition

Coronary CT angiography (CTA) is rapidly changing the patient-care algorithms used to detect coronary artery disease, as well as the approach we take in risk-factor assessment and in the triage of patients. The rapid adoption of coronary CTA into clinical practice has been fueled by significant yearly advances in CT technology, which have improved the spatial and temporal resolution of this technique while simultaneously decreasing radiation exposure.

The growing utilization of coronary CTA has created a need for comprehensive didactic texts that explain the numerous applications of this new technology with respect to the pathophysiology of coronary artery disease, while also providing information on the approach to patients who have undergone previous bypass surgery or percutaneous coronary intervention. I believe this book accomplishes both of these goals, and does so in a reader-friendly format. The image quality of the many figures that accompany each chapter is excellent and reflects the use of state of the art technology. The techniques described for plaque detection and characterization represent the current thinking pervasive in the coronary CTA community. The comprehensive reference list at the end of the book offers the reader a wealth of resources for further study.

There is no doubt that this book will be popular with radiologists, cardiologists, CT technologists and anyone else seeking to acquire a comprehensive understanding of coronary artery disease and its depiction using coronary CTA.

Galloway, October 2008　　　　　　　　　　　　　　　　David A. Dowe, MD

Contents

1   **Clinical Anatomy of the Coronary Circulation** 1
Massimo Fioranelli, Carlo Gonnella, Stefano Tonioni,
Fabrizio D'Errico and Mariantonietta Carbone

2   **Basic Techniques in the Acquisition of Cardiac Images
with CT** 13
Paolo Pavone

3   **CT Examination of the Coronary Arteries** 21
Paolo Pavone

4   **Image Reconstruction** 29
Paolo Pavone

5   **Coronary Pathophysiology** 41
Mara Piccoli, Serafino Orazi, Giovanna Giubilato
and Massimo Fioranelli

6   **Clinical Classification of Coronary Artery Disease:
Who Should Be Treated?** 47
Damien Casagrande, Jean-Jacques Goy, Mario Togni,
Jean Christophe Stauffer and Stéphane Cook

7   **Intravascular Ultrasound: From Gray-Scale
to Virtual Histology** 53
Giuseppe M. Sangiorgi, Luigi Politi, Chiara Leuzzi,
Luigi Mattioli, Fabiana Rollini and Massimo Fioranelli

8   **Identification and Characterization of the Atherosclerotic
Plaque Using Coronary CT Angiography** 63
Paolo Pavone, David A. Dowe and Roberto Leo

9   **Coronary CT Angiography: Evaluation of Stenosis
and Occlusion** 71
Paolo Pavone and Roberto Leo

10	**Current Strategies in Cardiac Surgery** 85
	Andrea Montalto and Francesco Musumeci

11	**Coronary CT Angiography: Evaluation of Coronary Artery Bypass Grafts** 91
	Carlo Nicola De Cecco, Gorka Bastarrika and Marco Rengo

12	**Coronary Stents** 101
	Enrica Mariano, Giuseppe M. Sangiorgi and Massimo Fioranelli

13	**CT Angiography of Coronary Stents** 115
	Gorka Bastarrika, Carlo Nicola De Cecco and U. Joseph Schoepf

14	**X-Ray Exposure in Coronary CT Angiography** 131
	Paolo Pavone and Roberto Leo

15	**Optical Coherence Tomography in the Cathlab** 137
	Francesco Prati and Luca Di Vito

16	**Triple Rule Out: the Use of Cardiac CT in the Emergency Room** 147
	Giulio Speciale and Vincenzo Pasceri

17	**Contraindications to Coronary CT Angiography** 153
	David A. Dowe

18	**Prognostic Value of Coronary CT** 157
	Bruno Pironi, Antonio Lucifero and Massimo Fioranelli

19	**Clinical Cases** 165
	David A. Dowe, Paolo Pavone and Massimo Fioranelli

Index 259

Contributors

Gorka Bastarrika Cardiothoracic Imaging Division, Department of Medical Imaging, Sunnybrook Health Sciences Centre, Toronto, Canada

Mariantonietta Carbone Interventional Cardiovascular Unit, San Carlo Hospital, Rome, Italy

Damien Casagrande Cardiology Service, Hôpital Cantonal, Fribourg, Switzerland

Stéphane Cook Cardiology Service, Hôpital Cantonal, Fribourg, Switzerland

Carlo Nicola De Cecco Department of Radiological Sciences, Oncology and Pathology, University of Rome "La Sapienza" Polo Pontino, Latina, Italy

Fabrizio D'Errico Interventional Cardiovascular Unit, San Carlo Hospital, Rome, Italy

Luca Di Vito CLI Foundation, Centro per la Lotta contro l'Infarto, Rome, Italy

David A. Dowe Coronary CTA Program Director, Atlantic Medical Imaging, Galloway, NJ, USA

Massimo Fioranelli Head of Heart Center, Casa di Cura Mater Dei, Rome, Italy. Scientific Director of the Centro Studi in Scienze della Vita, "Guglielmo Marconi" University, Rome, Italy

Giovanna Giubilato Heart Center, Casa di Cura Mater Dei, Rome, Italy

Carlo Gonnella Cardiology Department, "San Carlo di Nancy" Hospital, Rome, Italy

Jean-Jacques Goy Cardiology Service, Hôpital Cantonal, Fribourg, Switzerland

Roberto Leo Internal Medicine, University of Rome Tor Vergata, Rome, Italy

Chiara Leuzzi Interventional Cardiology, Policlinico Universitario, Modena, Italy

Antonio Lucifero Heart Center, Casa di Cura Mater Dei, Rome, Italy

Enrica Mariano Interventional Cardiology Unit, "Tor Vergata" University, Rome, Italy

Luigi Mattioli Department of Cardiology, Cardiac Cath Lab, "Tor Vergata" University, Rome, Italy

Andrea Montalto Department of Cardiac Surgery and Transplantation, San Camillo Hospital, Rome, Italy

Francesco Musumeci Department of Cardiac Surgery and Transplantation, San Camillo Hospital, Rome, Italy

Serafino Orazi Head of Cardiology Department, Ospedale Civile di Rieti, Rieti, Italy

Vincenzo Pasceri Interventional Cardiology, San Filippo Neri Hospital, Rome, Italy

Paolo Pavone Radiology Department, Casa di Cura Mater Dei, Rome, Italy

Mara Piccoli Cardiology Unit, Policlinico "Luigi di Liegro", Rome, Italy

Bruno Pironi Interventional Cardiology, "M.G. Vannini" Hospital, Rome, Italy

Luigi Politi Interventional Cardiology, Policlinico Universitario, Modena, Italy

Francesco Prati Interventional Cardiology, San Giovanni Hospital, Rome, Italy

Marco Rengo Department of Radiological Sciences, Oncology and Pathology, University of Rome "La Sapienza" Polo Pontino, Latina, Italy

Fabiana Rollini Interventional Cardiology, Policlinico Universitario, Modena, Italy

Giuseppe M. Sangiorgi Interventional Cardiology, University of Roma Tor Vergata, Policlinico Casilino, Rome, Italy

U. Joseph Schoepf Department of Radiology and Radiological Science, Division of Cardiology, Department of Medicine, Medical University of South Carolina, Charleston, South Carolina, USA

Giulio Speciale Chief Interventional Cardiology, San Filippo Neri Hospital, Rome, Italy

Jean Christophe Stauffer Cardiology Service, Hôpital Cantonal, Fribourg, Switzerland

Mario Togni Cardiology Service, Hôpital Cantonal, Fribourg, Switzerland

Stefano Tonioni Cardiology Department, "San Carlo di Nancy" Hospital, Rome, Italy

Clinical Anatomy of the Coronary Circulation

Massimo Fioranelli, Carlo Gonnella, Stefano Tonioni, Fabrizio D'Errico and Mariantonietta Carbone

1.1 Introduction

The classification of the American Heart Association, which divides the coronary arteries into 15–16 segments, is often used in the evaluation of the coronary anatomy with multi-slice computed tomography (Fig. 1.1) [1-5]. In this chapter, a more complex classification is used, as it provides a more detailed anatomic picture. We begin with a brief review of the coronary anatomy.

The right coronary artery (RCA) takes origin from the right aortic sinus of Valsalva and then divides to form two terminal branches, the posterior descending artery (PDA) and the posterolateral (PLV) branches. Along its course, the RCA gives off several branches: the sinus node artery, right ventricular (RV) branches, acute marginal (AM) branch, and the atrioventricular node artery.

The left coronary artery (LCA) arises from the left aortic sinus of Valsalva; the left main (LM) branch of the LCA ends in a bifurcation, giving rise to the left anterior descending artery (LAD) and the left circumflex artery (LCx). Sometimes a third ramus intermedius is present between these two branches.

The LAD gives off septal (SP) and diagonal (DIAG) branches and ends at the apex of the heart, sometimes reaching the posterior interventricular groove. The LCx has two or three obtuse marginal branches (OM), before either terminating or, in the case of left-dominant or balanced circulation, giving off a posterolateral branch or ending in the posterior atrioventricular groove.

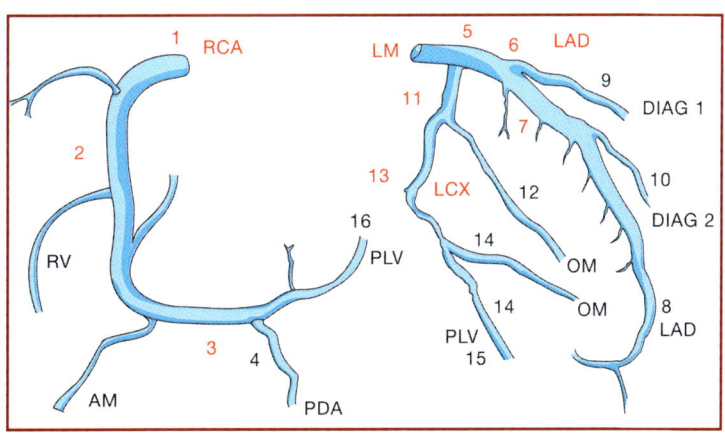

Fig. 1.1 Classification of the American Heart Association. *RC* right coronary artery, *RV* right ventricular branch, *AM* acute marginal branch, *PLV* posterolateral ventricular branch, *PDA* posterior descending artery, *LCA* left coronary artery, *LM* left main artery, *LAD* left anterior descending artery, *DIAG 1* first diagonal branch, *DIAG 2* second diagonal branch, *LCx* left circumflex artery, *OM* obtuse marginal branches

C. Gonnella (✉)
Cardiology Department
"San Carlo di Nancy" Hospital, Rome, Italy
e-mail: carlo.gonnella@tiscali.it

1.2 Angiographic Anatomy of the Coronary Circulation

The classification proposed in the Bypass Angioplasty Revascularization Investigation (BARI) trial reported by Alderman and Stadius (1992) divides the coronary arteries into 29 segments (Fig. 1.2).

The coronary trees have two principal components: the *subepicardial system* consists of the arteries and veins that course and ramify on the surface of the heart; the *intramyocardial system* comprises their perforating branches.

The subepicardial system is formed by the right and left coronary arteries, arising from the right and left aortic sinus of Valsalva, respectively. The RCA is divided into three segments. The first segment (BARI 1) extends from the coronary ostium to the first RV branch; if the latter is not present, the segment is usually identified between the ostium and the acute margin of the heart. The second segment (BARI 2) extends from the first RV branch to the acute margin of the heart, which usually coincides with the origin of the AM branch (BARI 10). This vessel is the most constant branch of the RCA and it runs on the surface of the free wall of the right ventricle in the direction of the apex, at an angle proportional to the proximity of its origin. The third segment (BARI 3) begins at the acute margin of the heart and courses to the origin of the PDA (BARI 4), at the level of the crux cordis. At this level, in right-dominant circulation (85% of cases), the RCA divides into two terminal branches, the PDA and PLV branches (BARI 5),

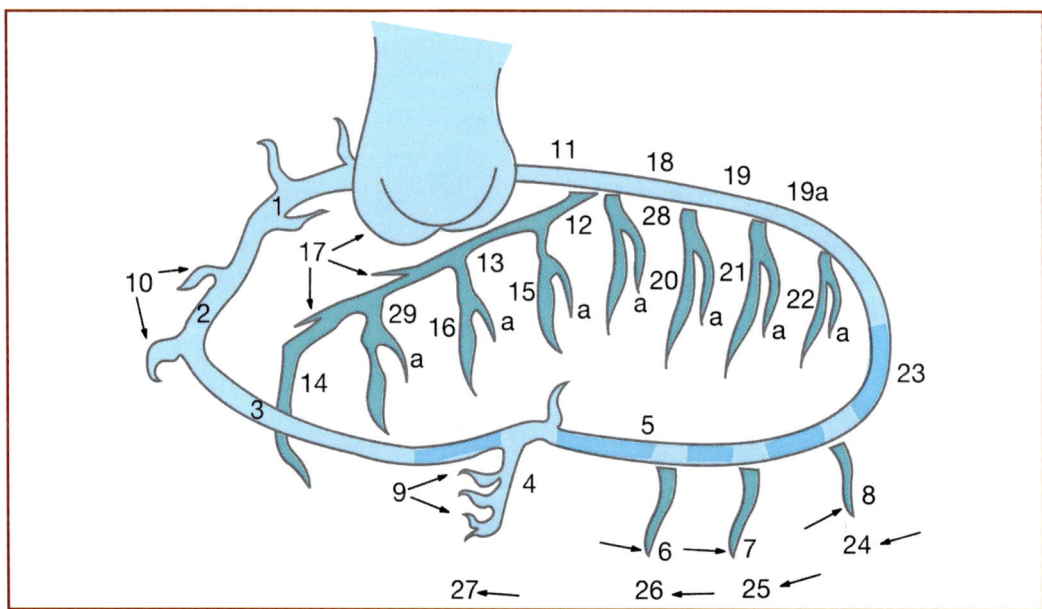

Fig. 1.2 Classification of the BARI Study Group: The coronary arteries are divided into 29 segments: *1* Proximal segment of the right coronary artery (RCA), *2* middle segment of the RCA, *3* distal segment of the RCA, *4* posterior descending artery (PDA), *5* posterolateral branch of the RCA (PLV), *6* first posterolateral branch of the RCA, *7* second posterolateral branch of the RCA, *8* third posterolateral branch of the RCA, *9* inferior septal branches, *10* acute marginal branches of the RCA, *11* left main of the left coronary artery (LM), *12* proximal segment of the left anterior descending artery (LAD), *13* middle segment of the LAD, *14* distal segment of the LAD, *15* first diagonal branch (DIAG), *15a* lateral first diagonal branch, *16* second diagonal branch, *16a* lateral second diagonal branch, *17* septal branches of the LAD (SP), *18* proximal segment of the left circumflex artery (LCx), *19* middle segment of the LCx, *19a* distal segment of the LCx, *20* first obtuse marginal branch (OM), *20a* lateral first obtuse marginal branch, *21* second obtuse marginal branch, *21a* lateral second obtuse marginal branch, *22* third obtuse marginal branch, *22a* lateral third obtuse marginal branch, *23* LCx continuing as the left atrioventricular branch, *24* first left posterolateral branch, *25* second left posterolateral branch, *26* third left posterolateral branch, *27* left posterior descending artery (PD) (in left-dominant circulation), *28* ramus intermedius, *28a* lateral ramus intermedius, *29* third diagonal branch, *29a* lateral third diagonal branch

perfusing the diaphragmatic wall of the left ventricle. In the remaining 15% of cases, the circulation may be left-dominant or balanced: in left-dominant circulation, the PLV and PDA originate from the LCx; in balanced circulation, the PDA originates from the RCA, and the PLV from the LCx.

The concept of dominance is defined by the relationship between the RCA and LCx, according to the origin of the PDA and in relation to the arterial supply of the inferior wall of the left ventricle, but independent of the extent of the circulatory system.

The PDA, also called the posterior interventricular branch, with its septal branches (BARI 9), is the most important branch of the RCA; it courses in the homonymous groove without reaching the apex of the heart, which is usually supplied by the recurrent branch of the LAD. The PLV immediately originates after the PDA, at the level of the crux cordis. It courses along the posterior atrioventricular sulcus, branching with its collateral vessels (BARI 6–8) at the diaphragmatic and inferioposterior walls of the left ventricle.

The RCA furnishes smaller branches such as the conus artery, sinus node artery, RV branches, and atrioventricular node artery (Fig. 1.3). The conus artery is the first vessel originating from the RCA. In 40% of the cases it directly originates from the right aortic sinus or from the aorta. The sinus node artery arises from the RCA (two-thirds of the cases); in 25% of cases, it may originate from the LCx, while in 10% the two vessels arise from both coronary arteries. The RV branches originate in the second segment of the RCA and run along the surface of the RV, anterior to the interventricular groove. The number of these branches varies greatly and is inversely proportional to the diameter of such vessels. In nearly all of the cases of right-dominant circulation and in 75% of the cases of balanced circulation, the atrioventricular node artery arises at the end of the third segment of the RCA. Its location is important in the angiographic identification of the crux cordis. In individuals with left-dominant circulation, it originates from the distal segment of the LCx. At the level of Koch's triangle is the subendocardial artery, situated between the septal cuspid of the tricuspid valve and the coronary sinus; it furnishes branches to the posterior interventricular septum and the atrioventricular node.

The LCA arises from the left aortic sinus, at a higher level than the RCA, and is divided into

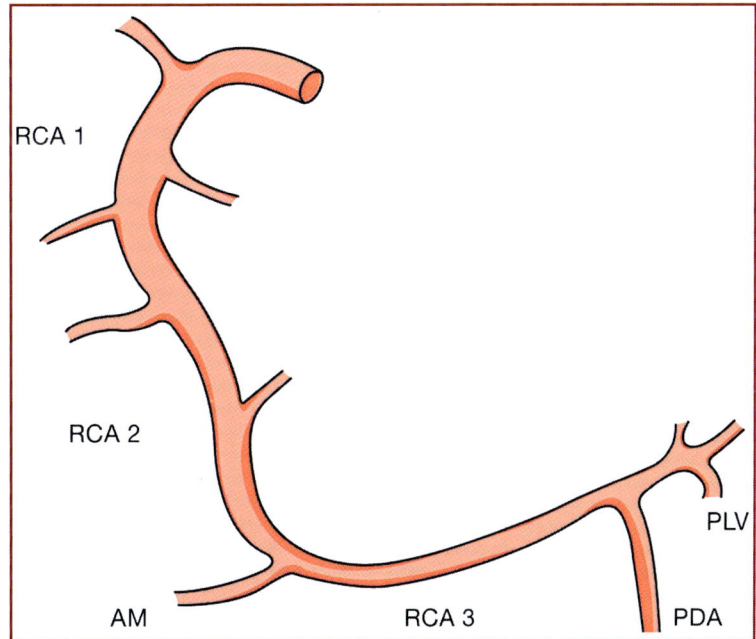

Fig. 1.3 Right coronary artery in left anterior oblique (LAO) view. *RCA* Right coronary artery (segments 1–3), *AM* acute marginal branch, *PLV* posterolateral branch, *PDA* posterior descending artery

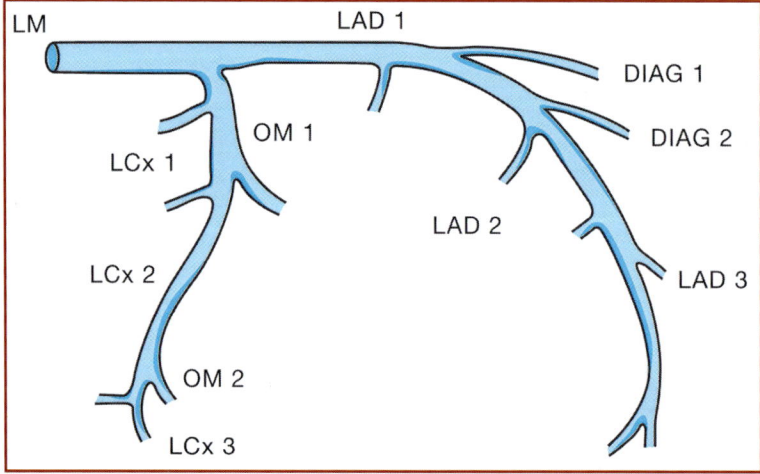

Fig. 1.4 Left coronary artery in caudal right anterior oblique (RAO) view. *LM* Left main artery, *LAD* left anterior descending artery (segments 1–3), *DIAG 1* first diagonal branch, *DIAG 2* second diagonal branch, *LCx* left circumflex artery (segments 1–3), *OM 1* first obtuse marginal branch, *OM 2* second obtuse marginal branch

three segments (Fig. 1.4). The LM branch of the LCA (BARI 11), also called the left main coronary artery (LMCA), extends for a varying length (generally 2 cm, diameter 3–6 mm) from the ostium to the bifurcation of the LAD and LCx. In 30–37% of the cases, the LM artery gives off three branches, one of which, the ramus intermedius (BARI 28), runs toward the apex and supplies the anterolateral wall of the left ventricle.

The LAD is the most constant, in origin and distribution, among all the coronary vessels. It originates from the LM artery and runs in the anterior interventricular groove to the apex of the heart. In 70% of the cases, the LAD extends up to the posterior interventricular groove such that it furnishes branches for perfusion of the inferior interventricular septum and the apex; otherwise, these arise along the length of the PDA. The first segment of the LAD (BARI 12) runs from the bifurcation of the LM artery to the origin of the first septal branch (SP, BARI 17). The second segment (BARI 13) extends from the origin of the first SP to the origin of the third septal or second DIAG branch. The third segment (BARI 14) ends at the apex, surrounding and sometimes traveling up to the posterior wall. When the third SP or second DIAG branch is not identified, the end of the second segment of the LAD is conventionally defined as the half-length between the first SP and the apex. The LAD furnishes branches for the anterior interventricular septum and the anterolateral wall of the left ventricle. There are generally three SP branches and they originate at right angles from the LAD.

The first SP branch is constant in its origin and course; thus, it is important to identify its passage between the proximal and middle segments of the LAD. Some segments may run intramyocardially but generally they develop caudally, along the interventricular septum, and supply the proximal two-thirds of the anterior septum. The second and third SP branches are more variable, with narrow diameters; they supply the distal third of the anterior septum. There are usually three DIAG branches (BARI 15, 16–29), each of which originates at an acute angle from the LAD; their pathway is to the anterolateral wall of the left ventricle. The diameter of these vessels is inversely proportional to the number of branches.

The LCx develops from the LM artery and runs in the posterior atrioventricular groove; after a short tract under the left atrium, it continues in the left posterior atrioventricular groove and contacts the mitral annulus. The LCx splits into three segments. The first (BARI 18) extends from the origin to the first marginal branch (OM, BARI 20). If the first OM is absent or not clearly identifiable, the zone of transition among the first and second segments is conventionally identified by a point corresponding to the half-length between the origin of the LCx and the origin of the second OM (BARI 21). The second segment (BARI 19) runs from the origin of the first OM to

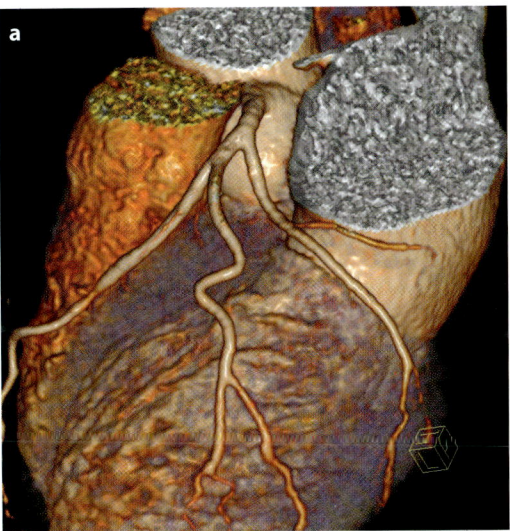 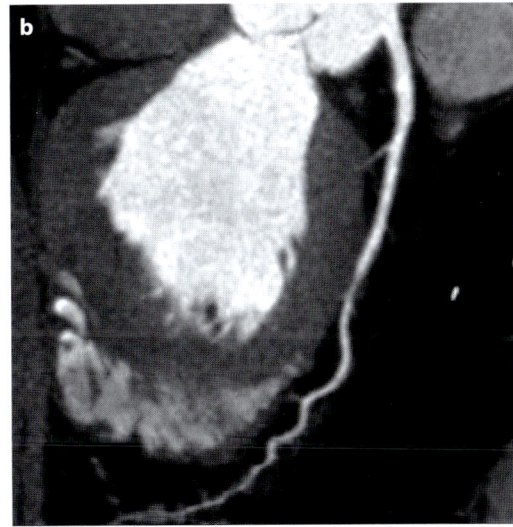

Fig. 1.5a, b Myocardial bridging of the left anterior descending artery reduces the arterial diameter

the origin of the second OM. If the second marginal branch is absent, the zone of transition is defined by the half-length between the origin of the first OM and the point where the circumflex artery terminates. The third segment (BARI 19a), in right-dominant circulation, extends from the origin of the second OM to the termination point of the vessel; in left-dominant or balanced circulation, to the point of origin of the left ventricular branch or the posterolateral branch in the posterior atrioventricular groove (BARI 23). In left-dominant circulation, the LCx gives rise to the left ventricular branch or PLV, with its side branches (BARI 24–26) and to the PDA (BARI 27), with its septal branches (BARI 9).

The LCx gives rise to the sinus node artery, left atrial branch, and marginal branches. In 25% of the cases, the sinus node artery arises from the proximal segment of the LCx, near the ostium. The atrial branch originates at the end of the proximal segment and runs to the inferoposterior wall of the left atrium. Of the three OM branches, the first one is usually larger and constant; it terminates on the posterolateral wall of the left ventricle toward the apex. Its development is inversely proportional both to the extent of the RCA on the posterolateral surface of the left ventricle and to the number and development of the diagonal branches of the LAD.

1.3 Intramyocardial Vascularization and the Venous Circulation

After oxygen and nutritional substrates have been extracted by the myocardium, a portion of the desaturated blood is transported directly into the ventricles through the Thebesian veins. Nevertheless, most of the blood, through the venules and myocardial veins, goes to the epicardial veins, which drain in the coronary sinus, located in the inferoposterior region of the right atrium.

The epicardial arteries are muscular vessels with a wall thickness of about 100 µm; they are made up of three overlapping layers: intima, media, and adventitia. These arteries, which transport oxygenated blood to the arteries, arterioles, and capillaries, traverse the surface of the heart covered by epicardium or sometimes by subepicardial adipose tissue. Muscular bridges of variable length, in which the epicardial vessels become intramyocardial, are present in 5–22% of the cases at the anterior LAD and in 86% in the other coronary arteries (Fig. 1.5).

Normal embryological development of the coronary circulation involves the formation of collateral vessels that link the different sections of the arterial circulation. The collateral circulation consists of four types of vessels: intramyocardial vessels originating from the same vessel (intracoronary

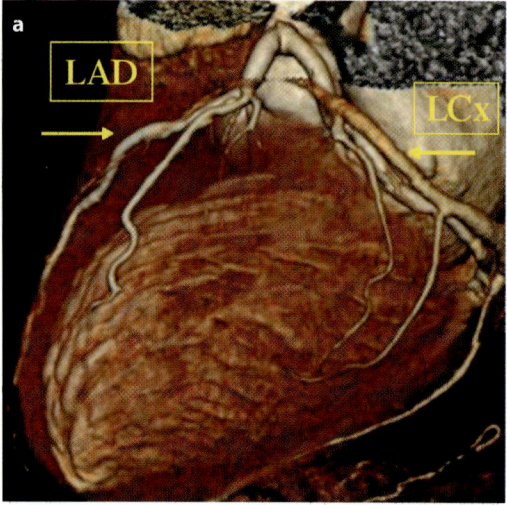 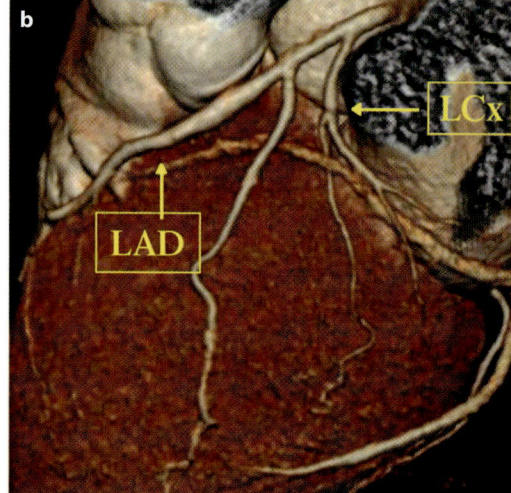

Fig. 1.6 a Hypertrophic left circumflex artery (*LCx*). **b** Hypoplastic LCx. *LAD* Left anterior descending artery

circulation), intramyocardial vessels originating from two or more coronary arteries (intercoronary circulation), atrial vessels connecting with the vasa vasorum of the aorta or other arteries (extracardiac circulation), and intramyocardial vessels that directly communicate with the ventricles (arteriolar luminal circulation). In the normal adult myocardium, the collateral circulation consists of small-caliber vessels (< 50 m in diameter) that contribute only marginally to coronary flow. In the presence of obstruction or myocardial ischemia, the diameter of the collateral vessels expands to 200–600 μm; the growth of a medial layer allows a significant quantity of blood flow. The development of collaterals results in the formation of connections among proximal and distal segments of a vessel crossing a stenosis.

1.4 Variability of the Coronary Artery Circulation

The native coronary artery circulation is highly variable. This is in contrast to other arterial vascular districts, which have a constant, readily identifiable anatomy, such as the carotid or iliac-femoral arteries, where, except for differences of caliber, the morphology, origin, and anatomic course are the same between individuals. Variations in the coronary arteries include the type of dominance, differences in caliber, and alternative branch morphologies. This aspect of the coronary circulation must be kept in mind during diagnostic evaluation of the arteries, to avoid considering an artery that is small and poorly developed as a stenosis.

The variability of the coronary circulation is such that two patients rarely have the same coronary vascular anatomy. In this context, the use of terminology such as "strongly developed branch" or "hypoplastic vessel" identifies the development of the vessel but does not denote the presence or absence of atherosclerotic lesions. For example, in some patients, the course and caliber of the LCx are highly developed, while in others the artery may be small and perfuses only a small portion of the myocardium. These differences are compensated for by the development of other vessels, which balance the perfusion of a myocardial region by a hypoplastic artery perfusion. The morphology of an artery and the extent of the territory it perfuses are very important considerations in therapeutic planning. The larger the myocardial region perfused by an artery, the greater the justification for a myocardial revascularization procedure in the presence of a critical stenosis.

As shown in Figure 1.6, there are some cases in which the LAD is more developed than the LCx, but in other situations the LCx is more developed and perfuses the largest part of the left ventricle. The caliber of the branches originating from these

1 Clinical Anatomy of the Coronary Circulation

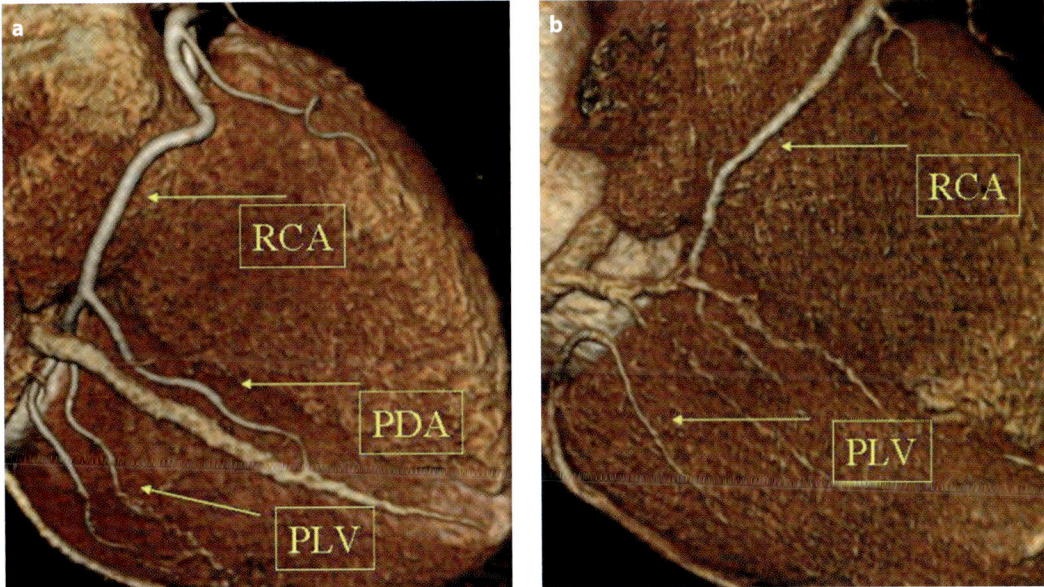

Fig. 1.7 a Right-dominant circulation. **b** Balanced circulation. *RCA* Right coronary artery, *PLV* posterolateral branches, *PDA* posterior descending artery

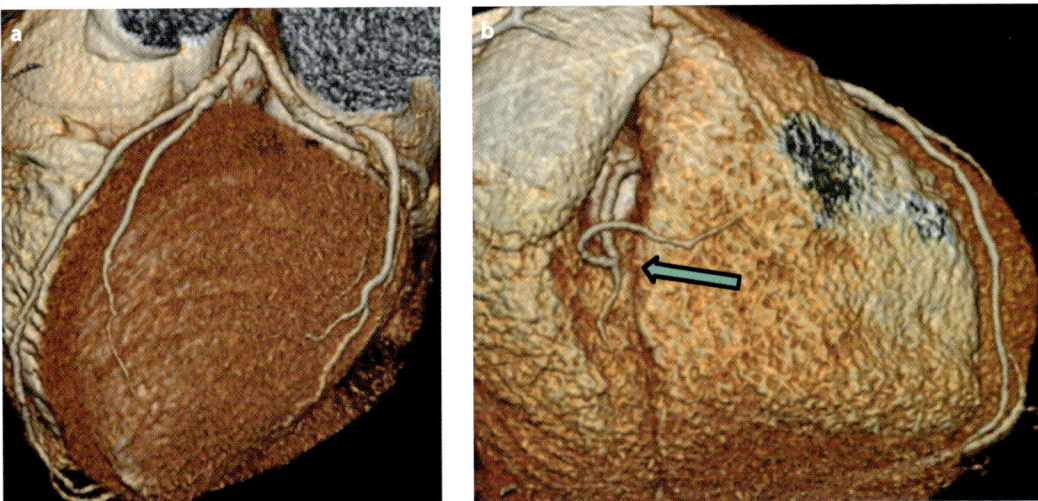

Fig. 1.8 a Left-dominant circulation. The left anterior descending and circumflex arteries are hypertrophic. **b** The right coronary artery (*arrow*) is hypoplastic and branches derive from the acute marginal branch

two arteries depends on the size of the artery from which they derive; that is, the DIAG branches will be of larger caliber than the OM branches when the LAD is more developed than the LCx, while the OM branches will be more developed if the caliber of the LCx is larger.

If the RCA is highly developed, its distal branches (PDA and PLV), in addition to vascularizing the right ventricle, will also perfuse the posterior wall of the left ventricle. In other cases, including right-dominant circulation, the PLV are poorly developed and the great part of the left ventricle is perfused by the LCx (Fig. 1.7).

Finally, the RCA can be hypoplastic, giving rise only to the conus artery after a single AM branch (Fig. 1.8).

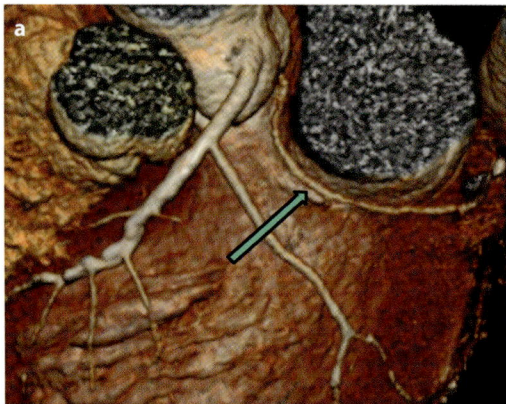 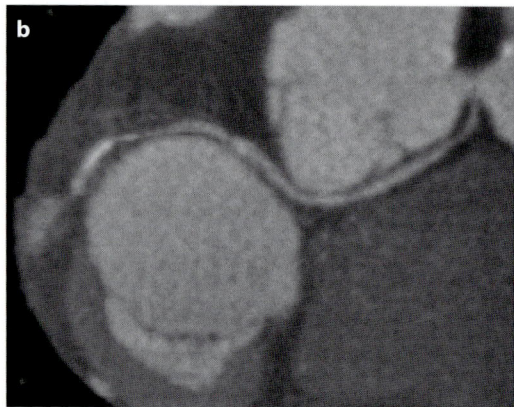

Fig. 1.9 Anomalous origin of the left circumflex artery from the right coronary artery. **a** In 3D view, the anomalous vessel (*arrow*) runs between the aorta and the pulmonary artery. **b** In 2D view, the origin and anomalous and tortuous course of the vessel are visible

These anatomic variations are normal and are not related to ischemic damage.

In the presence of atherosclerotic stenosis in a small vessel, the ischemic portion of the myocardium will be correspondingly small. However, when atherosclerosis develops in a main vessel of greater caliber, especially in the proximal segments, the clinical symptoms will be important and the ischemic area large.

The classical definition of single-, double-, or triple-vessel disease, referring to the number of vessels with critical stenosis, is tightly correlated with the prognosis and with therapeutic planning; nevertheless, the presence of coronary stenosis must be assessed in the context of the global coronary anatomy. Two-vessel coronary disease is similar to three-vessel disease if the third vessel is a hypoplastic or small artery rather than atherosclerotic.

1.5 Anomalous Coronary Arteries

An anomalous coronary artery can be found in 0.64–5.60% of patients who undergo coronary angiography (Fig. 1.9). Some of these variations have no clinical relevance, while others may represent an important pathology.

Separate origins of the RCA and conus artery occur in 40–50% of the cases and a separate origins of the LAD and LCx in 1%. The most important anomaly is a LM artery originating from the right sinus of Valsalva or from the RCA. The course between the pulmonary artery and the aorta can be the cause of vessel compression, and therefore of ischemia and sudden death, during or following physical effort. The same is true when the LAD originates from the RCA or from the right aortic sinus. By contrast, a circumflex artery originating from the RCA has no clinical consequences, because of its posterior course.

Some congenital cardiopathies are often associated with anomalous coronary arteries.

For example, in the tetralogy of Fallot, an anomalous coronary artery is present in 9% of the cases. The most common variation is a great conus artery, an anomalous LAD originating from the RCA or right sinus of Valsalva.

In transposition of the great vessels (D-type), the most frequent (60% of the cases) anomaly is a RCA that originates from the posterior surface of the right aortic sinus and a LAD originating from the posterior surface of the left aortic sinus. In 20% of the cases, the circumflex artery arises from the RCA. In 3–9% of the cases, the RCA arises from the left aortic sinus and the LCA from the right sinus or there is a single coronary artery that takes off from the right or left sinus of Valsalva; an intramyocardial course is frequent.

In the L-type transposition, the coronary arteries can derive from the originating sinus or from

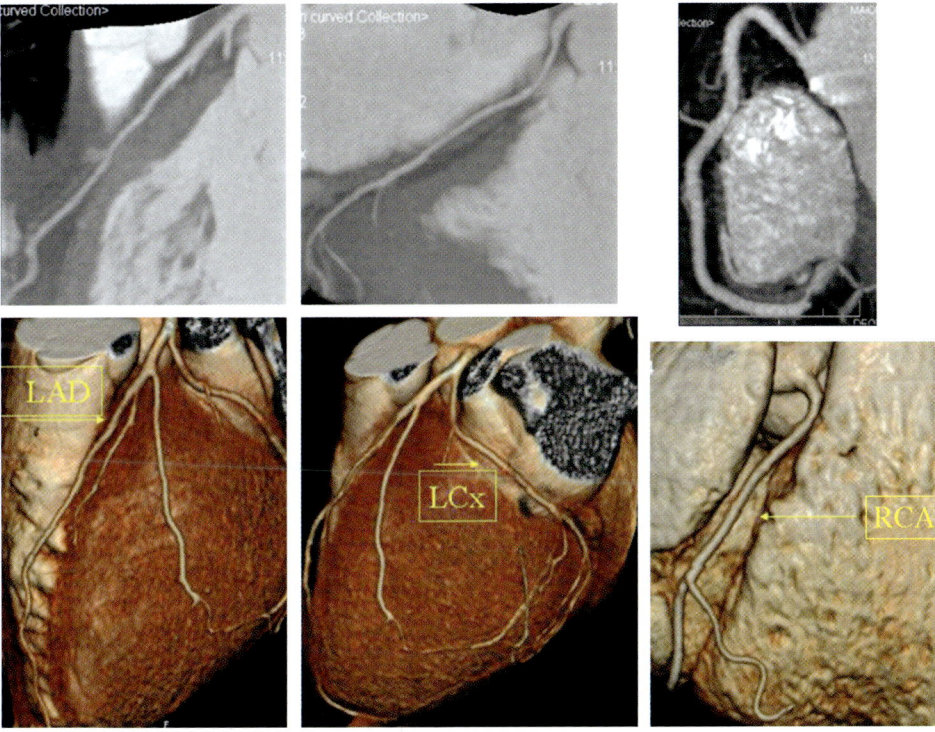

Fig. 1.10 Evaluation of the coronary anatomy with multi-slice computed tomography. *RCA* Right coronary artery, *LAD* left anterior descending artery, *LCx* left circumflex artery

the perfused ventricle. In this case, the RCA perfuses the left ventricle on the right side and divides into the LAD and LCx, and the LCA runs in the interventricular groove similar to the RCA.

The anomaly of one or more coronary arteries arising from the pulmonary artery is seen in 0.4% of patients with congenital cardiopathies.

The most frequent anomalous coronary artery is the LAD originating from the pulmonary artery (Bland-White-Garland syndrome).

Further coronary anomalies are aneurysms and fistulas. Aneurysm is an expansion of the coronary diameter by at least 1.5-fold more than an adjacent segment. Coronary fistulas are communications between the coronary arteries and the cardiac cavities or great vessels: these can be congenital or acquired following thoracic traumas, electrocatheter implantation, endomyocardial biopsies, etc. The most frequent location is the RCA (55%), LCA (35%), or both (5%); in 40% of these patients, the fistula is in the right ventricle, in 26% in the right atrium, and in 17% in the pulmonary artery.

1.6 Factors Determining Coronary Artery Size

Numerous independent factors, including age, sex, body surface area, physical activity, and some pathologies, influence the caliber of the coronary arteries.

For instance, with increasing age there is a reduction of the caliber of the coronary vessels, whereas in patients with myocardial hypertrophy the arteries are of increased caliber.

Generally, in females, the coronary arteries are narrower than in males, probably due to the difference in body surface area. The reduction in the caliber of the coronary arteries that occurs with age has many explanations: firstly, there is a high prevalence of concentric atherosclerosis (not visible with coronary angiography), which causes a homogeneous reduction of the arterial lumen. In most elderly subjects there is also subendothelial and medial hypertrophy. Angiographic examination of

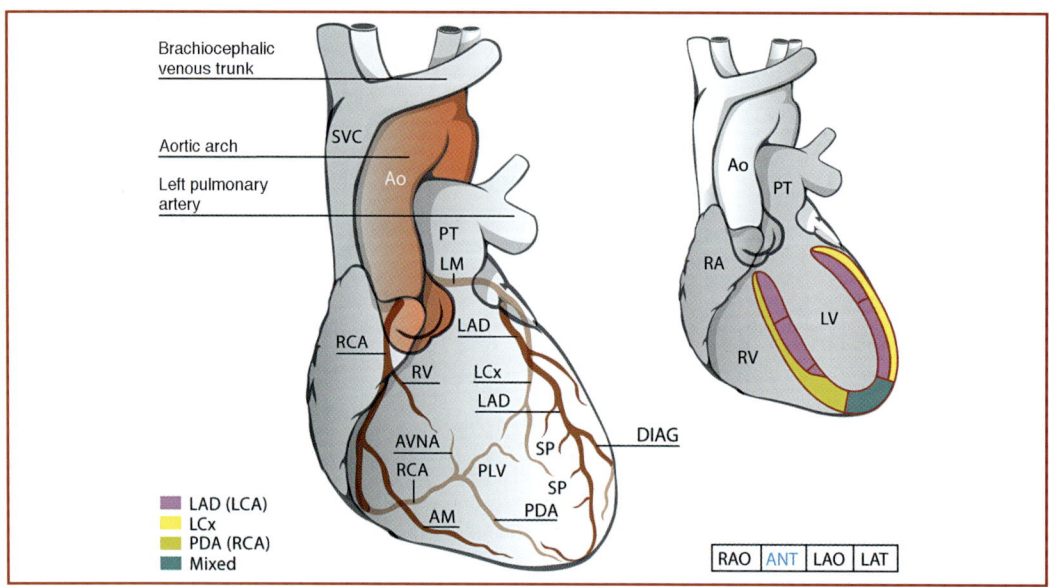

Fig. 1.11 Angiographic evaluation of the coronary circulation; anterior (*ANT*) view. The classification used by the BARI Study Group Investigators is in parentheses. *RCA* Right coronary artery (1), *RVB* right ventricular branches (10), *AM* acute marginal branches (10), *PDA* posterior descending artery (4), *PLV* posterolateral branches (5), *AVNA* atrioventricular nodal artery, *LCA* left coronary artery, *LM* left main artery (11), *LAD* left anterior descending: first segment (12), second segment (13), third segment (14), *SP* septal branches (*17*), *DIAG* diagonal branches (15, 16, 29), *LCx* left circumflex artery: first segment (18), second segment (19), third segment (19a), *OM* obtuse marginal branches (20–22), *Ao* aorta, *LV* left ventricle, *PT* pulmonary trunk, *RA* right atrium, *RV* right ventricle

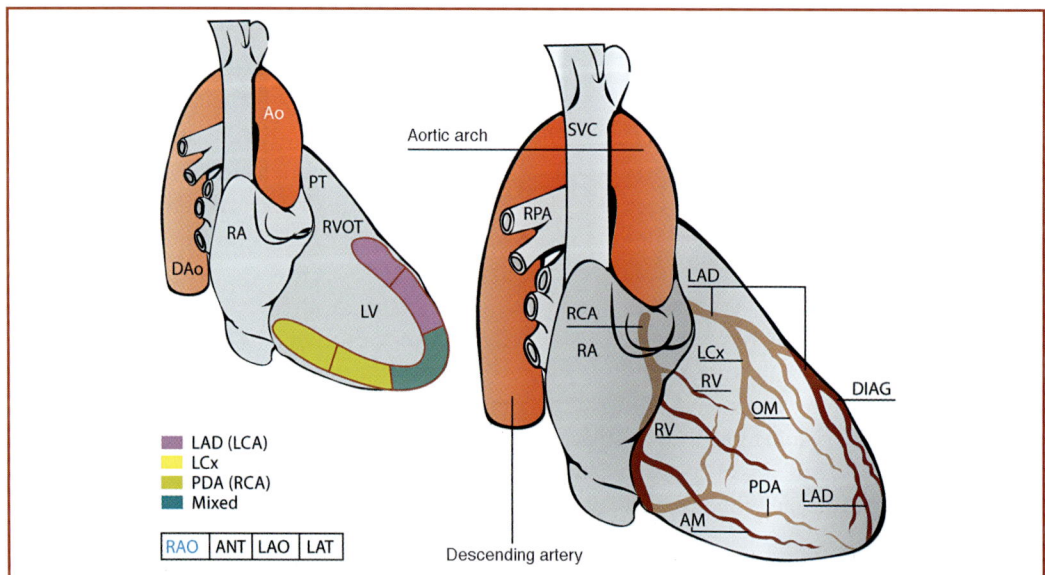

Fig. 1.12 Angiographic evaluation of the coronary circulation; right anterior view (RAO). *RCA* Right coronary artery, *RV* right ventricular branches, *AM* acute marginal branches, *PDA* posterior descending artery, *PLV* posterolateral branches, *LM* left main artery, *LAD* left anterior descending artery, *DIAG* diagonal branches, *LCx* left circumflex artery, *OM* obtuse marginal branches, *Ao* aorta, *Dao* descending aorta, *LV* left ventricle, *PT* pulmonary trunk, *RA* right atrium, *RPA* right pulmonary artery, *RVOT* right ventricular outflow tract, *SVC* superior vena cava

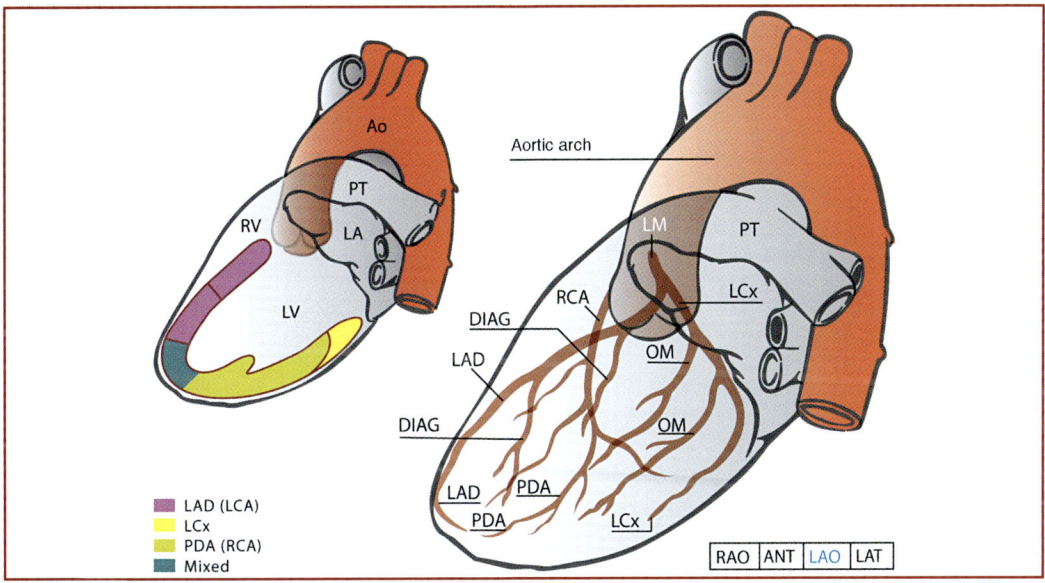

Fig. 1.13 Angiographic evaluation of the coronary circulation; left anterior oblique (LAO) view. *RCA* Right coronary artery, *RV* right ventricular branches, *PDA* posterior descending artery, *LCA* left coronary artery, *LM* left main artery, *LAD* left anterior descending artery, *DIAG* diagonal branches, *LCx* left circumflex artery, *OM* obtuse marginal branches, *Ao* aorta, *LA* left atrium, *LV* left ventricle, *PT* pulmonary trunk, *RV* right ventricle

the diameter of the coronary arteries often requires the use of nitrates to resolve vasospasm; however, with increasing patient age there is a reduction of the effects of nitrates. Furthermore, reduced physical activity and a prevalence of connective tissue in the myocardium are associated with a reduction in the caliber of the coronary arteries.

Physical exercise is a strong stimulus for increasing the caliber of the vessels and it potentiates the effects of nitroglycerin or endothelial-derived relaxing factor.

Cardiac pathologies that increase work by the heart or produce an increase in coronary flow increase the caliber of the coronary arteries. Thus, in the evaluation of the coronary anatomy it is useful to obtain anamnestic information from the patient.

Figures 1.10–1.13 provide examples of the coronary anatomy, as visualized by computed tomography (Fig. 1.10) or with traditional angiographic projections (Figs. 1.11–1.13), including the cardiac regions perfused by the larger coronary branches.

References

1. Alderman EL, Stadius ML (1992) The angiographic definitions of the Bypass Angioplasty Revascularization Investigation (BARI). Coron Artery Dis 3:1189-1220
2. Libby P, Bonow RO, Mann DL, et al (2008) Braunwald's heart disease: a textbook of cardiovascular medicine. 8th edn. WB Saunders, Philadelphia
3. Pavone P, Fioranelli M, Dowe DA (2009) CT evaluation of coronary artery disease. Springer-Verlag, Milan
4. Baim DS (2006) Grossman's cardiac catheterization, angiography and intervention. Lippincott, Williams & Wilkins
5. Topol EJ, Jacobs JJ (2008) A textbook of interventional cardiology, 5th edn. Saunders, Elsevier, Philadelphia

Basic Techniques in the Acquisition of Cardiac Images with CT

Paolo Pavone

2.1 Introduction

Computed tomography angiography (CTA) of the coronary arteries is a very fast and the most advanced imaging technique currently available for clinical use. Based on a multi-slice imaging approach together with specialized and dedicated software, CTA "freezes" cardiac movement, thereby acquiring static images of the rapidly moving heart. In addition, the same approach produces contrast-enhanced images of the coronary arteries, by employing a three-dimensional technique with high spatial and temporal resolution. This chapter informs the non-experienced reader about the CTA modalities that allow these images to be acquired. Specifically, the following topics are discussed: (a) the basic concepts of the equipment employed, (b) the technical procedures needed to image the coronary arteries, (c) the modalities for proper reconstruction of the three-dimensional images, and (d) the procedures allowing diagnostic analysis and image reproduction.

2.2 Technical Principles in the Acquisition of Cardiac Images by CT

"Freezing" moving organs has been one of the main goals of CT since its introduction. All of the apparatuses developed thus far are based on a simple principle: an X-ray tube (the same as employed elsewhere in radiology) rotates around the patient, who lies on a radio-transparent bed. A thin, collimated X-ray beam is sent towards the patient from one side while sensors (detectors) are located on the other. The amount of X-ray radiation absorbed by the patient at the anatomic level examined is then computed. Thus, from a simple perspective, CT consists (Fig. 2.1) of a large box, the gantry, which contains a circular track that allows fast rotation of the X-ray tube. On the other side of the tube, positioned along the same track, are the detectors, which rotate synchronously with the X-ray tube. The detectors transform the received signal (i.e., the X-ray beam after it has passed through the patient's body) into a weak but consistent electrical signal that is proportional to the amount of X-rays detected. Accordingly, the greater the absorption of the X-ray beam by the patient, the smaller the number of X-rays that hit the detector, and the weaker the electrical signal transformed and transmitted by the detector. Therefore, the electrical signal created by the detector is a direct measure of X-ray beam absorption. If the beam crosses an area containing bone (e.g., the vertebrae), X-ray absorption will be consistent and a weak signal will be produced by the detector (Fig. 2.2). If an anatomic area containing air (e.g., the lungs) is evaluated, X-ray absorption will be less and a strong, consistent signal will result as very little of the radiation is absorbed by the lungs.

At the same time that information on X-ray absorption is collected by the CT detectors during rotation of the tube around the patient's body, the de-

P. Pavone (✉)
Radiology Department
Casa di Cura Mater Dei
Rome, Italy
e-mail: paolo.pavone@materdei.it

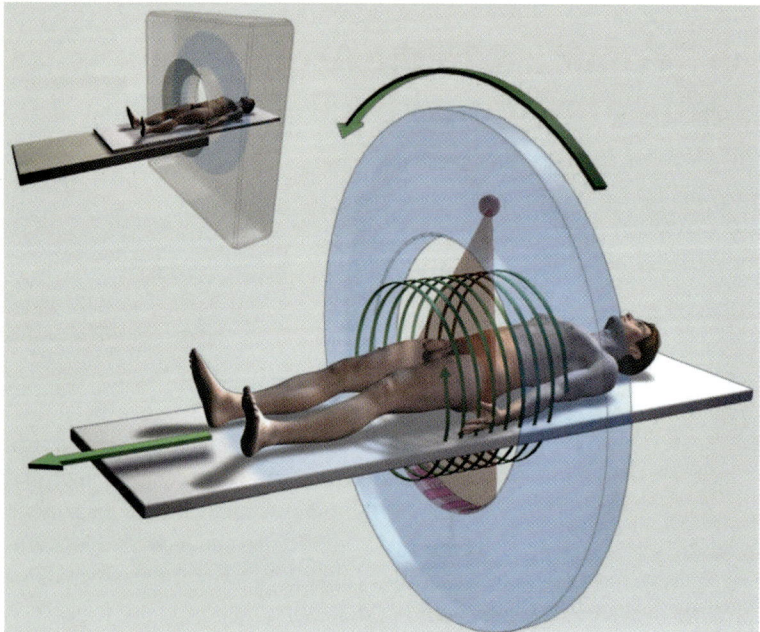

Fig. 2.1 Computed tomography (CT) equipment: basic principles. (Reproduced from Brenner and Hall, 2007. 2008 Massachusetts Medical Society, with permission)

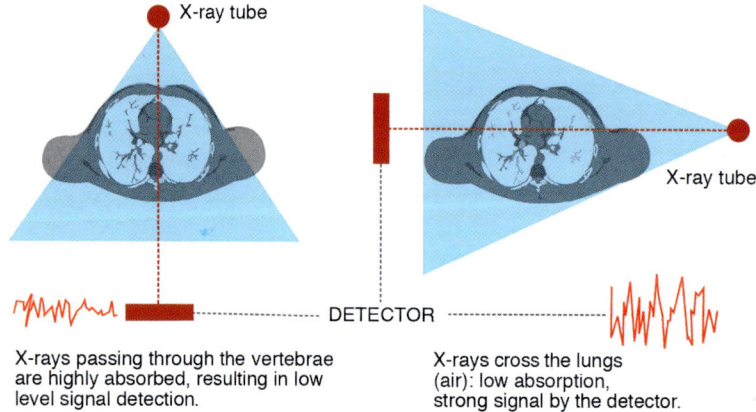

Fig. 2.2 X-ray absorption and signal detection. X-ray absorption is higher or lower depending on the anatomic area crossed by the X-rays. For example, when X-rays pass through the strongly absorbing vertebrae, the detector receives a weak signal. When they pass through the lungs, there is less absorption and the detector receives a much stronger signal

tectors are also continuously and rapidly sending electrical signals to a computer. In the process, these weak but significant electrical signals are immediately transformed into digital data that can be analyzed by the appropriate software. Complex reconstruction algorithms ultimately produce a series of diagnostic images, which are displayed on the console monitor and are thus readily accessible by the clinician.

As simple clinical users, it is not necessary to understand the mechanics of these analyses. It is important, however, to acknowledge those scientists who have been able to resolve the numerous technical problems such that CT image quality has constantly improved. Of interest is that the "inventor" of CT, Sir Hounsfield, succeeded in his efforts thanks in part to the Beatles, since EMI Records financed CT research and the construction of the first "commercial" CT unit. The volumetric (spiral) revolution was a product of the work of Willi A. Kalender. Due to these results and those of related scientific activities, today, CT is used almost as easily as digital photography. Indeed, the acquisition principles are the same: in CT, X-rays are absorbed by the anatomic region of interest; in digital photography, the brightness of the object is assessed by a kind of detector, the CCD (charge-coupled device), such that the light signal is transformed into numerical (digital) information.

ternal organs of the human body. Moreover, the development of spiral CT allowed the development of other techniques, such as virtual endoscopy and CTA, which have become routine tools in clinical practice.

2.3 From Conventional to Spiral CT

The speed of data acquisition in CT depends on two different factors: how fast the tube rotates around the patient and the amount of information that can be analyzed at the same time. Early CT machines needed 18–20 s for a single rotation; thus, the waiting time, in which the tube returned to its initial position ready to begin a new rotation, was as long as 1 min. A revolution in CT imaging of the abdomen occurred in the early 1980s, with a tube able to rotate around the body in 2 s, thereby minimizing all artifacts arising from motions of the abdominal organs. As a result, excellent static images of the liver, pancreas, and adjacent vessels could be obtained.

The next step was the introduction of spiral systems, in which the tube is able to move freely in the track contained in the gantry and does not return to its initial position after each rotation. In these machines, introduced in the early 1990s, the electrical power that supplies the X-ray tube is transmitted along the same rotational track, thus avoiding both the need for long cables and a return to the start position after each rotation. "Spiral" refers to the fact that, once a continuous rotation of the tube around the patient is started, movement of the bed along the longitudinal axis creates a spiral acquisition of images along the human body (Fig. 2.1) instead of the axial images acquired in conventional CT. There is dramatic improvement of image quality with spiral CT in terms of speed of data acquisition and the consistency of the diagnostic information. This is due to the fact that images are not acquired on a single imaging plane (axial); rather, data representative of an entire volume are reconstructed on the axial, coronal, sagittal, and curved planes of the target organ. The information provided by these three-dimensional images facilitates diagnostic evaluation of the in-

2.4 From Spiral to Multi-slice CT

Despite the advances made with the introduction of spiral CT, the acquisition times were still too long to allow cardiac imaging. The rotation time of the tube was about 1 s, not short enough to "freeze" cardiac movement. Moreover, the need remained to acquire more data within the same time frame, in order to include the anatomic area surrounding the heart. With multi-slice CT (MSCT) (Fig. 2.3), which became commercially available at the beginning of this century, an increase in the speed of data acquisition was achieved. The principle of MSCT is simple: in conventional CT, a collimated X-ray beam is emitted and data are collected by a row of detectors located on the other side of the patient, after attenuation of the beam through his or her body. In MSCT, there is a large data-acquisition system, composed of an array of detectors arranged in multiple parallel rows along the longitudinal axis. The larger collimation of the X-ray beam is such that all of the detectors are "hit" at the same time, allowing simultaneous evaluation of a larger anatomic area.

The first systems used in cardiac imaging had four rows of detectors, but the real clinical revolution in cardiac imaging came with the development of machines with 16 detector rows, as they were able to generate images of the coronary arteries with limited artifacts and improved resolution.

Currently, the most widely employed systems have arrays of 64 detector rows, although newer systems with 128, 256, and 320 detectors have since become available. It is easy to understand why the speed of acquisition is proportional to the number of detectors. Coverage of an anatomic volume such as the heart requires a certain number of rotations of the tube around the patient. Clearly, the larger the anatomic area covered by the detector rows, the fewer the number of rotations needed (Fig. 2.4).

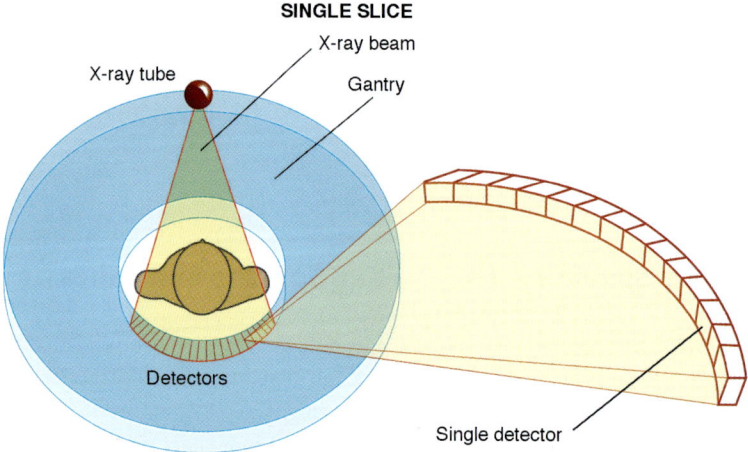
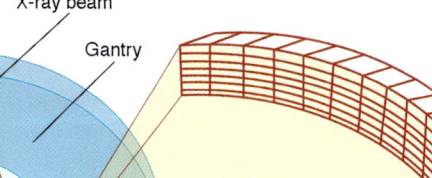
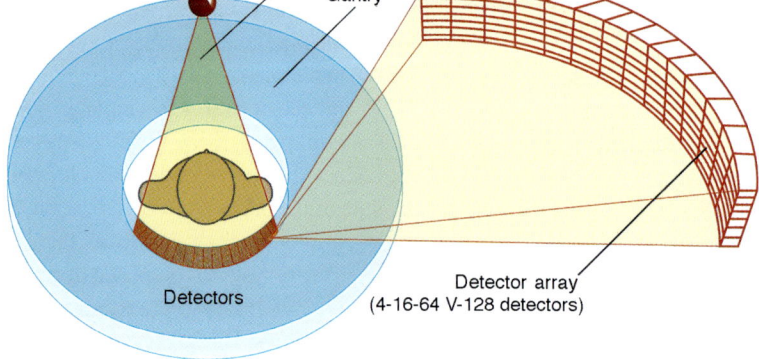

Fig. 2.3 Single slice and multi-slice (multi-row) detector CT

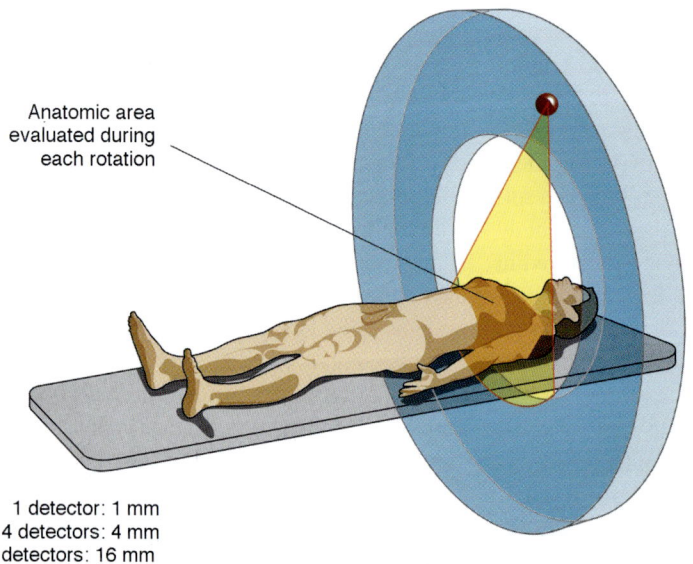

Fig. 2.4 Anatomic area evaluated in a single rotation of the X-ray tube. In MSCT, the higher the number of detectors, the wider the anatomic area evaluated during each rotation of the X-ray tube

2.5 Detector Number and Cardiac Imaging

It is worth emphasizing once more that the number of detectors used in MSCT corresponds to an array of defined width. The volume simultaneously evaluated by the X-ray beam equals the width of the detector array. In a 64-detector-row machine, the detector width and the anatomic area to be explored in a single rotation is in each case 4 cm. Thus, to fully cover the anatomic area of the heart (15–20 cm), four to five rotations are needed during each phase of the cardiac cycle (using cardiosynchronization, as discussed below). With 128 detectors, the number of rotations is reduced by one half, while with 320 detector rows it may be possible to evaluate the entire heart in a single rotation. It should be noted that with 320 detector rows the width of the volume acquired in one rotation corresponds to 16, not 20 cm, due to corrections needed for the so-called cone beam artifact. One rotation, carried out in the telediastolic phase of the cardiac cycle, allows for the simultaneous acquisition of data covering the entire heart. However, multi-cycle images of the heart can also be acquired in a single rotation, with the data reconstructed in the different cardiac phases.

2.6 Temporal Resolution in Cardiac Imaging

Together with progress achieved by MSCT regarding the simultaneous acquisition of more data, efforts have been made to reduce the rotation time of the X-ray tube. This technical parameter is of utmost importance, as it represents the real temporal resolution of cardiac CT. In fact, even with the largest detector array (i.e., 320), it would not be possible to "freeze" images of the heart if the rotation time of the X-ray tube was slow (e.g., 1 s, as was the case with the first generation of spiral scanners). In other words, it is not enough to simultaneously obtain as much data as possible; rather, data acquisition must be very fast if the goal is to generate consistent cardiac images.

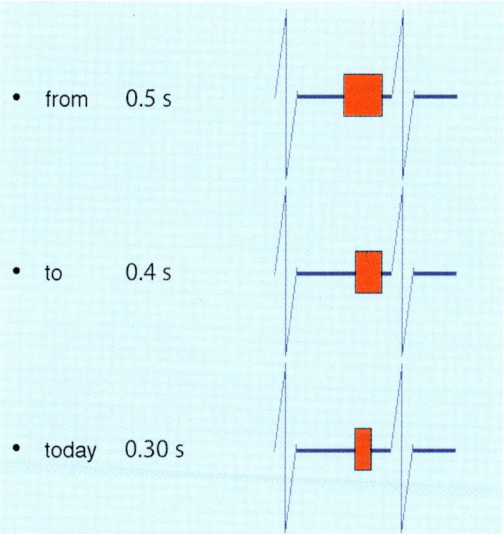

Fig. 2.5 Rotation time of the X-ray tube: during cardiac-gated image acquisition. The width of the red area in telediastole represents the imaging window (time) for data acquisition: the shorter the acquisition time, the fewer the motion artifacts

The rotation time of early MSCT equipment, 0.5 s, was too slow to completely "freeze" cardiac movement. Since the temporal resolution is equal to half of the rotation time, with 250 ms significant artifacts in the diagnostic images were produced and the images were of poor quality.

The rotation time of the X-ray tube has continuously improved in more recent equipment and currently ranges from 0.4–0.35 s to 0.3–0.27 s (temporal resolution < 150 ms). As would be expected, the faster rotation times have yielded cardiac images of much higher quality, greater reliability, and improved accuracy, as confirmed by world-wide clinical experience. The reason for this improvement lies in the fact that the width of the imaging "window" (Fig. 2.5) in the telediastolic phase (during which the heart is almost completely still) is limited; therefore, the faster the data are acquired, the fewer the movement artifacts.

Another approach to improve temporal resolution is the use of two perpendicular X-ray tubes. In dual-source technology, two different X-ray tubes are installed 90° to each other on the same rotational track, with two perpendicular detector

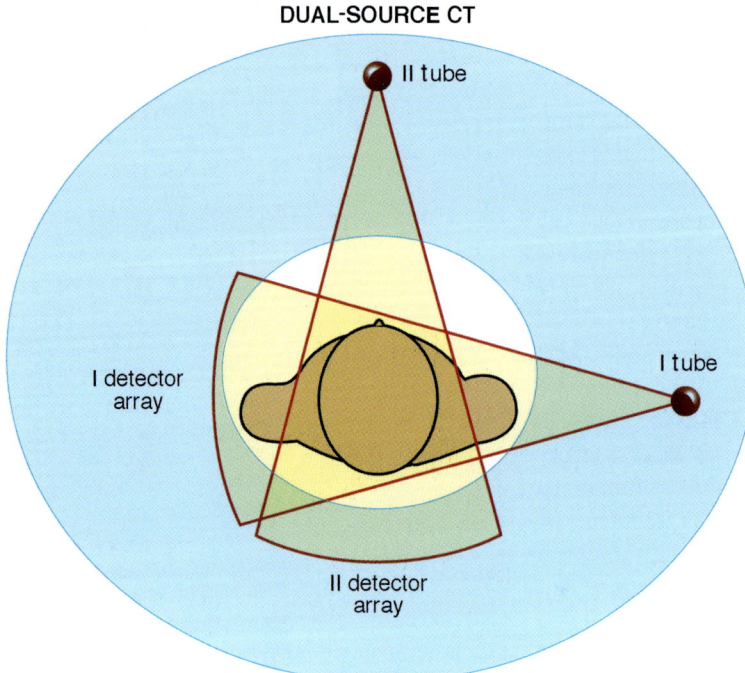

Fig. 2.6 In dual-source CT, the tubes are mounted perpendicular to each other and the data are obtained by two different detector arrays. The acquisition time for each rotation is therefore reduced by one half

arrays (Fig. 2.6). During X-ray emission and data acquisition, the two tubes and detector arrays operate independently and data are collected individually. The computer merges the information produced by the two tubes into a single data package, as if obtained by a single system. The end result is that data from the volume being evaluated are actually obtained in half the time and with a temporal resolution of 83 ms. Only this system generates images of the heart without significant artifacts, even in patients with faster heart rates, and without the need for bradycardic drugs.

2.7 Types of Equipment and Their Clinical Uses in Cardiac Imaging

Soon after the development of equipment with four detectors rows and a rotation time of 0.5 s, CTA of the coronary arteries was proposed. However, because of the long rotation time of the X-ray tube, the data were not satisfactory. Significant artifacts were present in almost all of the resulting images, which were of poor quality and exhibited limited anatomic definition of the coronary circulation. Nonetheless, this technology did find application in the evaluation of cardiac bypass grafts (CABG), since the reduced motion of the extracardiac vascular structures yielded fewer artifacts.

With 16 detectors rows and a rotation time of 0.4 s or less, the situation changed drastically. Clinical experience confirmed the improved accuracy of CT, while CTA of the coronary arteries became an established examination with a high degree of reliability, producing images of great clinical interest. This clearly defined the role of CTA in the assessment of patients with suspected atherosclerotic disease of the coronary arteries.

As noted above, the most widely diffused CT systems for imaging of the coronary arteries are those with 64 rows; however, there has not been the same degree of improvement as that achieved in moving from 4 to 16 slices. In a recent review of papers published in the international literature, the use of 16 and 64 detector rows has corresponded to an improvement in sensitivity (average from 83 to 93%) while there has been little change in the specificity (96%). The newer equipment does feature an improved spatial resolution, with better evaluation of stents (see chapter on this topic).

Newer equipment (128, 256, and 320 detector rows) provides improved spatial resolution and faster data acquisition, with complete coverage of the anatomic area containing the heart within 5–0.5 s. With an anatomic coverage of 16 cm, it is usually possible to capture the heart in a single rotation of the X-ray tube.

The current goal of CT research is the "imaging plate," that is, a device with 512 detectors. This would provide even more extended anatomic coverage and a definitive improvement in the image quality achieved with CTA. The major problem of imaging research is the cone beam artifact, i.e., conical divergence of the X-ray beam, which causes distortion in image reconstruction.

CT equipment with two X-ray tubes (dual-source technology) does not improve spatial resolution, because the acquisition technology is the same as that of machines with 64 detector rows. However, these systems do offer dramatic and unique improvement in temporal resolution, down to a value of 83 ms. The imaging window in telediastole is very short and for this reason, as discussed elsewhere in this volume, there is no need to administer beta-blockers to patients to induce bradycardia. The use of these systems is therefore recommended mostly in cardiology units with high patient turnover. They are also advantageous in the ICU, where patients must be quickly screened for coronary artery disease in cases of acute chest pain (so-called triple rule out) and there is no time, or opportunity, to wait for the bradycardic effect of beta-blockers.

A second generation of CT scanners, with two X-ray tubes, has been introduced into clinical practice. This dual-source CT scan can be used with a new ECG-triggered high-pitch protocol known as "flash spiral," which has been developed to acquire high-quality images with low radiation doses. This new technology can scan the entire cardiac volume in a single heartbeat. However in this setting the patient's heart rate should be decreased as much as possible, because the slower the heart beats the longer the duration of the R-R interval, thus allowing motion-free images to be acquired. Since this technology can acquire images with retrospective or prospective gating, and the rotation time has been accelerated to up to 280 ms, the actual temporal resolution reaches 70 ms.

With the fastest scanning speed in CT (i.e., 43 cm/s) and a temporal resolution of 70 ms, flash spiral enables, for example, complete scans of the entire chest region in just 0.6 s. Moreover, it operates at an extremely reduced radiation dose, such that a spiral heart scan can be performed with < 1 millisievert (mSv), whereas the average effective dose required for this purpose usually ranges from 8 to 20 mSv.

2.8 Other Factors That Improve the Image Quality of CT Technology

So far, our discussion has focused on the two most evident technical parameters of CT technology: the number of detectors in the array (64–320) and the rotation time of the X-ray tube (from < 0.4 to 0.3–0.27 s.). However, there are other ways to improve image quality, an important one being the speed of information capture. Detectors receive information (X-ray absorption through the patient's body) and then send it as an electrical signal to the computer. Since the tube rotates rapidly, the detectors must respond quickly enough to receive and process this information. This speed of data acquisition by the detectors influences an important parameter in spiral CT, the so-called pitch, i.e., the speed at which the patient can be advanced in the gantry, allowing all relevant data to be collected. A 256-detector system may have a slower pitch such that acquisition of the anatomic area containing the heart is achieved in 6 s, while a 128-detector system with faster detectors allows a more rapid pitch, with complete acquisition of the cardiac images in 4 s. Thus, the number of detectors is not the only parameter that determines the speed of data acquisition in CTA of the coronary arteries.

Another parameter currently targeted by CT manufacturers is spatial resolution. With more accurate and sensitive detectors along with proper and calibrated emission of the X-ray beam, spatial resolution has improved from the 0.6–0.5 mm of 64-detector technology to the 0.25–0.33 mm of today's technology. This improvement enables better evaluation of smaller, distal coronary arteries. Consequently, the results achieved with CTA of the coronary arteries may soon be on a par with the spatial resolution of catheter coronary angiography, i.e., < 0.2 mm.

Suggested Reading

Earls JP, Berman EL, Urban BA et al (2008) Prospectively gated transverse coronary CT angiography versus retrospectively gated helical technique: improved image quality and reduced radiation dose. Radiology 246:742–753

Leschka S, Stolzmann P, Schmid FT et al (2008) Low kilo- voltage cardiac dual-source CT: attenuation, noise, and radiation dose. Eur Radiol 18:1809–1817

Bischoff B, Hein F, Meyer T et al (2009) Impact of a reduced tube voltage on CT angiography and ra- diation dose: results of the PROTECTION I study. JACC Cardiovasc Imaging 2:940–946

Earls JP, Schrack EC (2009) Prospectively gated low-dose CTA: 24 months experience in more than 2,000 clinical cases. Int J Cardiovasc Imaging 25:177–187

Hara AK, Paden RG, Silva AC et al (2009) Iterative reconstruction technique for reducing body radiation dose at CT: feasibility study. AJR 193:764–771

Silva AC, Lawder HJ, Hara A et al (2010) Innovations in CT dose reduction strategy: application of the adaptive statistical iterative reconstruction algorithm. AJR Am J Roentgenol 194(1):191–199

CT Examination of the Coronary Arteries

Paolo Pavone

This chapter reviews the techniques needed to obtain high-quality diagnostic images of the coronary arteries by means of computed tomography angiography (CTA). The choice of imaging equipment, discussed in the previous chapter, involves the radiologist only once, at the moment that the CT equipment is purchased. By contrast, the choice of the optimal procedure for imaging of the coronary arteries involves the radiologist or technician in each exam, as the utmost care must be taken to always obtain images of optimal quality. It should be pointed out that this goal is unique for the coronary arteries, since in CT evaluation of the chest, abdomen, musculoskeletal system, or other static organs, suboptimal image quality may nonetheless allow a clinical diagnosis whereas for the coronary arteries the presence of movement artifacts may completely invalidate the diagnostic value of the examination.

chapter). Second, during the dynamic rapid acquisition of cardiac images there must be a high concentration of contrast agent in the coronary tree. Only the high density provided by the presence of contrast agent in the vessels allows for a proper evaluation of the coronary arteries and their walls. Third, to reduce imaging artifacts, the patient must be properly prepared for the imaging procedure; therefore, good patient cooperation is needed. In addition, in most cases (except with dual-source technology) the patient will be administered beta-blockers to reduce cardiac frequency, allowing a wider imaging window in telediastole.

In coronary CTA, images of a moving organ are rapidly acquired during the passage of contrast agent at high concentration (bolus). It is therefore crucial to define the procedures, including patient preparation, that will be performed prior to diagnostic CT examination of the coronary arteries.

3.1 Achieving Excellent Image Quality in CT of the Coronary Arteries

In performing CT of the coronary arteries, certain goals must be reached. First of all, the images must be obtained as fast as possible, using specific imaging protocols (which differ according to the type of equipment, as discussed in the previous

3.2 Patient Preparation

3.2.1 Informed Consent

Although CTA of the coronary vessels is a non-invasive procedure (no catheterization or other invasive modality is required), proper information must be obtained from the patient prior to the examination. The patient should not only fill out the informed consent documents (similar to those of any CT procedure using contrast agent), but should also be informed personally about the procedure, i.e., the cardiologist and radiologist must provide

P. Pavone (✉)
Radiology Department
Casa di Cura Mater Dei
Rome, Italy
e-mail: paolo.pavone@materdei.it

the appropriate information in person, clearly explaining the type of examination being performed, the indications for this procedure, whether it is aimed at ruling out a known clinical problem or serves as a screening procedure, as may be the case in mildly or non-symptomatic at-risk patients.

The informed consent documents contain generic information regarding, for example, the possibility that contrast agent may be the cause of allergic reactions; however, this information is very general and often not well-explained. Thus, the clinician must specify that, with the iodinated non-ionic contrast agent currently in use, such allergic reactions are extremely rare, as opposed to the situation 15–20 years ago, when ionic agents were employed. Furthermore, since patients are often alarmed by the prospect of iodine injection, the radiologist must reassure him or her that the iodine is encapsulated in a closed molecule of the contrast agent and therefore does not react with the human body, i.e., it does not affect iodine metabolism in the thyroid gland. For this reason, there are no contraindications for patients with thyroid gland disease; the contrast agent and its iodine component are rapidly eliminated through the kidneys after i.v. injection. Those allergic reactions that do occur are not related to iodine but to the molecule itself, and, as noted above, there has been a dramatic decrease in the incidence of allergic reactions following the switch from ionic to non-ionic, i.e., less reactive, molecules, despite the fact that both formulas contain three atoms of iodine per molecule. There is also no absolute contraindication to the use of contrast agent in patients with known allergic problems or in patients with previous allergic reactions to contrast agent. In these cases, however, pre-medication 3 days before the examination is indicated (usually corticosteroids per os).

In informing the patient, the clinician must also state that the examination is performed using ionizing radiation. Patient should be advised that X-ray exposure, mostly if repeated a short time after previous exposures, carries some risk. This topic is discussed elsewhere in this volume.

As for any other procedure involving contrast agent, patients undergoing CTA of the coronary arteries must fast for at least 5 h prior to the examination. Furthermore, the radiologists (or the anesthesiologist, who may be present during the examination) will review blood-test data (mostly referring to renal function) and evaluate the patient's ECG. The only real contraindications to CTA of the coronary arteries are severe renal dysfunction, which precludes the use of contrast agent, and not pharmaceutically controlled arrhythmia, which prevents "freezing" of cardiac movement during the examination.

3.2.2 Bradycardia

As the heart is a fast-moving organ, CT evaluation can be performed only by "freezing" cardiac motion, using software and protocols allowing rapid image acquisition. The temporal resolution of currently available equipment (150 ms) does not guarantee static images of the heart in three dimensions. Instead, to obtain dynamic images of the coronary arteries, pharmacologically controlled bradycardia, with an optimal cardiac frequency of 55–65 bpm, is required. Only by inducing bradycardia can an adequate temporal window in telediastole, during which the heart is practically completely still, be achieved (Fig. 3.1). In the absence of bradycardia, image quality will be impaired and, as noted above, a proper diagnosis will not be possible. In Fig. 3.2a, a bi-dimensional image of the anterior descending coronary artery is displayed on the

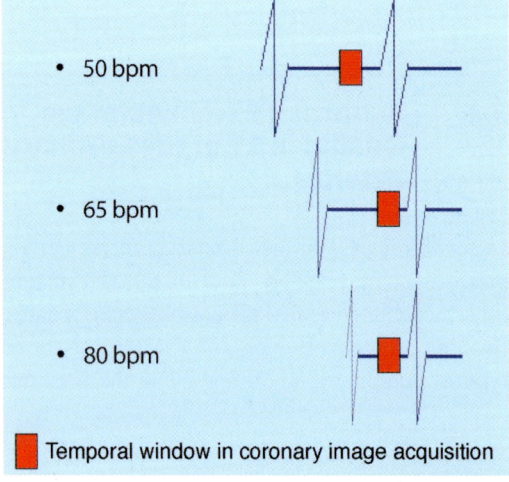

Fig. 3.1 Time imaging window in ECG gating procedures. The lower the heart rate, the larger the time imaging window, leading to a reduction of motion artifacts

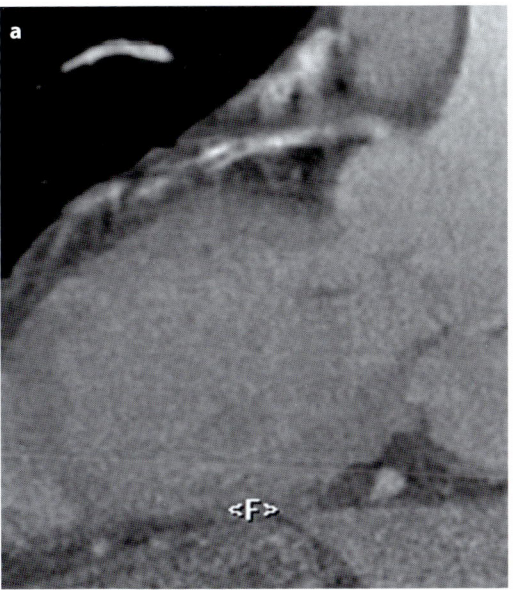
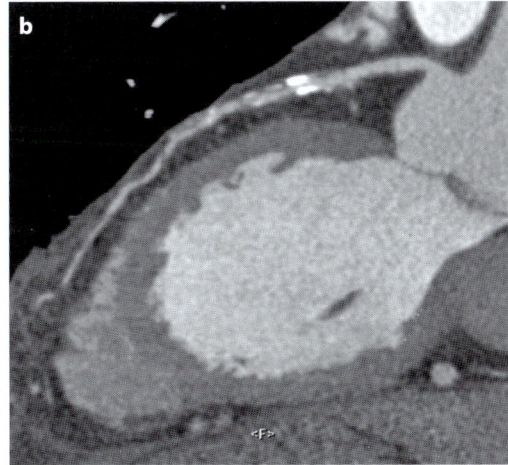

Fig. 3.2 Image acquired at 75 bpm (**a**) and afterwards, at 62 bpm, repeating the injection of contrast agent (**b**). Movement artifacts impair image quality and therefore the diagnostic value of the examination

left, with data acquired at 72 bpm. This image does not provide the diagnosis nor can the vessel contours or the presence of parietal pathology be defined. The image on the right was obtained after bradycardia was pharmacologically induced; there is clear definition of the vessel wall, with identification of the lumen and evidence of parietal thickening due to atherosclerotic involvement.

Pharmacological bradycardia is required if the cardiac frequency is > 65 bpm. While oral or i.v. administration of beta-blocker is possible, we prefer oral administration of a generic beta-blocker formula (e.g., metoprolol 100 mg) in tablet form 45–60 min prior to the examination. Usually, a frequency of 50–60 bpm is easily achieved, without any symptoms experienced by the patients (these drugs are currently widely used by general practitioners without major patient contraindications). As an alternative or in case of lack of pharmaceutical effect of the oral drug, i.v. formulas can be administered. These are injected at the moment of the examination in the same i.v. cannula prepared for contrast-agent injection, with cardiac frequency evaluated directly on the CT monitor.

Cardiac frequency is often influenced by the emotional status of the patient. Despite the efficiency of beta-blockers, once on the CT table and during contrast-agent injection, the patient often becomes tachycardic due to the emotional stress of the examination. We therefore suggest that an anxiolytic drug be provided i.v. just prior to contrast-agent injection. The short-lasting effects of these drugs do not interfere with consciousness at the end of the out-patient examination.

Finally, it should be noted that with dual-source technology there is no need for bradycardia, as the temporal resolution of 83 ms allows for a consistent image window even in tachycardic patients, without a decrease in the diagnostic quality of the images.

3.3 CT Angiography of the Coronary Arteries

3.3.1 Contrast-Agent Injection

The proper contrast-agent injection procedure is very important in CTA of the coronary arteries, as only by ensuring a consistent concentration in the vessels can good image quality be achieved. Visualization of the coronary arteries is made possible by increasing (temporarily, during passage of the bolus of contrast agent) the radiographic density of the blood plasma (blood mixed with contrast agent) that fills the coronary arteries at that moment. The radiographic density of the blood increases from 40–50 Hounsfield units (HU) to 300–400 and even 500 HU during the passage of contrast agent. Standard HU values are defined to allow the CT measurement of tissue density, with 0 HU corresponding to the CT density of pure water, -1000 to that of air, and +1000 to that of compact bone tissue. The higher the CT density of the coronary contents (blood mixed with contrast agent) during CT image acquisition, the better the quality of the coronary arterial images obtained.

3.3.2 Contrast-Agent Injection: Role of Resistance and Venous Anatomy

Different parameters determine the success of a consistently high concentration of contrast agent in the arterial lumen during CTA image acquisition, among them, the contrast-agent injection rate. This, in turn, is influenced by the amount of resistance encountered and the venous anatomy of the injection site, i.e., the forearm.

Contrast agent is injected through an automatic injector able to reach high injection rates (Fig. 3.3). In coronary CTA, better results are obtained with a double-syringe injector; here, contrast agent is injected with one syringe and,

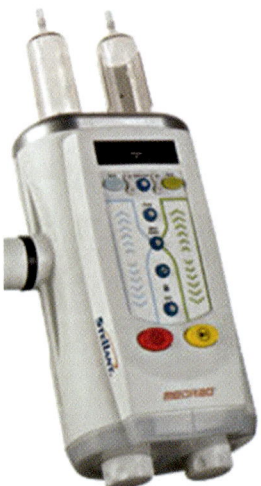

Fig. 3.3 Contrast-agent power injector (Stellant D, MEDRAD, USA, with permission)

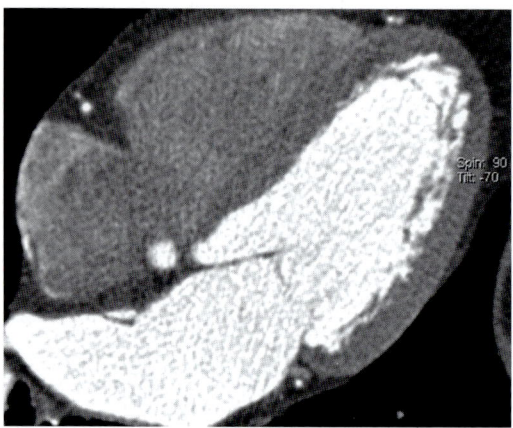

Fig. 3.4 A high concentration of contrast agent in the left chambers of the heart causes them to appear bright and hyperdense. The right chambers are "washed" by the chasing bolus and are therefore hypodense

immediately at the end of the injection, the second syringe is activated such that a second bolus, this time of saline, is injected. This saline bolus pushes the contrast-agent bolus towards the right cardiac chamber, thereby "washing" the peripheral veins, where the vascular flow is low; these vessels would otherwise stay filled with contrast agent. Accordingly, the dispersion of contrast agent in the peripheral veins is guaranteed and the bolus remains compact, thus yielding higher concentrations in the arterial bed. We prefer to inject the saline bolus at the same rate used for contrast-agent injection and as a large volume (80–100 ml), thus ensuring that all the contrast agent is washed out by the saline. In the example shown in Fig. 3.4, axial images acquired at the level of the cardiac chambers show the strong opacification of the left cardiac chambers due to high CT density values and a low density of the right chamber, washed out by the saline bolus.

An effective contrast-agent bolus injection speed is also related to the resistance that the bolus encounters during its passage in the i.v. cannula, given the high viscosity of these drugs. There are two ways to avoid local resistance: the first is to use a large-bore cannula in the antecubital vein. Based on our own experience, we recommend a 16G cannula (as opposed to the 18G or even 20G cannula usually proposed in the literature), which allows for a high injection rate without any local resistance. The sec-

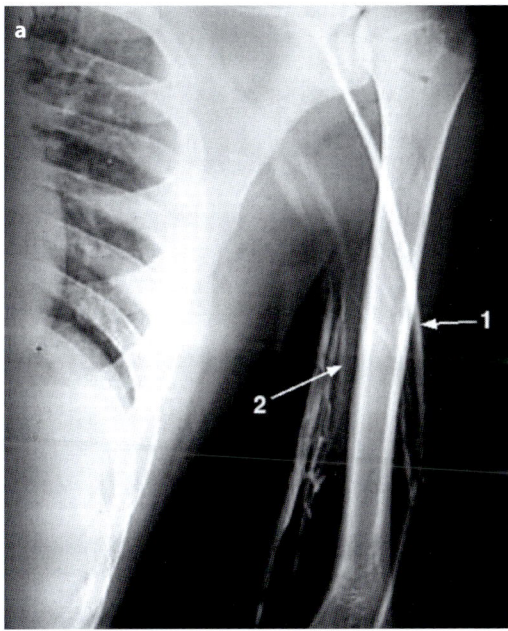
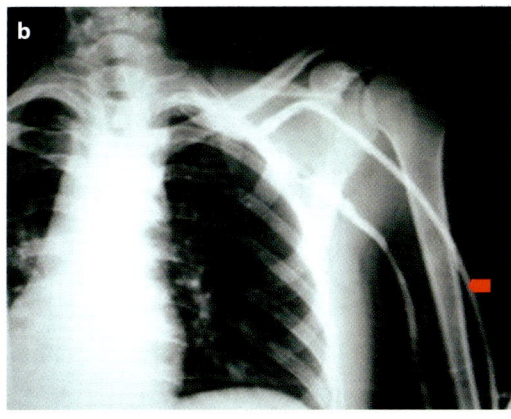

Fig. 3.5 a,b Anatomy of the veins of the arm. The basilic vein is medial and has a direct course towards the subclavian vein; the cephalic vein is lateral and has a steep angle at the confluence with the subclavian vein. *1* Cephalic vein, *2* basilic vein

ond is related to the anatomy of the veins of the forearm: the two main venous channels (in most cases) are the basilic vein, medially, and the cephalic vein, laterally. While the basilic vein (Fig. 3.5) follows a straight course, leading directly to the axillary and subclavian veins, the cephalic vein is more tortuous, contains valves, and drains in the axillary vein usually in an arch-wise fashion at an angle of 90°. Considering that the patient's arms are raised during CT examination, it can be readily appreciated that injection into the cephalic vein may cause the stagnant flow of contrast agent, leading to a less compact and more dilute bolus and thus to a lower concentration in the arterial bed. In Fig. 3.6, the effect of bolus dilution during the injection of contrast agent in the cephalic vein is evident. There is persistent opacification of the right chambers and a lower concentration of contrast agent in both the arterial bed and the left cardiac chambers (compare with Fig. 3.4).

3.3.3 Contrast-Agent Injection: Flow Rate and Amount

Contrast agent can be injected using an automatic injector at different flow rates, usually 3–5 ml/s. However, we routinely use a flow rate of 8 ml/s.

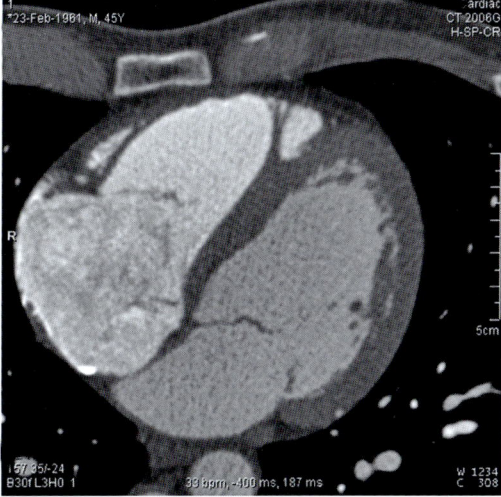

Fig. 3.6 Injection of contrast agent in the cephalic vein. The slower flow leads to a dilution of the contrast-agent bolus. There is evidence of residual opacification of the right chambers during 3D acquisition in an evaluation of the coronary arteries. Note the lower density in the left ventricle

This higher injection speed results in a more compact bolus and thus a higher concentration of contrast agent in the arterial bed (after passage through the capillary pulmonary bed and the left cardiac chambers). The average CT density of the coronary

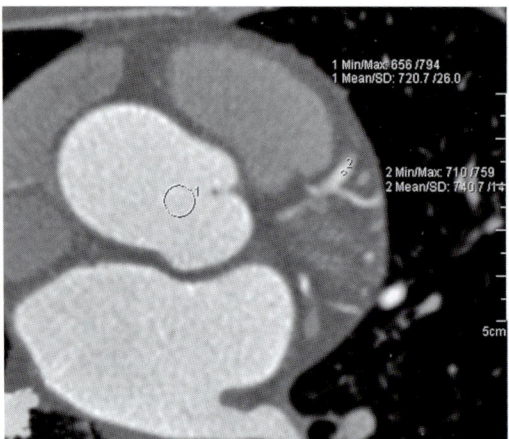

Fig. 3.7 Appropriate contrast-agent injection with high flow in the basilic vein. The CT density evaluated at the level of the aorta is 720 HU

tector rows, acquisition times are 15–18 s, therefore requiring a longer bolus to completely achieve a high density of contrast agent in these vessels throughout image acquisition (at least 120 ml are required to achieve a prolonged bolus of contrast agent). With faster systems, i.e., those with 64, 128, or 256 detector rows, the acquisition time decreases to 10, 6, and 4 s, respectively, thus necessitating a still compact but shorter bolus (70–80 ml of contrast agent). Data acquisition happens in real time such that, with experience, the radiologist will be able to determine the proper bolus size according to the equipment available and the nature of each case.

arteries as reported in the literature is 300–350 HU. Using faster injection rates and the procedures described above, we have been able to achieve an average density of ≥450–500 HU (Fig. 3.7).

Image quality is directly related to a higher concentration of contrast agent in the arterial bed and to a greater difference in density compared with the surrounding tissue. Our data are also in agreement with the results of Schueller et al., published in 2006. They were able to show that higher injection rates (8 ml/s) improved the evaluation of pancreatic tumors. In coronary CTA, the higher arterial density allows better evaluation of these vessels in three-dimensional reconstructions.

The amount of contrast agent to be injected varies between 70 and 120 ml, depending on the equipment employed. In CT systems with 16 de-

3.3.4 Contrast Agents for CT Angiography of the Coronary Arteries: Characteristics and Concentrations

An important element in defining proper image quality of the coronary vessels is the concentration of the contrast agent employed: the higher the concentration of contrast agent, the higher the CT density (measured in HU) of the blood in the coronary arteries. The contrast agent clinically used for i.v. injection is an iodinated non-ionic solution based on a tri-iodated benzene ring; iodated double benzene rings are also available (Fig. 3.8).

The iodine concentration of the contrast agent employed in CTA of the coronary arteries should be in the range of 350–400 mg iodine per 100 ml of solution. This high iodine concentration has been suggested because it provides an even higher CT density in the coronary vessels. In fact, for the same

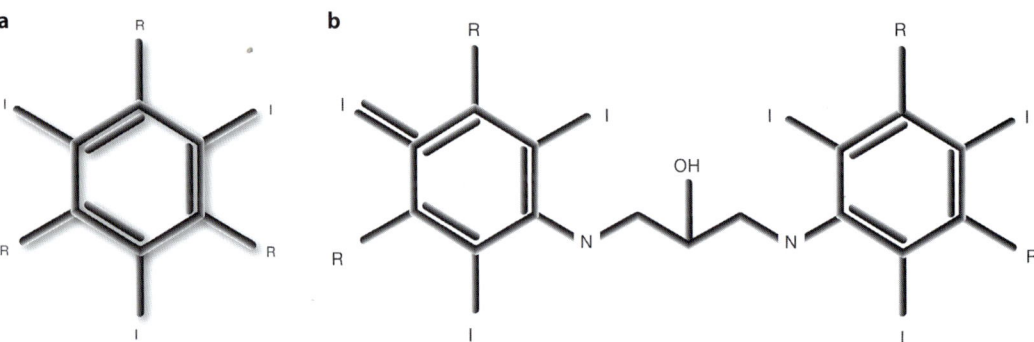

Fig. 3.8 Non-ionic contrast agents with single (**a**) and double (**b**) benzene rings

conditions in terms of contrast-agent volume and flow rate of the injection, higher CT densities in the vessels will be reached with higher concentrations of the contrast-agent solution. The viscosity of these solutions increases in parallel with concentration; however, if the proper injection procedure is used and the solution is injected through a large-bore cannula, viscosity should not pose a problem as resistance at the injection site will be minimal.

Currently employed contrast agents are extremely stable and safe molecules; they are rapidly eliminated through the kidney after i.v. injection. Non-ionic contrast agents are also characterized by a low osmolarity (~600 mOsm/l vs. 1200 mOsm/l for the ionic solutions previously employed). The decreased osmolarity has reduced the patient's heat sensation as well as allergic reactions to the contrast agent. Contrast agents based on an iodated double benzene ring have an even lower osmolarity (300 mOsm/l, similar to that of blood plasma) but have not reduced the incidence of allergic reactions any further. Although they have been successfully used for imaging, their viscosities are definitely higher and resistance at the injection site may be a problem in coronary CTA.

3.3.5 Optimizing the Imaging-Acquisition Window in CT Angiography of the Coronary Arteries

All coronary CTA equipment includes an automated procedure that recognizes the arrival of contrast agent (injected in a peripheral vein) at the level of the coronary arteries. Three-dimensional acquisition of the anatomic area including the heart should, in fact, start only when the bolus of contrast agent reaches the arterial system and creates a temporary but strong increase in the CT density of the arterial vessels. The automated procedure, referred to as "bolus tracking," requires the placement of a cursor that measures CT density in the center of the ascending aorta, after which single low-dose images are acquired every second following the start of contrast-agent injection. As soon as the cursor measures a density >100 HU, the acquisition of three-dimensional images is automatically started. This assures that an optimal high density of the vessels is achieved during image acquisition.

3.3.6 Cardiosynchronized Acquisition

Imaging data are acquired in real time, during the dynamic passage of contrast agent through the coronary arteries. In a cardiosynchronized procedure, the ECG data are available to the computer, which synchronizes them with the imaging data (Fig. 3.9). In a second phase, data related only to telediastole are reconstructed to create artifact-free cardiac images. Data referring to more than one telediastolic phase are needed to completely reconstruct the volume containing the heart. In CT systems consisting of 64 detectors rows, the volume reconstructed in each telediastolic phase corresponds to the width of the detector array (4 cm); therefore, four to five cardiac cycles must be evaluated for a complete set of information regarding the volume of interest, including the heart (15–20 cm).

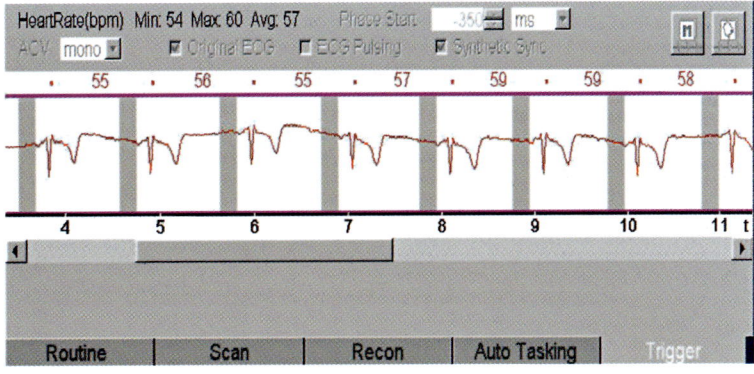

Fig. 3.9 ECG gating as shown on the CT console during data acquisition. *Gray vertical lines* represent the telediastolic temporal windows of data reconstruction for coronary CT angiography

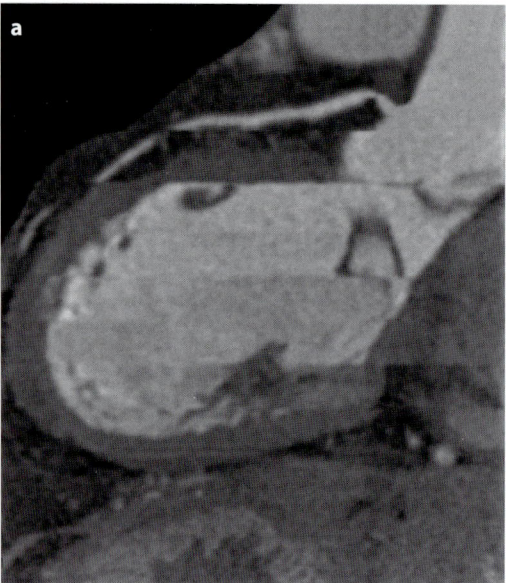 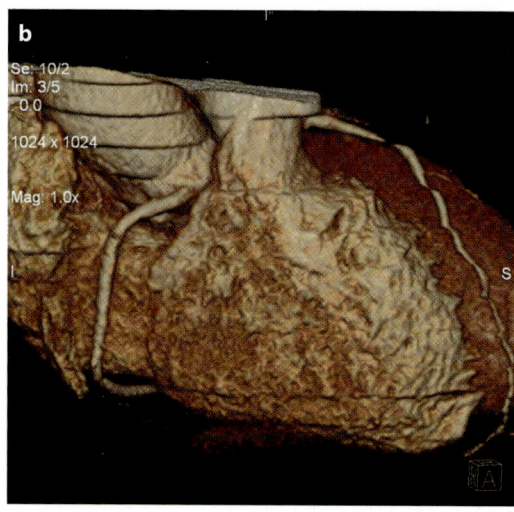

Fig. 3.10 a,b Images acquired in an arrhythmic patient show typical step artifacts

A three-dimensional image of the heart is an artificial single volume since in reality it is composed of a number of single smaller volumes placed one over the other and corresponding to succeeding telediastolic phases. Consequently, step artifacts are often present in the area of overlapping single volumes (Fig. 3.10).

As far as the radiation dose is concerned, the procedure described herein has the disadvantage that the patient is irradiated for the entire time of the procedure, during all cardiac cycles, while only data related to telediastole are used for data reconstruction. As explained in the chapter on dose exposure, there are a number of way to reduce or eliminate this problem. One of the techniques uses non-spiral data acquisition, with single, small axial volumes (each 4 cm) acquired during telediastole, without X-ray emission in the other cardiac phases. The reduction in X-ray exposure achieved with this procedure is in the range of 80%.

Suggested Reading

Lu JG, Lu B, Chen XB et al (2010) What is the best contrast injection protocol for 64-row multidetector cardiac computed tomography? Eur J Radiol 75(2):159-165. Epub May 21 2009

Mahabadi AA, Achenbach S, Burgstahler C et al; Working group "Cardiac CT" of the German Cardiac Society (2010) Safety, efficacy, and indications of beta-adrenergic receptor blockade to reduce heart rate prior to coronary CT angiography. Radiology 257(3):614-623

Weininger M, Barraza JM, Kemper CA et al (2011) Cardiothoracic CT angiography: current contrast medium delivery strategies. AJR Am J Roentgenol 196(3):W260-W272

Zhu X, Chen W, Li M et al (2011) Contrast material injection protocol with the flow rate adjusted to the heart rate for dual source CT coronary angiography. Int J Cardiovasc Imaging. DOI: 10.1007/s10554-011-9950-y

Image Reconstruction

Paolo Pavone

Coronary CT angiography (CTA) is a three-dimensional imaging technique. The data obtained during image acquisition, however, are not immediately evident to the radiologist, as the huge amount of digital information acquired is used to reconstruct three-dimensional images of the coronary arteries, according to dedicated and complex software and protocols. The coronary arteries are tortuous, moving objects and are thus often not easily visualized. For this reason, in CTA the movements of these arteries must be "frozen," through cardiosynchronization, during image acquisition.

In order to visualize the coronary arteries in CTA, a very high density of the internal lumen must be created. As specified in the previous chapter, this is accomplished by the dynamic injection of contrast agent. The vessels become evident because of the large difference in the density of the vessel lumen (high density: 300–500 HU, due to the iodine content of the blood during passage of contrast agent) and that of the surrounding tissues, such as epicardial fat (low density: -50–100 HU). The difference is important because during three-dimensional image reconstruction only structures with a very high density will be clearly visualized. The higher the density, the more evident the anatomic structures will be. This is the reason why the first three-dimensional images presented for clinical use were related to bone, a structure with a very high radiologic density.

Starting from volume data, there are two ways to construct three-dimensional images of the anatomic structures of interest: the first is to explore the volume using curved or orthogonal bi-dimensional planes with so-called planimetric technique; the second is to consider and image the entire package of three-dimensional data, using so-called volumetric techniques. In this chapter, we offer a simple explanation of the difference in these visualization techniques and their relative importance in clinical use for the evaluation of coronary artery disease.

4.1 Planimetric Techniques

4.1.1 Axial Images

During data acquisition in coronary CTA, the console automatically displays axial images of the slices of the anatomic area under investigation, usually at 1-mm intervals (Fig. 4.1). These images confirm that the procedure has been correctly performed and that the acquisition timing, as far as opacification of the vessels by contrast agent is concerned, has been optimally achieved. In fact, segments of the coronary arteries can already be evaluated from these axial images, together with the myocardial walls and the contrast-agent-filled cardiac chambers. For non-experts, these axial images may not offer a clue in the identification of the coronary arteries; however, radiologists are well-acquainted with the CT evaluation of anatomic structures in the axial plane and thus may already gain early information regarding the presence of

P. Pavone (✉)
Radiology Department
Casa di Cura Mater Dei
Rome, Italy
e-mail: paolo.pavone@materdei.it

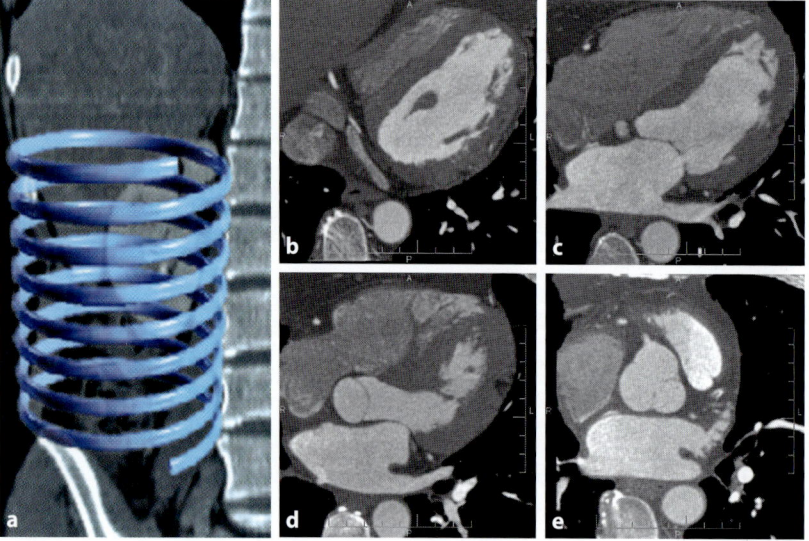

Fig. 4.1 3D volume acquisition using spiral technique: direct evaluation of single axial images slice by slice. **a** Scheme employed in spiral acquisition. **b–e** Slices reconstructed at different anatomic levels

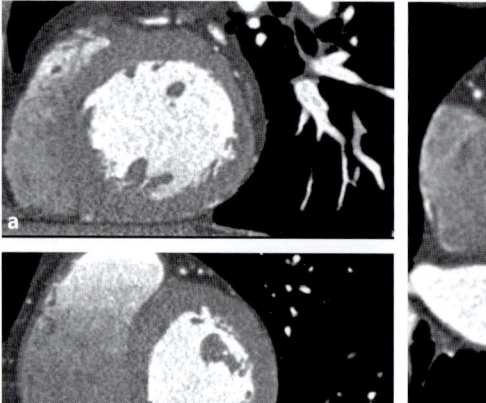
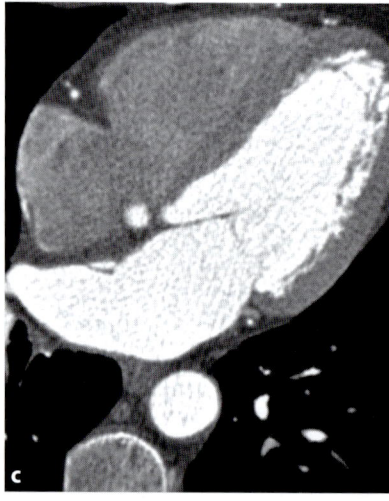

Fig. 4.2 Planimetric analysis (multi-planar reformatting, MPR) during 3D imaging. Reconstruction of images on the three different anatomic planes: **a** sagittal, **b** coronal, short axis, **c** axial, long axis

coronary artery disease simply by evaluating the images reconstructed in these anatomic planes. (Fig. 4.2). In the oblique plane, the course and location of the coronary arteries can be identified.

4.1.2 Multi-planar Reformatting

Three-dimensional reconstruction software provides direct access to images displayed in the three orthogonal planes, axial, sagittal, and coronal. This reconstruction technique is generically referred to as multi-planar reformatting (MPR). Moreover, the orthogonal images can be moved within the imaging volume and planes, such as the short or long axis, simplifying, anatomic evaluation of the heart

4.1.3 Reconstruction of the Curved Plane: Curved MPR

The same three-dimensional software that enables MPR allows reconstruction of curved planes (curved reformatting), according to the course and location of the coronary arteries. The course of each coronary artery can therefore be followed point by point and image by image. Direct reconstruction of a curved plane yields an image of the vessel of interest, from

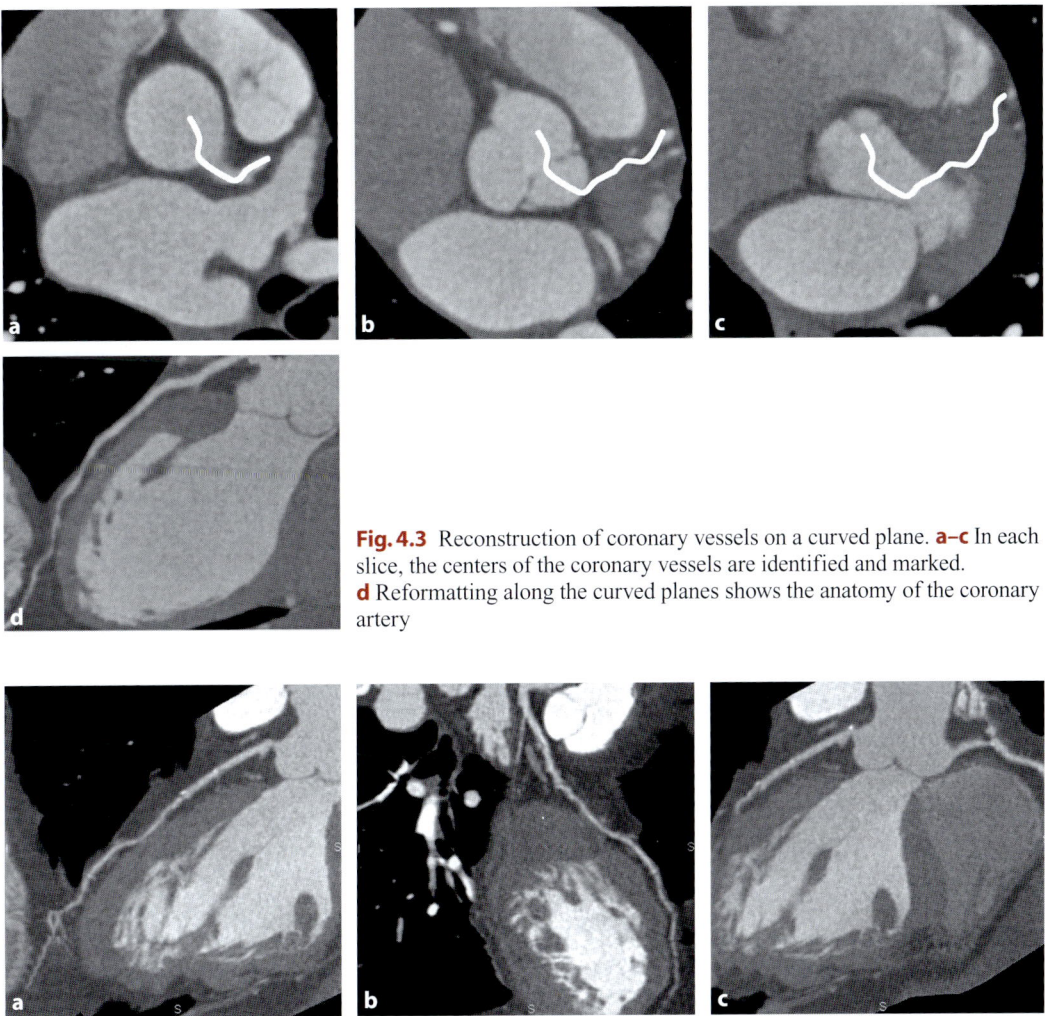

Fig. 4.3 Reconstruction of coronary vessels on a curved plane. **a–c** In each slice, the centers of the coronary vessels are identified and marked. **d** Reformatting along the curved planes shows the anatomy of the coronary artery

Fig. 4.4 a-c 3D imaging: planimetric analysis using curved-plane reformatting

its origins and extending to its more distal segments, according to specifications that are provided by the radiologist. These images may be obtained, manually or automatically, with reconstruction software that identifies the coronary arteries based on their higher CT density (Fig. 4.3). This image reconstruction technique is essential in the evaluation of coronary artery disease (Fig. 4.4). It allows clear differentiation between the vessel lumen (high density due to contrast agent in the blood and thus bright CT images), the surrounding epicardial fat tissue (darker, due to the lower CT density), and the myocardium (intermediate gray level, intermediate CT density). Furthermore, only these images clearly show the vessel wall, especially in the presence of pathologies such as fibrolipidic plaques (hypodense in CT, dark in reconstructed images) and calcific plaques (hyperdense, bright in CT images).

Bi-dimensional and planimetric images of the coronary arteries "slice" the vessel lumen in an orthogonal plane. The aim of the evaluation is to identify the vessel wall; therefore it is always important to image the vessels in two perpendicular orthogonal planes. Figure 4.5 very clearly demonstrates that in the case of an eccentric atherosclerotic plaque an orthogonal plane reveals the plaque, while the image reconstructed on a plane passing parallel to the fibrolipidic plaque does not show either the parietal plaque or the lumen stenosis. At least two planes for each coronary artery must therefore be

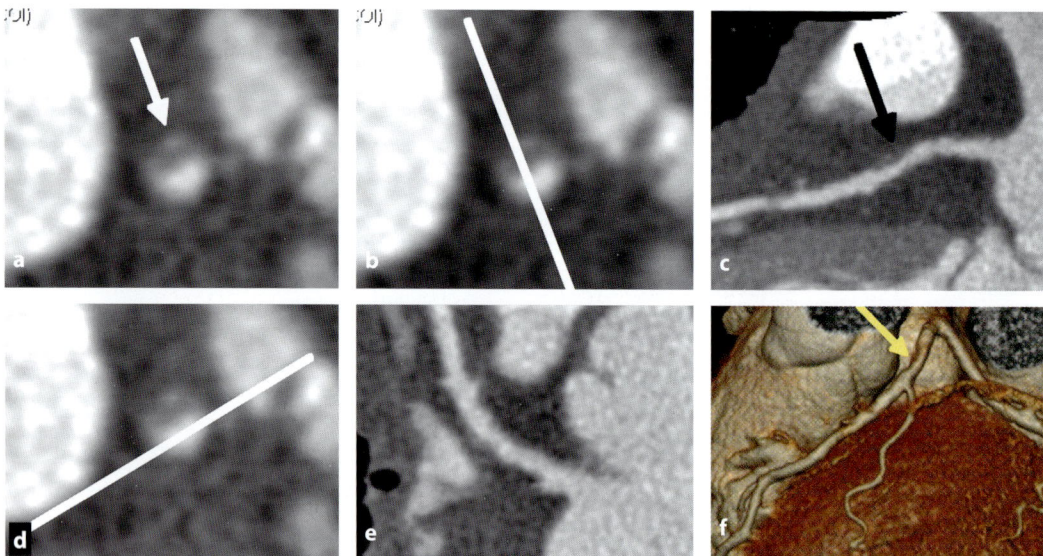

Fig. 4.5 Marginal eccentric plaque of the left anterior descending artery. **a** In the axial image, the eccentric fibrolipidic plaque is well evident (*arrows* in **a**, **c**, and **f**); the reduction in caliber is 50%. Visualization is possible only in one reconstruction plane (**b**, *white line* shows the reconstruction plane; **c** is the resulting image). In the orthogonal plane, the vessel seems to be of normal caliber (**d**, *white line* shows the reconstruction plane; **e** is the resulting image). **f** 3D image using volume-rendering technique allows a clear evaluation of the stenosis

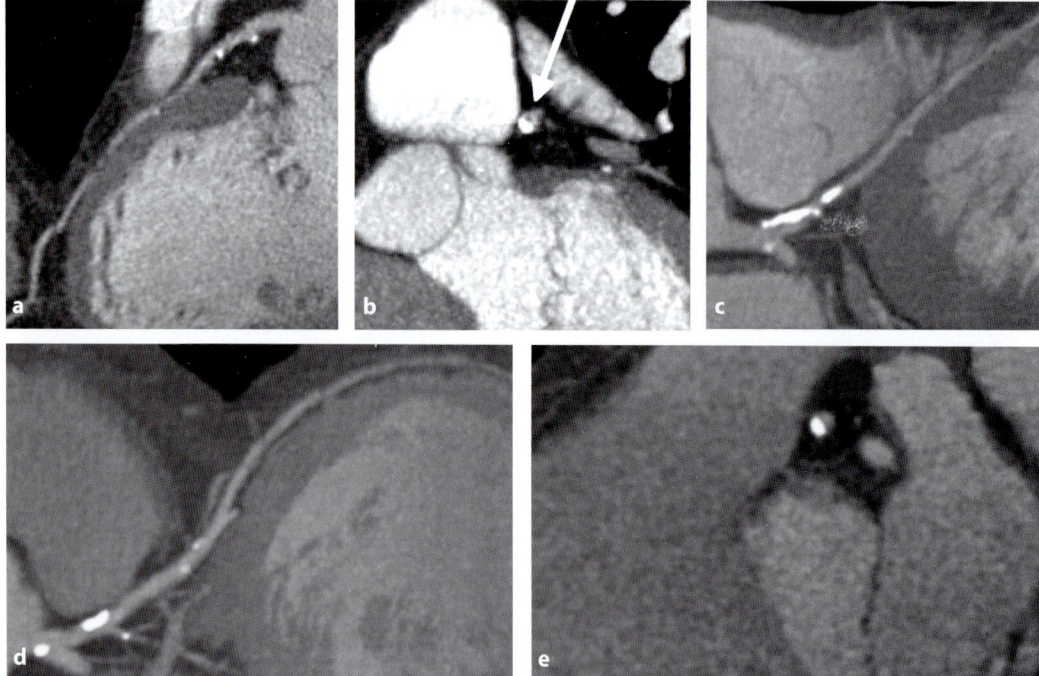

Fig. 4.6 Marginal plaque of the LAD with a calcific core and fibrolipidic cap (**a**, **b**), both of which are well-evident in the axial reconstruction (**b**, *arrow*). **a–e** Eccentric calcified plaque without a hypodense component

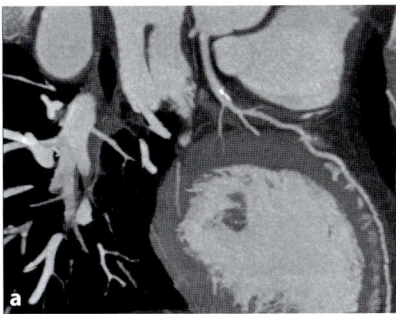 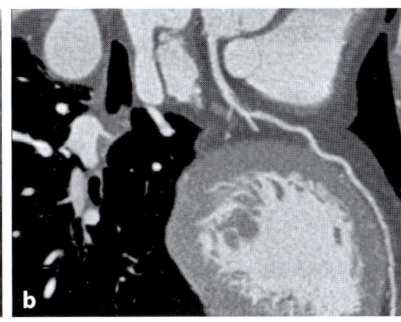

Fig. 4.7 3D imaging: planimetric analysis (MPR). **a** Reconstruction with thick slices (5 mm) allows better evaluation of the anatomic course of the LAD along the wall of the left ventricle. **b** The same artery evaluated using a thin slice (1 mm)

reconstructed and imaged (six images for three coronary arteries); depending on the specific anatomic variation, orthogonal images of other vessels will also be required, such as the intermediate, diagonal, and obtuse marginal branches.

Together with reconstruction of the vessel in curved longitudinal images, axial images, perpendicular to the imaging plane of the arteries, must be evaluated. Clear evidence of the location of the plaque (concentric or eccentric) and the degree of stenosis can be provided, including information on the presence of remodeling (as discussed later) (Fig. 4.6). Most of the currently available software allows direct evaluation of the vessels along their longitudinal axes, in addition to the possibility to interact with the images and rotate them along the different orthogonal planes. At the same time, axial images for the chosen view are displayed on the same console, allowing evaluation of the plaque burden at that specific level.

Usually, MPR curved images have a thickness of 1 mm or less. Depending on the amount of epicardial fat surrounding the arteries, the thickness can be increased to 3–5 mm, yielding anatomically reconstructed images of a more consistent quality (Fig. 4.7). However, these thicker images may hide small parietal plaques, which can be reconstructed and displayed only by the evaluation of thinner slices.

4.1.4 Clinical Use of Planimetric Techniques

Planimetric techniques do not provide direct evidence of the entire data volume acquired, as they are reconstructed according to the three-dimensional data set. These images are very important to define the parietal atherosclerotic plaque burden, identify the plaque, and properly characterize the plaque components. Software that "straightens" the vessels along their longitudinal axes is also available. It can be used to visualize the different sides of the vessel wall, since eccentric plaques may be evident on one side of the artery but not on the other side. Other types of software may also use planimetric images for quantitative evaluation of the vessel lumen, allowing measurement of the degree of stenosis in areas involved by atherosclerosis. Despite these numerous possibilities, in coronary CTA direct evaluation of the coronary vessels by the clinician may be necessary (Fig. 4.8). In calcific plaques, for instance, the so-called blooming artifact leads to an image in which the volume of the plaque is increased such that a false degree of stenosis is estimated by the computer. An expert radiologist, however, is able (using other reconstruction filters) to estimate the real extent and importance of the atherosclerotic involvement. Thus, regardless of the improvements in software for direct evaluation of the coronary vessels, a proper direct interface of the clinician with the console will always be needed to confirm the clinical diagnosis.

4.2 Volumetric Techniques (Volume Rendering)

Image analysis using volumetric techniques creates a color, three-dimensional image that allows direct interactive evaluation of the coronary vessels. The software employed in this application was initially developed mostly for military (aerospace) purposes and was later used in the film industry in virtual-

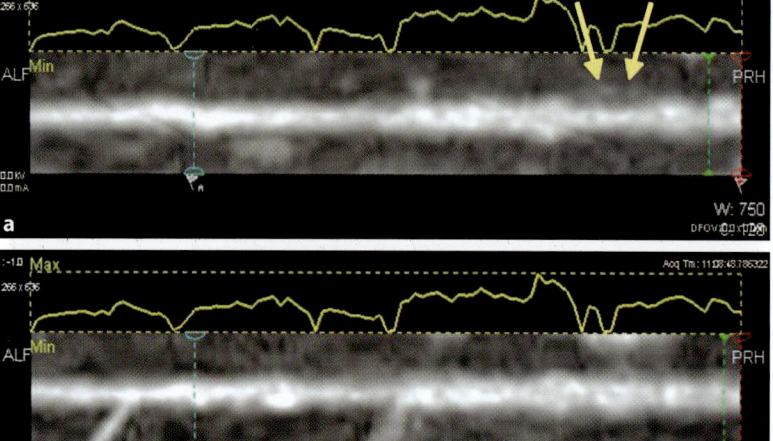

Fig. 4.8 Coronary artery "straightening" using special software. Rotation along the central axis reveals evidence of plaque (*arrows*, **a**), which is not seen in **b**

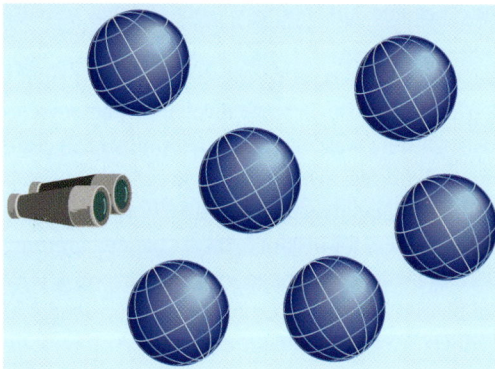

Fig. 4.9 Orthogonal view: all the globes are of the same size

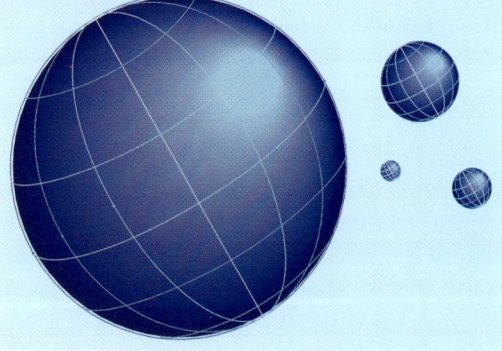

Fig. 4.10 Perspective view. As seen through a virtual eye (the binoculars in Fig. 4.9), there is true 3D evaluation. As in real life, the globes that are closer appear larger than those that are more distant

reality cartoons. The medical and radiology fields have taken advantage of the progress made in these animation techniques, as they have contributed to improvements in CT image reconstruction.

4.2.1 Orthogonal and Perspective Imaging

In order to understand the concept of volumetric imaging, a distinction must be made between the traditional concept of images (radiologic, artistic, etc.) and the newer one introduced by 3D imaging. In conventional radiologic images, the anatomic area under evaluation is perceived orthogonally, as if an infinite distance has been created between the viewer and the object being evaluated. In the example shown in Fig. 4.9, a series of round objects, all of the same diameter, is shown. In orthogonal view they all appear to be of the same size and dimension. In a routine X-ray, the abdomen, kidneys, vertebrae, and all other structures are visualized in a dimension that reflects their original size in the real world. By interacting with a volume data set in 3D imaging, we can move the volume, making it closer to us (the viewer), therefore modifying our relationship to it, i.e., the closer the object is to us, the larger it will appear. In the example of Fig. 4.10, our

4 Image Reconstruction

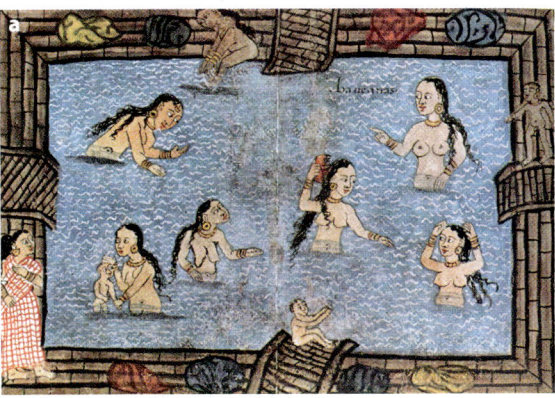 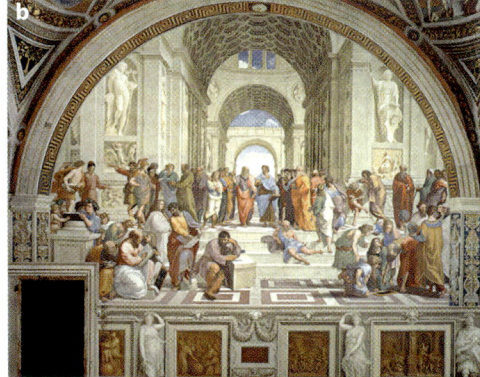

Fig. 4.11 a Orthogonal and **b** perspective views in art. Raffaello's *La scuola di Atene* (Rome, Vatican Museum) is an example of the perspective view in Renaissance art

eye is the binocular, such that the rounded structure is viewed from very near. Thus, objects very close to the binocular (our eye) are very large, while those progressively more distant become proportionally smaller. This phenomenon is referred to as the perspective view of a volumetric object.

In early paintings, the figures in a work of art are always of the same size, as if the viewer was at an infinite distance from them. During the Renaissance, painters, particularly Italian painters, became experts in realizing perspective views of human figures and landscapes, with attention to small details that made the depicted objects closer to our visualization of them in the real world (Fig. 4.11). The size of the figures in the painting became proportional to the distance from the painter or the viewer. In the same way, in volumetric CT imaging, a perspective vision is created in which the closer the object is, the larger it appears. Moreover, while a painting is a static object, the viewer of a CT image is able to adjust the distance between his or her eyes and the object under evaluation (the 3D volume of images) by direct interaction with the computer console.

4.2.2 Volume Rendering of Human Anatomy

Data sets acquired in CT include all the information contained in the anatomic area under investigation, with the risk that overlapping structures, or structures with different densities may create confusion, e.g., due to distension of the anatomic object (in our case, the coronary vessels) being evaluated. Volume-rendering technique allows the imaging display parameters to be set so that the structure of interest can be readily identified. For example, to evaluate the surface of the body, the density values are set such that they correspond to those of the skin; by progressively enhancing the density values, muscular structures, internal parenchymal organs, bones or, as in our case, vessels filled with contrast agent (density values of 300–500 HU) are visualized (Fig. 4.12). In effect, the image is restricted to the contrast-agent-filled coronary artery of interest, which is viewed in 3D images that have been reconstructed using volume-rendering techniques. The only overlapping components in the arteries are thus related to the presence of calcified plaques, which have a density even higher than that of the contrast agent. Images of the coronary arteries reconstructed with these techniques are extremely informative and of great diagnostic value, as discussed in other chapters of this book.

4.2.3 Color and Virtual Lighting

Three-dimensional images reconstructed using volume-rendering techniques became more realistic following the introduction of color (albeit, in effect, a false color) and by the use of virtual lighting to create shading effects that enhance the three-dimensional information. Similar effects

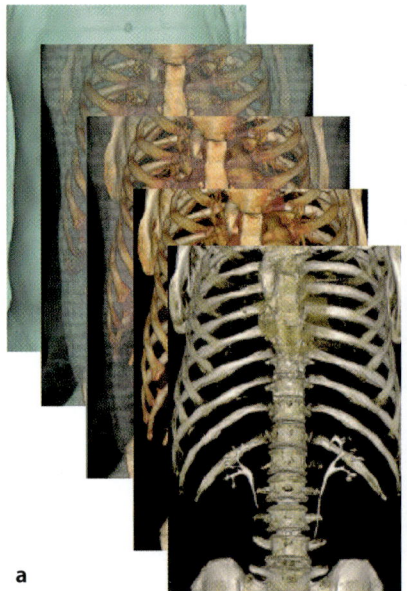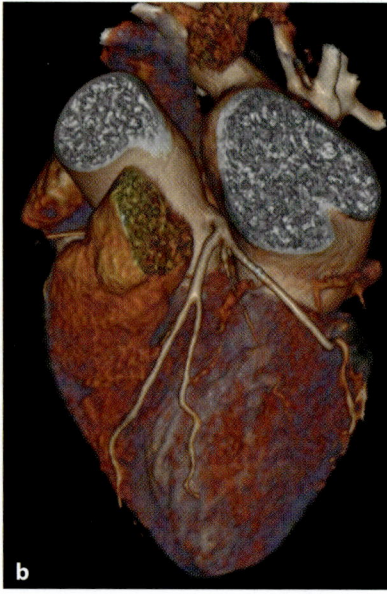

Fig. 4.12 Volume-rendering technique. **a** In evaluations of the body based on changing transparency values, deeper structures become evident, from the skin to the bones. **b** In cardiac imaging, a 3D setting is used that is already optimized for evaluating vascular structures opacified by means of contrast agent

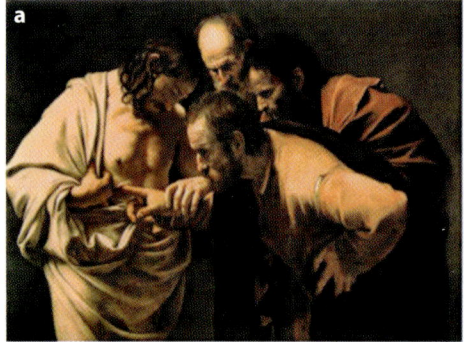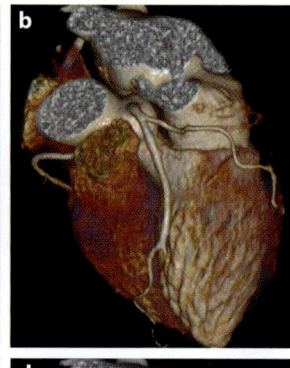
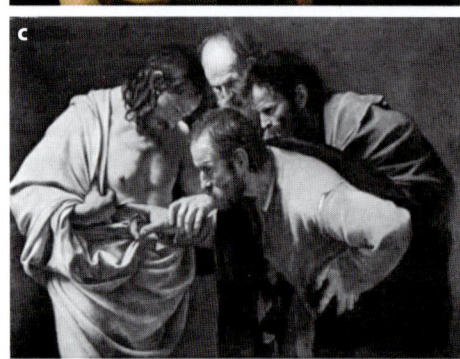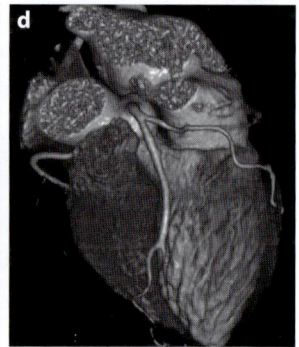

Fig. 4.13 Use of false color. The 3D effect, both in *Caravaggio's Incredulità di Tommaso* (Potsdam, Bildgalerie) (**a**) and in the image of the coronary artery (**b**), is enhanced by the use of color, as seen by a comparison with the respective black and white images (**c, d**)

(use of color and the proper use of lateral lighting) were used masterfully by the Italian painter Caravaggio, who more than any other artist of his time was an expert in using external light to make figures appear more realistic, including in their three-dimensional aspect (Fig. 4.13).

Modern three-dimensional image reconstruction techniques, such as those employed in radiology and in movie animation, are based on the same fundamental concepts but adapted to be standard, reproducible, and accessible at the computer console. Moreover, there is the additional advantage

4 Image Reconstruction

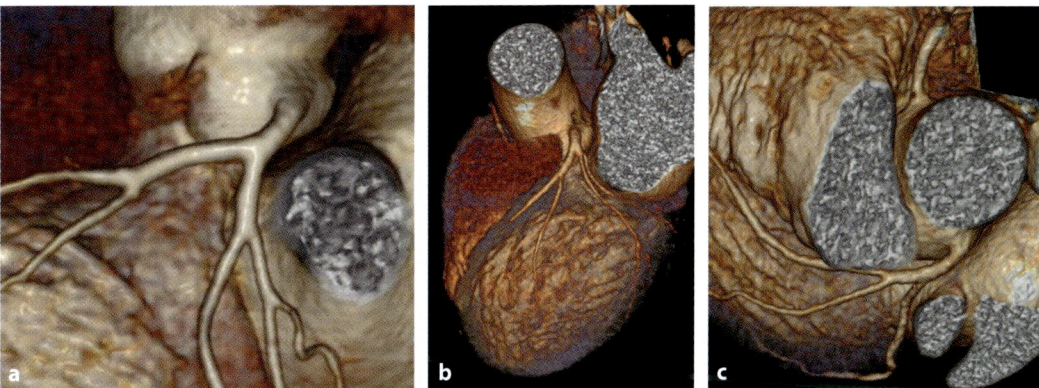

Fig. 4.14 a–c Examples of coronary vessels evaluated by means of volume-rendering technique

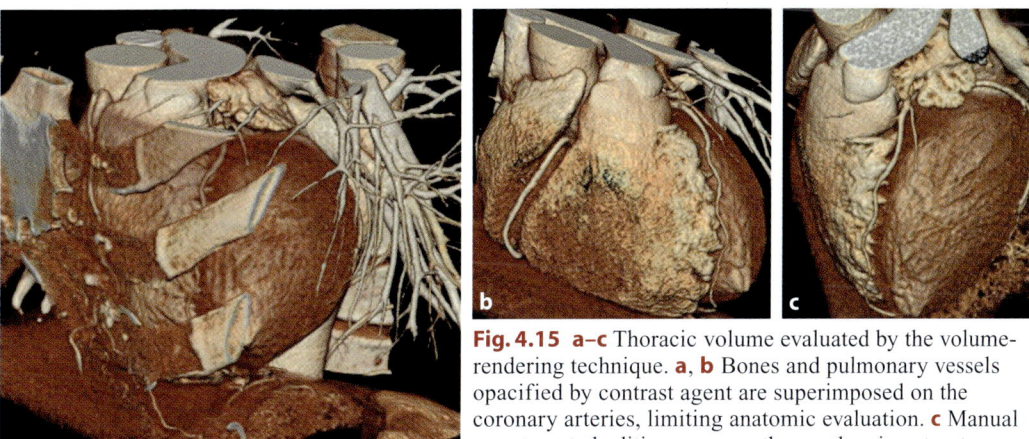

Fig. 4.15 a–c Thoracic volume evaluated by the volume-rendering technique. **a, b** Bones and pulmonary vessels opacified by contrast agent are superimposed on the coronary arteries, limiting anatomic evaluation. **c** Manual or automated editing removes the overlapping structures, revealing the coronary vessels

of direct interaction with the object being evaluated, which allows for a point by point evaluation that enhances the areas of interest in order to define the presence of disease, etc.

Once again, it must be emphasized that it is not the coronary arteries that are being seen, but the contrast agent contained within them. Likewise, a surface image of the myocardium and cardiac chambers is achieved only due to the higher density conferred by the presence of contrast agent (Fig. 4.14). Three-dimensional reconstruction of a volume of data acquired at the level of the heart without contrast agent injection would produce a useless evaluation of the soft tissues (the myocardium), which would be visible only because they are surrounded by the very low density of the air present in the lungs, but any evidence of the coronary arteries would be absent.

Other structures with high radiologic density overlap the coronary arteries, such as the pulmonary vessels and the bony thoracic cage. These structures can be excluded by "editing" the images (either automatically or manually), thereby providing direct and exclusive evidence of the coronary vessels (Fig. 4.15).

4.2.4 Clinical Use of Volume-Rendering Images

Three-dimensional reconstructed images are of foremost importance as they provide direct and

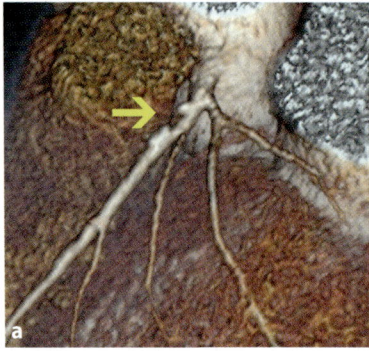 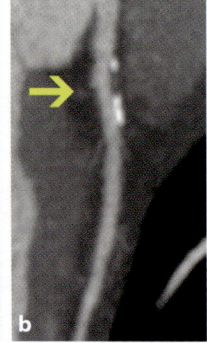

Fig. 4.16 a Fibrolipidic plaque evaluated using three-dimensional volume-rendering technique. **b** Evaluation using bi-dimensional technique. Note the central hypodense component of the plaque and the calcific spots (*arrows*)

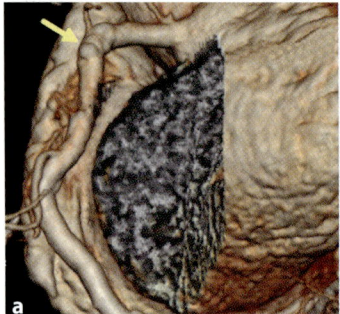 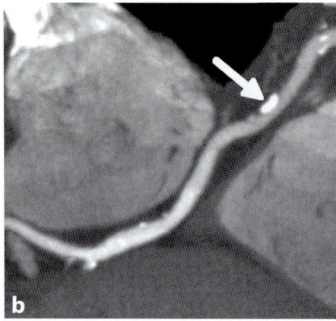 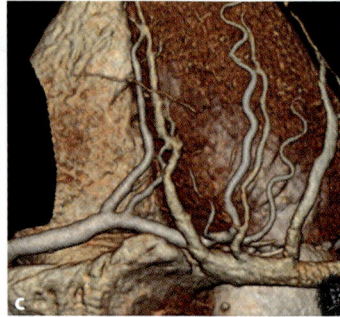

Fig. 4.17 Calcific plaque evaluated using volume-rendering technique. **a** The plaque is hyperdense (*arrow*). **b** A detailed evaluation of the vessel lumen is not possible but can be achieved by instead using bi-dimensional images (*arrow*). **c** There is marked hypertrophy of the distal branches of the right coronary artery

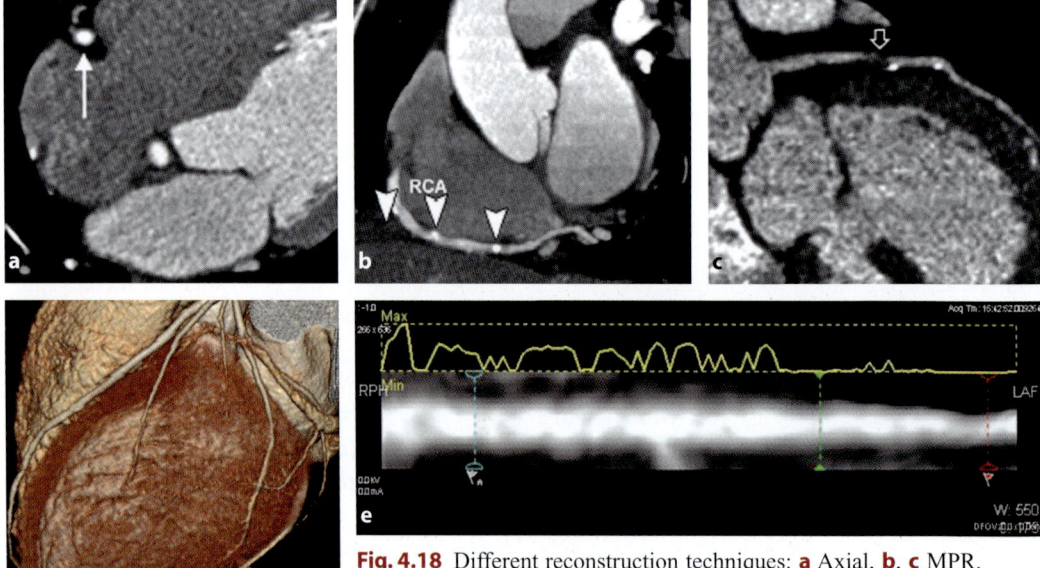

Fig. 4.18 Different reconstruction techniques: **a** Axial, **b**, **c** MPR, **d** volume rendering, **e** straightened vessel

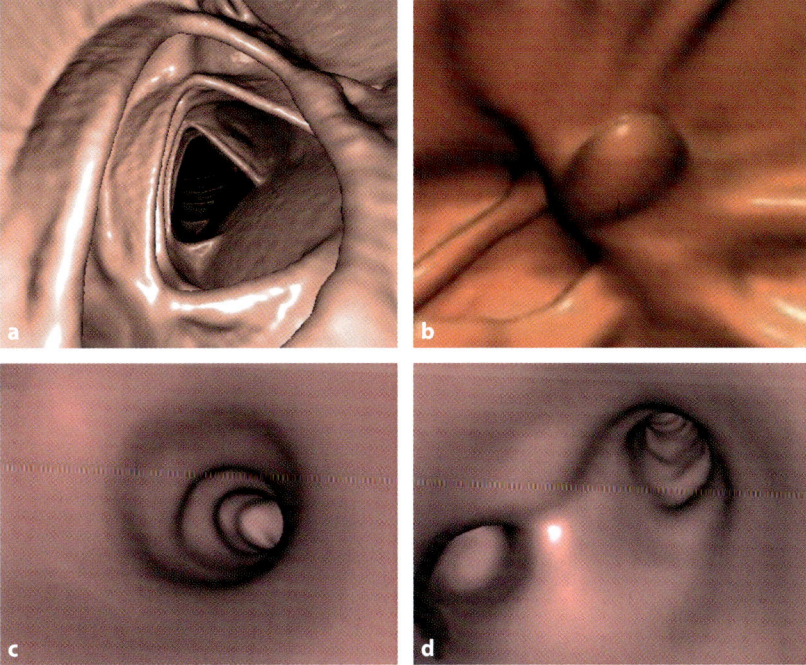

Fig. 4.19 a-d Virtual endoscopy of the coronary arteries

immediate evidence of the anatomy of the coronary tree (see Chap. 1 for a discussion of the variability of the coronary anatomy). Moreover, this technique allows for a complete and simultaneous evaluation of the entire volume acquired. Nonetheless, care must be taken in evaluating volume images reconstructed with volume-rendering techniques as, in fact, they provide a superficial evaluation from outside of the vessels (Fig. 4.16). In a patient with parietal atherosclerotic involvement, stenosis can be visualized only when a fibrolipidic low-density plaque is present; if the plaque is calcific, the higher density of the plaque material will overlap with the density of the vessel lumen, prohibiting proper visualization and analysis of a possible stenosis (in addition to the previously mentioned blooming effect) (Fig. 4.17). Therefore, in every case and for every vessel, images generated by the two types of reconstruction must be evaluated and compared. This will result in proper anatomic definition and correct identification of the atherosclerotic involvement (Fig. 4.18).

4.3 Virtual Endoscopy

We conclude this chapter with a brief discussion of another three-dimensional visualization technique, albeit one that is seldom used to evaluate the coronary arteries: virtual endoscopy. The principles and software needed to acquire virtual endoscopy images are the same as those for volume-rendering images. The difference is that the virtual eye moves from a surface evaluation to an internal examination of the anatomic 3D data sets. To do so, specific settings have to be used, such that the density contained in the lumen (contrast agent) becomes transparent while other densities are made evident. This procedure is carried out by a mouse click at the computer, as these settings are already among the many available to the clinician. Once "inside" the vessel of interest, the viewer can move his or her virtual eyes along the course of the vessels and the area of stenosis, then move on to the origin of the side branches (Fig. 4.19). Although fascinating, this technique does not add any further information to

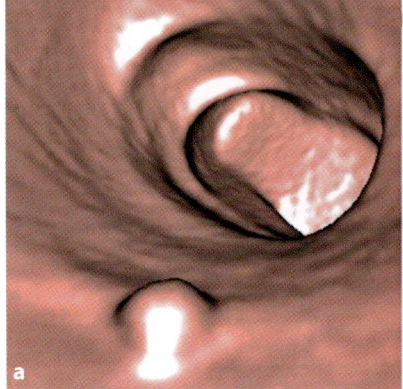 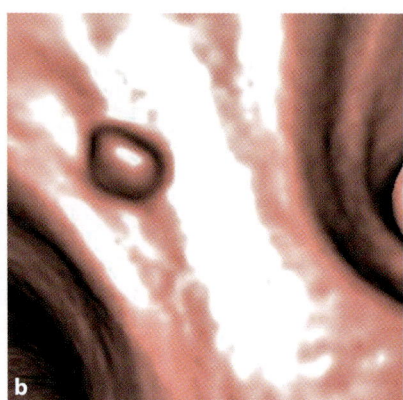

Fig. 4.20 Virtual endoscopy of the colon (**a**): a parietal 5-mm polyp is easily detected (**b**)

that already provided by the other above-described procedures and is therefore seldom employed. Virtual endoscopy is more useful in other settings, e.g., in the evaluation of pre-cancerous polyps of the colon (virtual colonoscopy) (Fig. 4.20).

Suggested Reading

Araoz PA, Kirsch J, Primak AN, Braun NN, Saba O, Williamson EE, Harmsen WS, Mandrekar JN, McCollough CH. Optimal image reconstruction phase at low and high heart rates in dual-source CT coronary angiography. Int J Cardiovasc Imaging. 2009 Dec;25(8):837-45

Brenner DJ, Hall EJ (2007) Computed tomography. An increasing source of radiation exposure. N Engl J Med 357:2277-2284

Diederichs CG, Keating DP, Glatting G, Oestmann JW: Blurring of vessels in spiral CT angiography: effects of collimation width, pitch, viewing plane, and windowing in maximum intensity projection. J Comput Assist Tomogr 1996;20:965–974

Herzog C, Nguyen SA, Savino G, Zwerner PL, Doll J, Nielsen CD, Flohr TG, Vogl TJ, Costello P, Schoepf UJ. Does two-segment image reconstruction at 64-section CT coronary angiography improve image quality and diagnostic accuracy? Radiology. 2007 Jul; 244(1):121-9. Epub 2007 May 10. PubMed PMID: 17495177

Matsuura N, Horiguchi J, Yamamoto H, Hirai N, Tonda T, Kohno N, Ito K. Optimal cardiac phase for coronary artery calcium scoring on single-source 64-MDCT scanner: least interscan variability and least motion artifacts. AJR Am J Roentgenol. 2008 Jun;190(6):1561-8. PubMed PMID: 18492907

Coronary Pathophysiology

Mara Piccoli, Serafino Orazi, Giovanna Giubilato and Massimo Fioranelli

5.1 Introduction

The heart pumps approximately 5 L of blood per minute at rest and up to 24 L per min during vigorous exercise. Accordingly, it consumes more energy than any other organ, cycling about 6 kg of ATP, which is 20–30 times its own weight, every day. To acquire this enormous amount of energy, the heart converts chemical energy stored in fatty acids and glucose into mechanical energy, in the form of actinomyosin myofibrillar interactions. Fatty acids, through β-oxidation, account for about 70% of ATP synthesis, and glucose, through aerobic glycolysis, for the remaining 30%. Due to this dependence on oxidative energy production, increases in cardiac activity require instantaneous parallel increases in oxygen availability [1].

Energy supplied to the myocardium is used for mechanical activities, i.e., contraction (65%) and relaxation (15%), and for electrical activity (5%); the rest is spent on basal metabolism (15%) Under anoxic or ischemic conditions, the myocardium uses anaerobic glycolysis to produce energy. However, this pathway is inefficient as it consumes a large amount of glucose and leads to the production of lactate and only 2 ATP molecules for every molecule of glucose, whereas oxidative phosphorylation produces 36 molecules of ATP for the same amount of glucose. Moreover, lactate reduces intracellular pH, which inhibits glycolysis, β-oxidation, and protein synthesis.

Oxidative phosphorylation is carried out in the mitochondrial respiratory chain and accounts for almost 90% of the energy (ATP) derived from substrate utilization. Recent findings [2] have shown that resting cardiac energy metabolism is inversely associated with heart rate, which may explain the prognostic role of heart rate as evidenced by epidemiological studies.

During coronary ischemia, the degradation of ATP results in the production of ADP and then AMP and adenosine. Consequently, adenosine diffuses from myocytes into the interstitial fluid and the coronary venous effluent. Adenosine is a powerful coronary dilator and the rise in its interstitial concentration parallels the increase in coronary blood flow. However, the loss of adenosine from myocytes can lead to the permanent injury of these cells. In fact, during a prolonged ischemic event (> 30 min) as much as 50% of the adenosine reserve may be depleted. Since the de novo synthesis of adenosine is very slow, about 2% every hour, ischemia lasting more than 30 min can have catastrophic consequences for the myocardium.

The coronary arteries supply the myocardium with oxygen and nutrients; only the innermost layer of the endocardium (about 0.1 mm thick) is supplied directly from the blood within the heart chambers. From the epicardial coronary arteries, and then via intramuscular and subendocardial vessels, blood flows to the myocardial capillaries. The coronary microcirculation is crucial in providing oxygen to cardiomyocytes and in maintaining myocardial metabolism, and thus to myocardial contraction and re-

M. Piccoli (✉)
Cardiology Unit, Policlinico "Luigi di Liegro"
Rome, Italy
e-mail: mandimara@libero.it

laxation The cardiomyocytes are surrounded by reticular capillaries, which feed into arterioles and venules, thereby forming intramyocardial microcirculatory units that regulate the coronary circulation [3]. The myocardial oxygen supply rises and falls in response to the oxygen demands of the myocardium. At rest, myocardial oxygen extraction is almost maximal (about 70%), facilitated by a high capillary density of 3,000-4,000/mm^2. Thus, an increased metabolic demand can only be met by augmented coronary flow. The resting coronary flow rate is 220–250 ml/min (70–90 ml per 100 g myocardial tissue per min), which is about 5% of cardiac output. In response to physiologic or pharmacologic stimuli, coronary flow to the myocardium is increased from its basal level to a maximal flow of 280 ml per 100 g/min, without any signs of under- or overperfusion. During systole, blood flow through the myocardial capillaries is very low due to cardiac contraction and ventricular ejection. In a normal heart, blood flow is controlled by the vascular tone of the coronary microcirculation (vessels with diameters < 400 μm). Kaneko et al. [3] suggested that the precapillary and capillary sinuses together comprise a micropump that utilizes cardiomyocyte contraction and relaxation to maintain uniform perfusion of the myocardial parenchyma.

Exercise is the most important physiological stimulus for increasing myocardial oxygen demand and supply [4-6]. An increase in oxygen demand induces an increase in contractile activity, principally attributed to an increase in heart rate (60%), but also to the augmentation of contractility and ventricular work. The increased blood supply derives from enhanced coronary blood flow that in turn is the result of coronary vasodilation (decreased coronary resistance) and an increase in mean arterial pressure. In the normal heart, exercise induces adaptations by coronary resistance vessels, manifested as an increase in basal tone and in vasodilator influences (elevated NO production and K$^+$ channel activity). These adaptations are thought to contribute to the improved perfusion observed after exercise training, but further studies are required to identify the system of vasodilatory components that mediate exercise hyperemia.

A pressure drop across a stenosis causes compensatory vasodilation at rest, thereby diminishing the ability of the coronary circulation to adapt to an increase in oxygen demand. Resting coronary flow is not impeded by mild or moderate stenosis and is maintained by normal vasodilatory regulation of the microcirculation, remaining constant until epicardial coronary constriction exceeds 85–90% of the normal segment diameter. By contrast, maximal hyperemic coronary blood flow begins to decline when the diameter of the stenosis exceeds 45–60%, leading to myocardial ischemia and angina.

5.2   Coronary Flow Reserve

The capacity to increase coronary blood flow in response to a hyperemic stimulus is referred to as coronary flow reserve, defined as the ratio of maximal to basal coronary flow. It is a measure of the ability of the two components of myocardial perfusion, namely, epicardial stenosis resistance and microvascular resistance, to achieve maximal blood flow. Since flow resistance is mainly determined by the microvasculature, coronary flow reserve reflects the microvascular response to a stimulus and therefore presumably the function of the small vessels.

Coronary flow reserve is determined by measuring coronary or myocardial blood flow and taking measurements both at rest (basal flow) and with maximal hyperemia, which is achieved with an intracoronary or intravenous infusion of adenosine or an intravenous infusion of dipyridamole. Normal coronary flow reserve in young patients with normal arteries commonly exceeds 3.0; in patients undergoing cardiac catheterization with angiographically normal vessels, coronary flow reserve averages 2.7±0.6. In patients with coronary artery disease, the extent of the reduction in coronary flow reserve is directly related to the severity of the stenosis, whereas in individuals with angiographically normal arteries it is a marker of microvascular dysfunction. A coronary flow reserve of < 2.0 is often considered abnormal. However, the dependence of coronary flow reserve on hemodynamic conditions and cardiac function limits its use as a reliable and reproducible tool of microvascular disease [7].

Instead, measurement of fractional flow reserve (FFR), introduced in 1996, allows accurate eval-

5 Coronary Pathophysiology

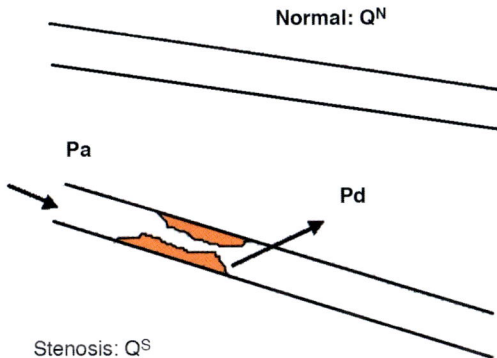

Fig. 5.1 Definition of FFR. FFR = $Q^S/Q^N \simeq$ Pd/Pa during maximum hyperemia; PaPd, hyperaemic distal coronary pressure; Pa, mean aortic pressure; Q^S, maximum myocardial blood flow in the presence of stenosis; PdQ^N, normal maximum blood flow

uation of the severity of a stenosis [8-10]. FFR is defined as the maximum myocardial blood flow in the presence of a stenosis divided by the theoretical maximum blood flow in the same region in the absence of stenosis (Fig. 5.1). In the presence of a stenosis, there is a decrement in the distal pressure that is proportional to its severity. To maintain resting myocardial perfusion, arteriolar resistance decreases to compensate for the pressure drop caused by the epicardial stenosis. FFR estimates coronary blood flow through a stenotic artery and it is calculated by measuring the coronary pressure distal to a stenosis at constant and minimal myocardial resistances (i.e., maximal hyperemia) obtained during intracoronary adenosine infusion. Since it is calculated only at peak hyperemia, FFR differs from coronary flow reserve by being largely independent of basal flow, driving pressure, heart rate, systemic blood pressure, myocardial contractility, or status of the microcirculation.

The theoretical FFR value of a normal coronary artery is 1, with pathology indicated at FFR < 0.75 and in the presence of an identified coronary stenosis in patients with inducible ischemia. The FFR has a high sensitivity (88%), specificity (100%), and overall accuracy (93%). For example, dividing the pressure value distal to the stenosis, e.g., 52 mmHg, by the value obtained proximal to the stenosis, e.g., 101 mmHg, yields FFR = 0.51, which is obviously indicative of a pathology [11, 12].

5.3 Definition and Evaluation of Coronary Stenosis

On 30 October 1958, the first coronary angiography was performed by Sones. Shortly thereafter, the technique became the gold standard in the evaluation of coronary artery disease as it allowed a visual estimation of the percentage of stenosis. The presence and degree of a coronary stenosis can be assessed by different approaches: by evaluating lumen reduction (anatomo-pathological section or CT imaging) or by measuring the reduction in longitudinal diameter (angiography imaging) (Fig. 5.2).

Coronary angiography provides information about the reduction in diameter and quantifies coronary lesions in terms of the percentage stenosis and minimal lumen diameter. The percentage

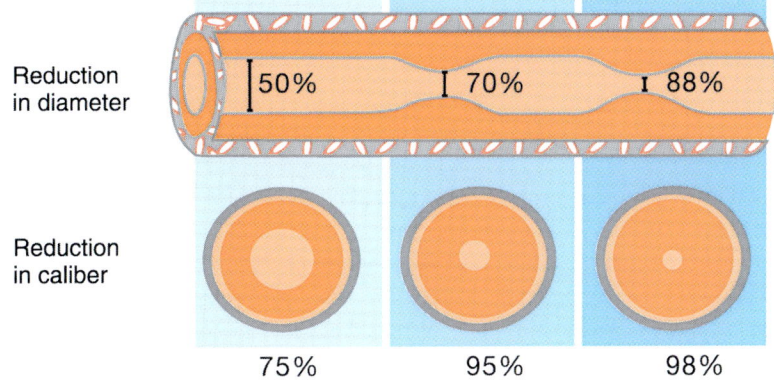

Fig. 5.2 Relationship between diameter and caliber (lumen) reduction in coronary stenosis

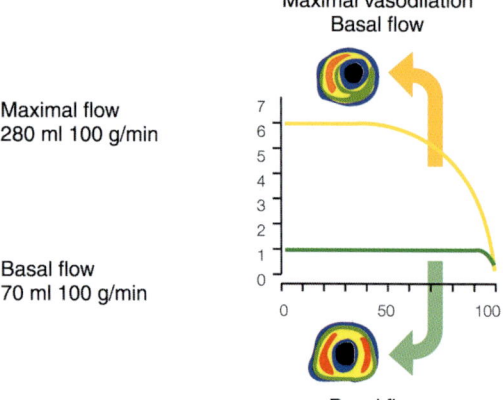

Fig. 5.3 Coronary flow reserve. Relationship between stenosis and microvasculature [15]

stenosis is given by the relationship between the minimal lumen diameter resulting from the stenosis and the reference diameter upstream or downstream of the lesion, identified as normal. Minimal lumen diameter is calculated in millimeters and is an absolute value. While it is more reliable and more consistent than percentage stenosis it is of limited value in the precise determination of coronary stenosis [13, 14].

Hyperemic flux, in the animal model proposed by Gould et al. [15] (Fig. 5.3), begins to decrease when an atherosclerotic plaque causes a 50% reduction in diameter, implying a 75% stenosis of the luminal area (Fig. 5.2). Accordingly, an atherosclerotic plaque is defined as obstructive when the vessel diameter is decreased by > 50%. However, this does not mean that the lesion will certainly cause ischemia; rather, it is a threshold value over which the stenosis has ischemic potential. Coronary blood flow at rest is not significantly decreased until the diameter of the lumen is reduced by about 90%. In the absence of coronary microcirculation dysfunction or hypertrophy, coronary blood flow during exercise is reduced when the stenosis is severe (diameter reduction between 50 and 80%).

In patients with coronary artery disease, any revascularization strategy needs to be discussed not only in anatomic terms but also regarding the functional severity of the stenosis. Thus, it is extremely important to evaluate patients non-invasively, since the angiographic degree of stenosis is not always of prognostic value. When there is moderate stenosis (between 50 and 80%) and non-invasive tests have confirmed myocardial ischemia, if medical therapy is unable to stop the symptoms then the patient is referred for percutaneous revascularization. If non-invasive testing does not detect myocardial ischemia, even in patients with chest pain, then a functional evaluation of the stenosis should be obtained through a battery of functional tests, including measurements of FFR and Doppler flow velocity (the velocity of the blood before and after the stenosis, measured using a Doppler probe).

5.4 The Limits of Coronary Angiography

Coronary angiography is able to identify the number, extent, and degree of stenosis. However, one of its limitations is that it only visualizes the lumen, whereas coronary artery disease usually affects the arterial wall. Intravascular ultrasound (IVUS) provides information not only about the arterial lumen but also about the thickness and tissue characteristics of the arterial wall. In fact, IVUS data together with anatomo-pathological studies have shown that angiographically normal coronary artery segments often have an atherosclerotic burden. The disadvantages of IVUS, as opposed to other imaging modalities, are that it is invasive, such that it is currently performed only in conjunction with selective coronary angiography, and the fact that it visualizes only a limited portion of the coronary tree [16]. Moreover, many trials have shown that most coronary thromboses occur in a non-occluding plaque, and often in the presence of mild or moderate stenosis. In addition, positive remodeling, which is caused by an atherosclerotic plaque that extends outwardly from the vessel wall, decreases the accuracy of coronary stenosis evaluation by coronary angiography.

Coronary stenosis is most commonly evaluated according to the degree of vessel diameter reduction compared to apparently normal proximal and distal vessel segments; but since coronary artery disease is usually pervasive it is highly likely that the reference segment also contains plaque [13, 14]. Thus, the amount of stenosis is generally underestimated, as the atherosclerotic burden is present throughout the vessel. In the evaluation of coronary artery disease, it is of pivotal importance to determine the atherosclerotic burden as well as the biological qualitative composition of the plaque. As many vulnerable plaques prone to rupture are non-obstructive, they are often missed by coronary angiography. Several studies on patients with sudden death or who died from myocardial infarction have clearly established that the most important prognostic factor is the extent of atherosclerotic disease and not the degree of stenosis. Indeed, only 26% of vulnerable plaques cause > 50% stenosis, whereas about 50% of healed plaques rupture and acute ruptures result in severe stenosis [17].

The findings of coronary plaque characterization are highly variable because atherosclerosis is an active process involving the intima. The vulnerability of a plaque to rupture is typically indicated by the presence of a necrotic core. This is a region of the fibroatheroma that is largely devoid of viable cells and consists of cellular debris and cholesterol clefts, a thin fibrous cap (< 65 mm), and macrophage infiltration, with rare smooth cells and the variable presence of T lymphocytes [18, 19]. The identification of vulnerable plaques, i.e., those likely to rupture due to a disruption of the fibrous cap, is an important clinical goal. Although current guidelines do not recommend the evaluation of coronary plaques for risk stratification, patients considered to be at high clinical risk should undergo individualized risk assessment of their atherosclerotic burden.

References

1. Westerhof N, Boer C, Lamberts RR, Sipkema P (2006) Cross-talk between cardiac muscle and coronary vasculature. Physiol Rev 86:1263-1308
2. Fragasso G, De Cobelli F, Spodalore R (2011) Resting cardiac energy metabolism is inversely associated with heart rate in healthy young adult men. Am Heart J 162(1):136-141
3. Kaneko N, Matsuda R, Toda M, Shimamoto K (2011) Three-dimensional reconstruction of the human capillary network and the intramyocardial necrosis. Am J Physiol Heart Circ Physiol 300:H754-H761
4. Deussen A, Ohanyan V, Jannasch A et al (2011) Mechanisms of metabolic coronary flow regulation. J Mol Cell Cardiol 52:794-801
5. Duncker DJ, Bache RJ, Merkus D (2011) Regulation of coronary resistance vessel tone in response to exercise. J Mol Cell Cardiol 52:802-813
6. Duncker DJ, Bache RJ (2008) Regulation of coronary blood flow during exercise. Physiol Rev 88:1009-1086
7. Knaapen P, Camici PG, Marques KM et al (2009) Coronary microvascular resistance: methods for its quantification in humans. Basic Res Cardiol 104:485-498
8. Uren NG, Melin JA, de Bruyne B et al (1994) Relation between myocardial blood flow and the severity of coronary artery stenosis. NEJM 330:1782-1788
9. Gould KL, Lipscomb K, Hamilton GW (1974) Physiologic basis for assessing critical coronary stenosis: instantaneous flow response and regional distribution during coronary hyperemia as a measure of coronary flow reserve. Am J Cardiol 33:87-94
10. Pijls NHJ, de Bruyne B, Peels K et al (1996) Measurement of fractional flow reserve to assess the functional severity of coronary artery stenosis. NEJM 334:1703-1708
11. Hau WK (2004) Fractional flow reserve and complex coronary pathologic conditions. Eur Heart J 25:723-727
12. Tonino PA, Fearon WF, de Bruyne B et al (2010) Angiographic versus functional severity of coronary stenosis in the FAME study: Fractional flow reserve versus angiography in multivessel evaluation. JACC 55:2816-2821
13. White CW, Wright CB, Doty DB et al (1984) Does visual interpretation of the coronary arteriogram predict the physiological impor-

tance of coronary stenosis? NEJM 310:819-824
14. Topol EJ, Nissen SE (1995) Our preoccupation with coronary luminology. The dissociation between clinical and angiographic findings in ischemic heart disease. Circulation 92; 2333-2342
15. Gould KL (2009) Does coronary flow trump coronary anatomy? JACC Cardiovasc Imaging 2(8):1009-1023
16. Rickenbacher PR, Pinto FJ, Chenzbraun A et al (1995) Incidence and severity of transplant coronary artery disease early and up to 15 years after transplantation as detected by intravascular ultrasound. J Am Coll Cardiol. 25:171-177
17. Kolodgie FD, Virmani R, Burke AP et al (2004) Pathologic assessment of the vulnerable human coronary plaque. Heart 90:1385-1391
18. Falk E (1999) Stable versus unstable atherosclerosis: clinical aspects. Am Heart J 138:S421-S425
19. Virmani R, Burke AP, Farb A, Kolodgie FD (2002) Pathology of the unstable plaque. Prog Cardiovasc Dis 44:349-356

Clinical Classification of Coronary Artery Disease: Who Should Be Treated?

Damien Casagrande, Jean-Jacques Goy, Mario Togni, Jean Christophe Stauffer and Stéphane Cook

6.1 Introduction

Coronary heart disease affects 2–6% of the general population; in the USA, it is responsible for more than 400,000 deaths each year. Epidemiological data show that, annually, approximately 785,000 Americans experience a heart attack [1], underlining the urgency of detection, quantification, and the prompt initiation of treatment of ischemic heart disease. Obstructive coronary disease causes an imbalance between oxygen supply and oxygen consumption, leading to the various clinical syndromes described below. Atherosclerotic plaque growth proceeds from the accumulation of fatty deposits, cholesterol, and cellular waste products in the inner layer of the coronary arteries. Other substances, such as calcium, can also be found in the fatty streaks. Over time, fibrous atherosclerotic plaques develop, narrowing the arteries and thereby limiting coronary blood flow. At this stage, coronary artery disease can be asymptomatic or associated with angina pectoris, and it is typically accompanied by calcification of the atherosclerotic plaque. Calcification is an active process, a part of the atherosclerotic burden, similar to metaphysis in bone formation. In addition, the plaque may rupture, due to the atherosclerotic burden, leading to vessel occlusion, blood flow interruption, and acute coronary syndrome.

J.J. Goy (✉)
Cardiology Service, Hôpital Cantonal
Fribourg, Switzerland
e-mail: jjgoy@goyman.com

6.2 Epidemiology and Natural History

The prevalence of coronary artery disease increase with age in both genders, from approximately 1% in women age 45–55 to 15% in women age 65–75, with corresponding values in men of 5% and 20% [1, 2]. Therefore in Western countries, 2–4% of the population suffers from coronary artery disease, albeit with great geographic variations; for example, the incidence of angina is approximately two-fold higher in Ireland than in France. Both the natural history of the disease and the prognosis vary with the mode of disease presentation. Annual mortality ranges from 1 to 1.5%, with the incidence of myocardial infarction ranging from 0.5 to 2.5% in patients with stable angina pectoris. In patients with acute coronary syndrome, mortality studies carried out in the pre-reperfusion era reported an in-hospital fatality of 16%. With the use of coronary revascularization, (fibrinolytic agents, antithrombotic therapy, and secondary prevention), the overall 1-month mortality has been reduced to 4–6%. Prognostic assessment is important in the management of patients with coronary artery disease.

Even if several different clinical syndromes are associated with obstructive coronary artery disease, angina pectoris, an expression of myocardial ischemia, remains the cornerstone of the diagnosis. Chest pain is typically felt during physical exercise, emotional stress, cold weather, or after a heavy meal. Patients usually describe middle-chest constrictive pain with irradiation into the left arm, neck, jaw, and back. Additional symptoms, including pangs of anx-

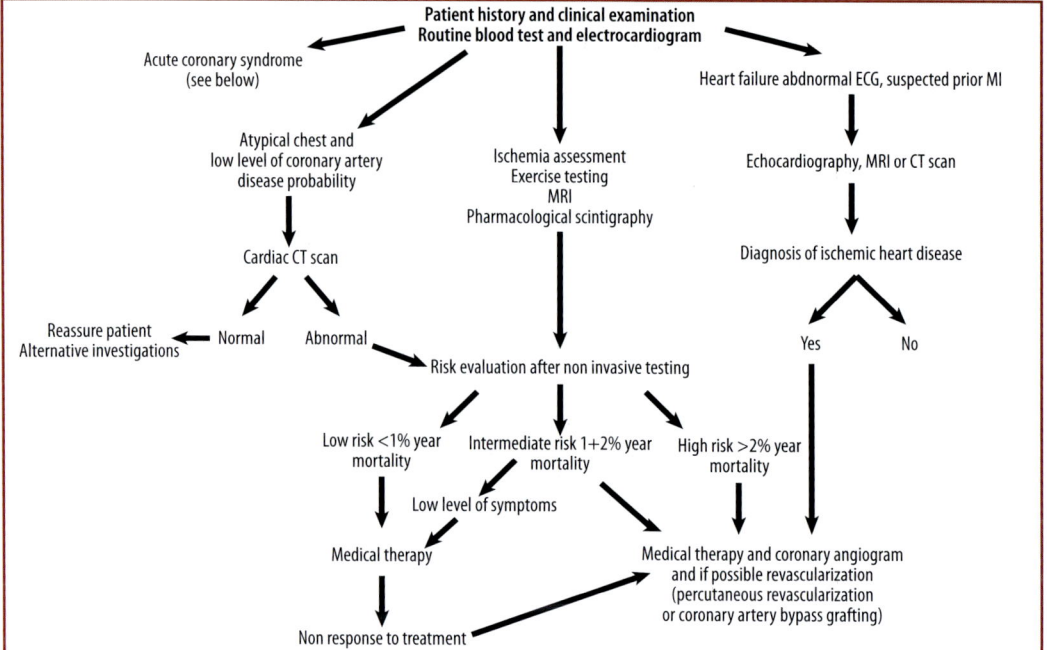

Fig. 6.1 Algorithm for the management of patients with chest pain

iety and feelings of numbness, pressure, and suffocation, are also reported by many patients.

6.3 Specific Clinical Conditions

6.3.1 Silent Ischemia

The term "silent ischemia" is used in asymptomatic patients with clinical evidence of obstructive coronary artery disease. As long as the disease does not restrict routine daily activities and, to a lesser extent, exercise, coronary narrowing develops unnoticed. Particular attention must be paid to patients with diabetes, because of the high incidence of silent ischemia in this cohort. The management of these patients should not differ from that of patients with stable angina pectoris [3]. Non-invasive risk assessment should therefore be performed in patients at high risk.

6.3.2 Stable Angina

Stable angina is the main expression of chronic coronary insufficiency. According to the definition, it manifests as angina pectoris that is present for at least 1 month without any recent major aggravation. It is generally caused by emotional stress or physical exercise. Patients describe a recurrent consistent type of pain that typically disappears with rest or with medication. Persistent pain or changes in pain intensity suggest unstable angina pectoris. The goal of medical management is pain relief and, if possible, to improve prognosis, which depends on disease severity [3]. Risk stratification, i.e., with respect to death and myocardial infarction, serves to inform patients and to determine the most appropriate treatment. Several non-invasive and invasive tests allow risk stratification and patient management [4], as summarized in Fig. 6.1.

6.3.3 Medical Treatment for Patients with Stable Angina and Silent Ischemia

The goal of medical treatment in patients with stable angina is to improve the quality of life and the prognosis. It is an alternative to invasive strategies for many patients since the efficacy of percuta-

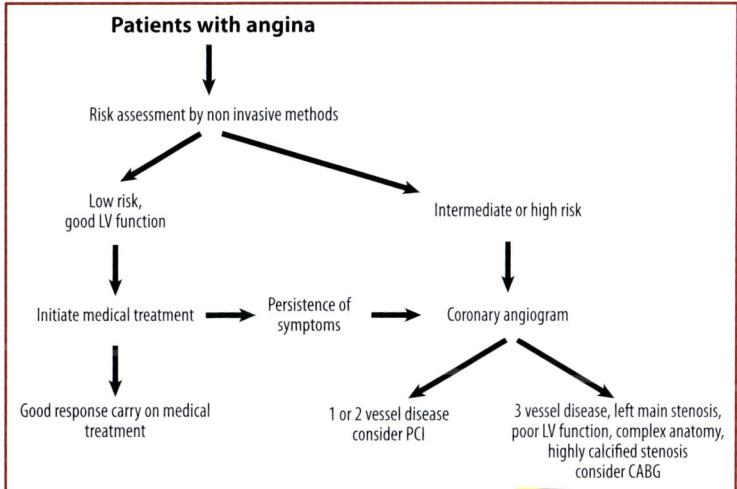

Fig. 6.2 Algorithm for the management of patients with stable angina pectoris

neous coronary intervention (PCI), while associated with less need for repeat revascularization, has no mortality benefit [5]. Thus, PCI should be reserved for patients at high risk or those poorly controlled with medical treatment [6]. Medical treatment can be divided into:

1. Treatment aimed at improving prognosis: aspirin 100 mg/day, statin (titrate dose to achieve target cholesterol [7, 8]), β-blockers in patients post-myocardial infarction, and angiotensin conversion enzyme inhibitors for patients with heart failure or low ejection fraction.
2. Treatment aimed at symptom relief: short-acting nitrates, long-acting nitrates, calcium antagonist, potassium channel openers.

PCI reported no differences in mortality and myocardial infarction but a decreased rate of additional revascularization in favor of CABG [9, 10]. Thus, PCI is considered for low-risk patients with one- or two-vessel disease poorly controlled with medical therapy. CABG can be performed in all patients requiring revascularization, but is the preferred approach for patients with left disease, multivessel disease, and proximal LAD stenosis. To facilitate decision-making, angiographic prognostic scores have been developed, such as the currently favored Syntax score (www.syntaxscore.com). The algorithm for the management of patients with stable angina pectoris or silent ischemia who require revascularization is shown in Fig. 6.2.

6.4 Myocardial Revascularization

Myocardial revascularization for patients with silent ischemia or stable angina pectoris can be achieved by PCI or coronary artery bypass grafting (CABG). The objectives of these approaches are an improvement in survival or the eradication of symptoms. Proximal left anterior descending (LAD) stenoses, left main disease, and multivessel disease are strong indications for revascularization. The individual merits of CABG and PCI differ according to the pattern of coronary disease. Meta-analyses of trials comparing CABG with

6.5 Acute Coronary Syndrome: Unstable Angina Pectoris, STEMI and Non-STEMI

Unstable angina or acute coronary syndrome is the expression of an acute coronary insufficiency and is a life-threatening form of coronary artery disease. Experimental and clinical evidence have confirmed that unstable plaques are involved in the pathogenesis of acute coronary syndrome [11-13]. Plaque rupture with thrombosis, elevated levels of systemic markers of inflammation and thrombosis, and coagulation system activation have been documented in these patients [14].

The cause of acute coronary syndrome is partial or complete thrombotic vessel occlusion. Symptoms include typical chest pain, shortness of breath, swelling, and dizziness. Most patients have persistent ECG modifications, with persistent ST-segment elevation myocardial infarction (STEMI). However, some patients with acute chest pain do not show ST-segment elevation but T-wave inversion or pseudo-normalization of T waves or even the absence of ECG modifications (non-STEMI). A diagnosis of non-STEMI is more difficult to establish than a diagnosis of STEMI, but the prognosis of patients with either condition is comparable in terms of both the incidence of myocardial infarction in the 6 months following the acute event and mortality. Elevated biological markers such as troponin and creatine kinase are part of the diagnosis of STEMI and non-STEMI. However, the management of STEMI patients differs from that of non-STEMI patients since STEMI represents a true medical emergency [10, 15]. The initial strategy in these patients is to alleviate ischemia and symptoms. Coronary angiography should be performed as quickly as possible and arrhythmia monitoring is mandatory.

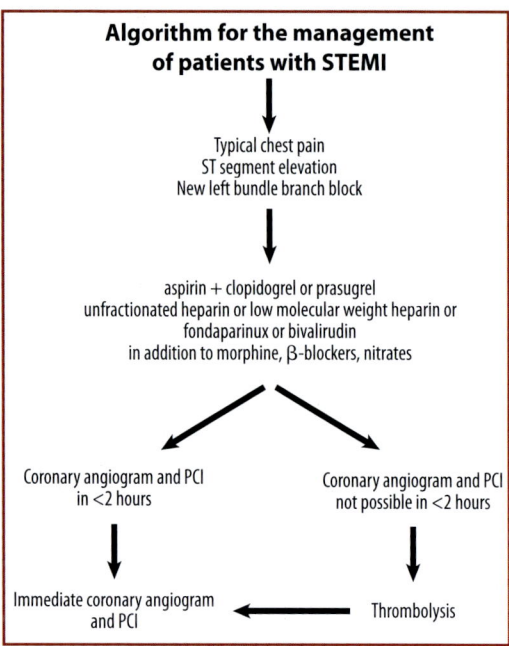

Fig. 6.3 Algorithm for the management of patients with STEMI

with a fibrinolytic agent and then transferred for PCI, with the procedure performed within 3 to 24 h. The algorithm for the management of STEMI patients is shown in Fig. 6.3.

6.6 Management of Patients with Acute Coronary Syndrome

6.6.1 Recommendation for Patients with STEMI

The true medical emergency posed by STEMI makes it essential to minimize the treatment delay, especially within the first 6 h of chest pain. Patients admitted to hospitals with catheterization facilities should be immediately transferred to the catheterization laboratory in order to benefit from primary PCI. Patients admitted to hospitals without such facilities but with a transfer duration < 90 min should be transferred to hospitals with PCI capability. Fibrinolytic agents should not be administered [15]; however, if the time needed for transfer to a hospital with PCI facilities is expected to be more than 90 min, patients should be treated

6.6.2 Recommendation for Patients with Non-STEMI

Medical treatment, including anti-ischemic agents (β-blockers, nitrates, and calcium channel blockers), anti-coagulants (unfractionated heparin, low molecular weight heparin, fondaparinux, and bivalirudin), and antiplatelet agents (aspirin, clopidogrel, prasugrel, and IIb/IIIa blockers), should be initiated as soon as possible [10]. All patients should be referred for coronary angiogram and revascularization in addition to receiving medical treatment. In high-risk patients (high troponin level and ST-segment modifications), an angiogram must be performed as soon as possible. In low-risk patients, coronary angiography can be delayed up to 72 h after the beginning of symptoms. The algorithm for the management of these patients is shown in Fig. 6.4.

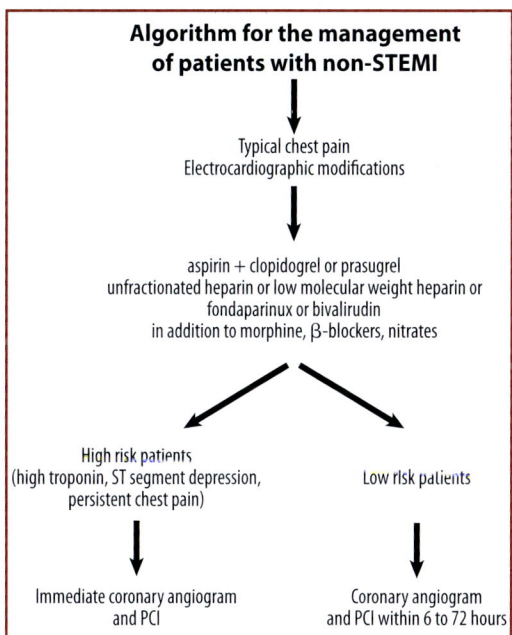

Fig. 6.4 Algorithm for the management of patients with non-STEMI

6.7 Angina with Normal Coronary Arteries

6.7.1 Syndrome X

As suggested by its name, the definition of this condition is still unclear. According to the classical description, it includes typical chest pain, a positive stress test, and a normal coronary angiogram. It can mimic chronic stable angina pectoris but the mechanism of the chest pain is not understood and controversy persists regarding the pathogenesis of this syndrome. Exaggerated vasoconstrictor response, as well as impaired endothelial function, and coronary flow have been demonstrated. The prognosis is good, without excess mortality, although morbidity is significant and the quality of life is diminished, with recurrent hospital admissions.

6.7.2 Vasospastic or Variant Angina

Patients with variant angina report typical chest pain that occurs at rest, with ST-segment elevation on some occasions (Prinzmetal angina). Nitrates usually relieve the pain. Obstructive coronary artery disease is diagnosed in a substantial proportion of patients with variant angina, and there is clearly some overlap between patients with variant angina and those with syndrome X. The mechanism that leads to coronary spasm has not been identified. The hyper-reactivity of smooth muscle cells is thought to play a role, as is endothelial dysfunction. The prognosis of variant angina is good provided there is no underlying obstructive coronary disease.

The treatment of patients with variant angina or syndrome X can be disappointing due to the persistence of symptoms in spite of the well-conducted prescription of anti-ischemic agents. Treatment includes short-acting nitrates during crisis events, and calcium channel blockers as the first option in chronic treatment; molsidomine can sometimes be helpful. By contrast, β-blockers are not recommended although in some patients they can be useful. In a few patients with drug-resistant vasospastic angina or syndrome X, the relief of symptoms can be obtained by implantation of a medullary stimulator.

6.8 Conclusions

Despite many therapeutic advances, the management of patients with coronary disease remains challenging and risk determination is a key feature. Among the many non-invasive and invasive tests that are available, the ability of coronary CT scan to risk-stratify patients has been demonstrated. The coronary calcium score, determined by CT, has been shown to be superior to other tests in the detection of atherosclerosis [16-18]. However, personalized strategies have to be established in order to minimize disease progression, improve symptoms, and slow disease progression, thus allowing secondary prevention [19, 20].

References

1. Roger VL, Go AS, Lloyd-Jones DM et al (2011) AHA Statistical Update, Heart Disease and Stroke Statistics – 2011 Update: A Report From the American Heart Association. Circulation 123:e18-e209
2. Pelberg R, Mazur W (2007) Cardiac CT angiography manual. Springer, Heidelberg, pp 3-16
3. Fox K, Alonso Garcia MA, Ardissino D et al (2006) Guidelines on the management of stable angina pectoris: The Task Force on the Management of Stable Angina Pectoris of the European Society of Cardiology. Eur Heart J 27:1341-1381
4. Gibbons RJ, Abrams J, Chatterjee K et al (2003) ACC/AHA 2002 Guideline Update for the Management of Patients With Chronic Stable Angina: A Report of the American College of Cardiology/American Heart Association Task Force on Practice Guidelines. J Am Coll Cardiol 41:159-168
5. Danchin N, Coste P, Ferrières J et al (2008) Comparison of thrombolysis followed by broad use of percutaneous coronary intervention with primary percutaneous coronary intervention for ST-segment-elevation acute myocardial infarction. Circulation 118:268-276
6. Smith SC, Feldman TE, Hirshfeld JW et al (2006) ACC/AHA/SCAI 2005 Guideline Update for Percutaneous Coronary Intervention. A Report of the ACC/AHA Task Force on Practice Guidelines, ACC/AHA/SCAI Writing Committee to Update the 2001 Guidelines for Percutaneous Coronary Intervention. J Am Coll Cardiol 47:e1-e121
7. Expert Panel on Detection, Evaluation, and Treatment of High Blood Cholesterol in Adults (2001) Executive summary of the third report of the National Cholesterol Education Program (NCEP) Expert Panel on Detection, Evaluation, And Treatment of High Blood Cholesterol in Adults (Adult Treatment Panel III). JAMA 285:2486-2497
8. Karalis DG (2009) Intensive Lowering of low-density lipoprotein cholesterol levels for primary prevention of coronary artery disease. Mayo Clinic Proceedings 84:345-352
9. Singh AK (2010) Percutaneous coronary intervention vs coronary artery bypass grafting in the management of chronic stable angina: A critical appraisal. J Cardiovasc Dis Res 1:54-58
10. Bassand J-P, Hamm CW, Ardissino D et al (2007) Guidelines for the diagnosis and treatment of non-ST-segment elevation acute coronary syndromes: The Task Force for the Diagnosis and Treatment of Non-ST-Segment Elevation Acute Coronary Syndromes of the European Society of Cardiology. Eur Heart J 28:1598-660
11. Kojima S, Nonogi H, Miyao Y et al (2000) Is preinfarction angina related to the presence or absence of coronary plaque rupture? Heart 83:64-68
12. Hort W (1991) Arteriosclerotic plaque rupture: Its significance for myocardial infarct, sudden heart death and unstable angina. Versicherungsmedizin 43:151-154
13. Kragel AH, Gertz SD, Roberts WC (1991) Morphologic comparison of frequency and types of acute lesions in the major epicardial coronary arteries in unstable angina pectoris, sudden coronary death and acute myocardial infarction. J Am Coll Cardiol 18:801-808
14. Avanzas P, Arroyo-Espliguero R, Cosín-Sales J et al (2004) Markers of inflammation and multiple complex stenoses (pancoronary plaque vulnerability) in patients with non-ST segment elevation acute coronary syndromes. Heart 90:847-852
15. Kushner FG, Hand M, Smith SC Jr et al (2009) 2009 Focused Updates: ACC/AHA Guidelines for the Management of Patients With ST-Elevation Myocardial Infarction and ACC/AHA/SCAI Guidelines on Percutaneous Coronary Intervention: A Report of the ACC/AHA Task Force on Practice Guidelines. J Am Coll Cardiol. 54:2205-2241
16. Greenland P, LaBree L, Azen SP et al (2004) Coronary artery calcium score combined with Framingham score for risk prediction in asymptomatic individuals. JAMA 291:210-215
17. Budoff MJ, Diamond GA, Raggi P et al (2002) Continuous probabilistic prediction of angiographically significant coronary artery disease using EBCT. Circulation 105:1791-1796
18. Knez A, Becker A, Leber A et al (2004) Relation of coronary calcium scores by EBCT to obstructive disease in 2,115 symptomatic patients. Am J Cardiol 93:1150-1152
19. Kajinami K, Seki H, Takekoshi N et al (1997) Coronary calcification and coronary atherosclerosis: site by site comparative morphologic study of electron beam computed tomography and coronary angiography. J Am Coll Cardiol. 29:1549-1556
20. Budoff MJ, Gul KM (2008) Expert review on coronary calcium. Vasc Health Risk Manag. 4:315-324

Intravascular Ultrasound: From Gray-Scale to Virtual Histology

Giuseppe M. Sangiorgi, Luigi Politi, Chiara Leuzzi, Luigi Mattioli, Fabiana Rollini and Massimo Fioranelli

7.1 Introduction

For over a decade, coronary angiography has been the "gold standard" in the appraisal of the coronary anatomy and the diagnosis of coronary artery disease. However, the introduction of percutaneous coronary revascularization, along with increasing evidence of the prognostic importance of atherosclerotic plaque composition, has fostered the concept that simple coronary angiography is limited in estimating the distribution and extent of coronary pathology. Indeed, angiography only shows the vessel lumen, a perspective that is insufficient in representing the complex nature of coronary disease.

Since its introduction at the end of the 1980s, intravascular ultrasound (IVUS), as the most modern application of diagnostic ultrasound, has supplied important information about the composition of atherosclerotic plaques. IVUS is an invasive technique that yields tomographic images of the vascular structures and allows direct visualization of both the luminal area and vessel wall composition. Since angiography only provides planar, map-like information about the coronary anatomy, it is also limited in estimating the mechanisms and progression of atherosclerotic disease. By contrast, IVUS visualizes the artery in cross-sections through tomographic appraisal of the plaque, its extent, and its composition below the endothelial surface. Moreover, IVUS can also supply qualita-

G.M. Sangiorgi (✉)
Interventional Cardiology, University of Rome,
Tor Vergata, Policlinico Casilino, Rome, Italy
e-mail: gsangiorgi@gmail.com

tive information regarding the risk of plaque progression/destabilization and quantitative data about the dimensions of the lumen and vessel.

The IVUS console is made up of three components: a catheter with a transducer, a pullback system, and a computer containing the software and the hardware able to convert the ultrasound signal into gray-scale imaging. The IVUS catheters currently available for clinical use have external diameters between 2.6 and 3.5 French (0.87–1.17 mm coronary and peripheral arteries, respectively). The probe is available as either a mechanical or an electronic device, with the spatial resolution of the latter lower than that of the former. To acquire the IVUS image, the target vessel should be selectively cannulated with a guiding catheter. After a 0.014-inch angioplasty wire has been positioned in the vessel, the IVUS probe is advanced distally to the level of the target area and withdrawn proximally by an automated pullback device (with a speed of 0.5 or 1.0 mm/s) into the ostium of the guiding catheter.

Ultrasound gray-scale images of a normal coronary segment show a circular lumen surrounded by three layers. The inner layer is relatively echolucent and represents the intima and inner elastic lamina in normal arteries, or the atherosclerotic plaque in atherosclerotic arteries. The middle layer is usually transparent and dark, and represents the media. The external layer is more echolucent and represents the external elastic lamina, the adventitia, and the periadventitial tissue. The different echolucencies of these layers are due to their different histological composition; for example, the collagen-rich adventitia is very echolucent whereas the media, rich in smooth muscle cells, is relatively less echolucent.

Validation studies have demonstrated that the atherosclerotic plaque can be differentiated according to its prevalent characteristic, i.e., lipidic, fibrotic, or calcific, which can also be distinguished echogeneically. Thus, on the basis of the echogenicity of the plaque, three different types of coronary lesions can be distinguished: (1) hyperechoic regions with acoustic shadow, corresponding to calcific deposits; (2) hyperechoic regions without acoustic shading, corresponding to fibrotic components of the plaque; and (3) hypoechoic regions, corresponding to lipid lakes or thrombotic material. However, the sensitivity and specificity for calcific and fibrotic tissues are much greater than for lipidic tissue. Thus, calcium is very well visualized as a highly echolucent, distinct area such that the diagnostic accuracy is much higher than obtained with conventional angiography. Initially, the classic IVUS pattern of a low echolucent area with a sharp border was misinterpreted and sometimes confused with the echotransparency (gradual acoustic shadow) typical of dense fibrous tissue; however, the use of 40-MHz probes has improved the identification of lipid "pools," as documented by in-vitro and in-vivo studies (with a spatial resolution of 150–300 µm).

Gray-scale images provide a relatively precise image of vessel anatomy and, above all, of plaque morphology. Indeed, it is possible to obtain detailed information about intimal surface ulcerations, vessel remodeling (compensatory expansion of the media during plaque development), plaque distribution and, especially, the type of plaque composition. All of this information is extremely important in the planning of interventional procedures, such as the choice of stent design, in optimizing acute results (by stent apposition to the arterial wall and uniform circumferential expansion of the stent), and in identifying complications (such as plaque dissection or re-stenosis).

7.2 From Gray-Scale to Color-Coded IVUS: The Virtual-Histology Revolution

Today, clinical and laboratory data have challenged classical notions of the pathogenesis of acute coronary syndromes. Several independent lines of clinical evidence have shown that critical stenosis causes only a fraction of this group of pathologies. Rather, the rupture of a thin fibrous cap covering a large, lipid-rich, necrotic or superficial intimal erosion frequently triggers acute coronary thromboses at sites of non-critical narrowing of the coronary arteries. This shift in our thinking has fostered the notion of the "vulnerable" or "high-risk" plaque and spawned manifold attempts to develop methods for its detection, a quest predicated on the postulate that local intervention could preclude plaque thrombosis and thus acute coronary syndromes. This approach may prove applicable to patients already targeted for invasive diagnosis or treatment in whom the identification of non-stenotic lesions unseen by traditional angiography might guide a local intervention aimed at the prevention of a coronary event. Patients presenting with acute coronary syndromes are at a high short-term risk of recurrence, which justifies an aggressive approach such as this one.

The typical vulnerable plaque has been clearly defined in autopsies of patients who died of acute myocardial infarction. It is mostly constituted by a necrotic core, rich in cholesterol crystals and lipids, with an overlying thin fibrous cap that separates this highly thrombogenic material from the blood stream. Such lesions are referred to as thin-cap fibroatheromas (TCFAs).

Several imaging modalities, including gray-scale IVUS, are under investigation by extensive clinical testing in order to identify the one that is the most reliable in discovering the "vulnerable plaque." However, some studies have reported that, according to gray-scale IVUS analysis, stable and unstable plaques share several characteristics that reduces the ability of IVUS to clearly differentiate among them. Moreover, IVUS resolution is about 200–300 µm, a threshold far above the thickness of the typical thin fibrous cap of a vulnerable plaque (40–80 µm). Another limitation is that the gray-scale code is not useful for clearly differentiating between the different histological components of the vulnerable plaque (i.e., necrotic core vs. fibrous material and calcium microcrystals), thus reducing the diagnostic accuracy of the methodology in detecting vulnerable TCFAs.

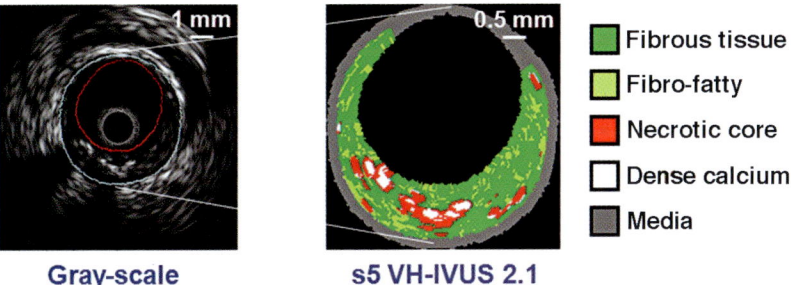

Fig. 7.1 Comparison between gray-scale and virtual-histology. A moderately calcific deposit can be clearly seen in the intravascular ultrasound (IVUS) gray-scale image on the left at 6 and 7 o'clock. In addition, IVUS-virtual histology (IVUS-VH) identifies lipid lakes associated with the calcium deposit. This is sometimes a characteristic of the necrotic core

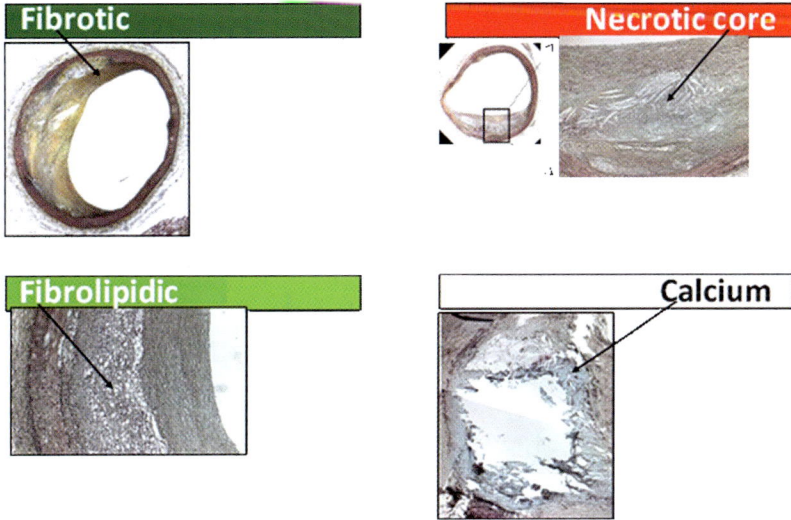

Fig. 7.2 The four color-coded plaque components classified by virtual histology and their corresponding histopathologies

The development of IVUS-virtual histology (IVUS-VH) is a promising step, as the technique can be used in the catheterization lab to identify vulnerable plaques. IVUS-VH discriminates among different tissues with high sensitivity and specificity, thus improving the diagnostic accuracy for any single plaque and, prospectively, distinguishing between vulnerable (rupture prone) and non-vulnerable (non-rupture prone) atherosclerotic lesions.

IVUS-VH images color-code four different tissue types (Figs. 7.1, 7.2):
- Lipid: displayed in yellow
- Fibrolipids: displayed in green
- Necrotic core: displayed in red
- Calcium: displayed in white.

IVUS-VH image acquisition and processing are very different than in standard gray-scale IVUS. VH uses the frequency and amplitude from tissue-reflected ultrasound. Moreover, the analysis, which is performed on backscatter signals and based on all data acquired by the ultrasound beam, uses complex mathematical equations (blind deconvolution, autoregressive modeling, three-component classification algorithm) to extract the required information. "In vitro," the diagnostic accuracy in identifying the four different tissue types ranges from 93 to 99%. The "in vivo"

Table 7.1 Sensitivity and specificity of virtual histology (VH) for the different tissue types

	Accuracy	Sensitivity		Specificity	
Type		%	CI	%	CI
Fibrous	93.5%	95.7%	94–98	90.9%	88–94
Fibrolipids	94.1%	72.3%	65–80	97.9%	97–99
Core necrotic	95.8%	91.7%	87–96	96.6%	95–98
Calcific	96.7%	86.5%	81–92	98.9%	98–100

CI confidence interval.

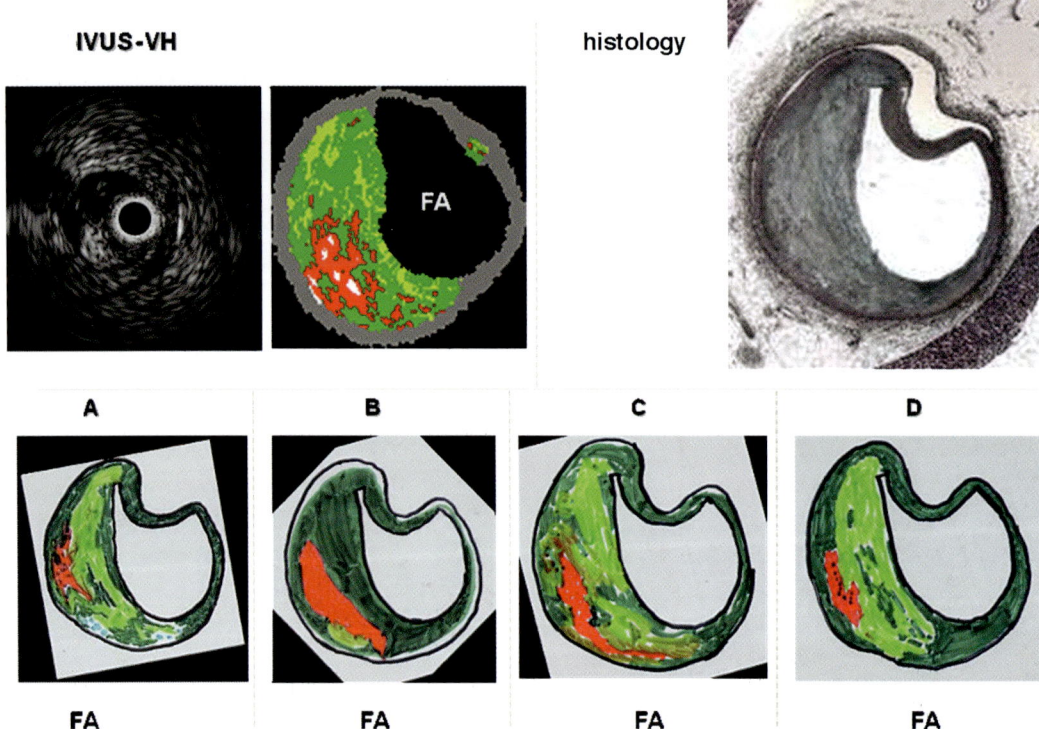

Fig. 7.3 Comparison between histology and IVUS-VH. Hand-drawn reconstructions by four different pathologists (**a-d**) using the same colors as in VH. Note the excellent correlation with the three classifications by VH. In the reconstruction of an IVUS-VH image, the 300-μm field of interest is essentially the sum of many histological 4-μm slices and therefore is not perfectly super-imposable. *FA* Fibroatheroma

diagnostic accuracy is also extremely high (Table 7.1, Fig. 7.3). Of note is the observation that a typical virtual histology slice is 3- to 4-μm thick in contrast to the 300-μm thickness of an IVUS slice. This means that slices obtained during IVUS analysis do not perfectly correlate with histological slices; instead, IVUS-VH images represent the mean of values acquired from more than one histological segment (Fig. 7.4a).

7.3 Lesion Classification Using IVUS-VH

Coronary lesions can be classified as stable (pathological intimal thickening, fibro-atheroma; calcific fibro-atheroma) and unstable (TCFA, superficial erosions, superficial microcalcifications). The most representative of this latter group,

Fig. 7.4 Comparison between histologic cross-sections and those obtained with virtual histology (*VH*) (**a**). Since the former are usually 4-μm and the latter 300-μm thick, the two image sets may not be perfectly matched. Instead, a single VH image corresponds (when utilized for comparison with histology) to the sum of several histologic cross-sections. **b** Classification of the different atherosclerotic plaque types by intravascular ultrasound IVUS-VH.
FA Fibroatheroma

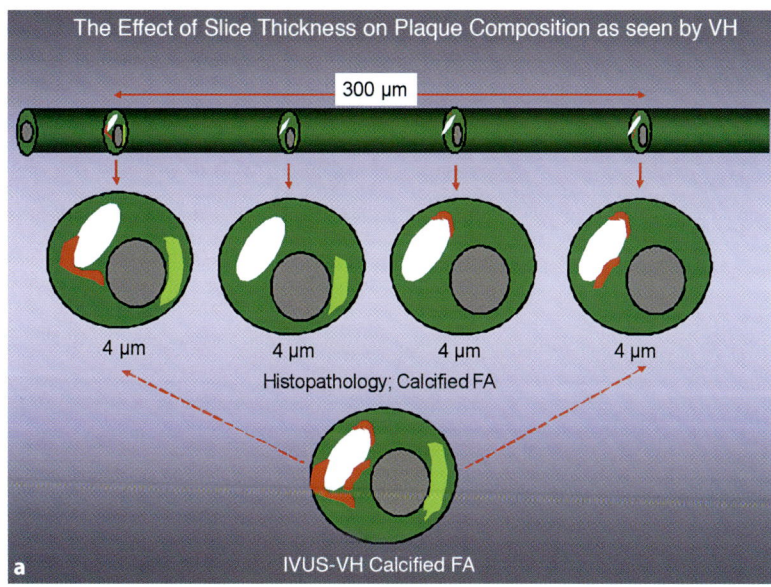

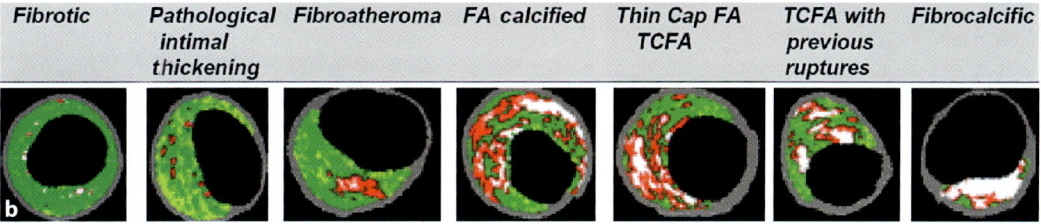

Table 7.2 Specificities, sensitivity, and diagnostic accuracy of virtual histology for different types of atherosclerotic lesions

Type of plaque	Accuracy	Sensitivity	Specificity	Total (n)
FACa	72.4%	32.5%	93.0%	40
TCFACa	96.1%	90.0%	97.1%	20
FA	85.9%	54.1%	96.9%	37
FCa	85.5%	87.1%	84.5%	31
PIT	83.4%	88.5%	82.0%	26
TCFA	99.4%	75.0%	100%	4

FACa fibroatheroma calcified, *TCFACa* thin cap calcific fibroatheroma, *FA* fibroatheroma, *FCa* fibrocalcific, *PIT* pathological intimal thickening, *TCFA* thin-cap fibroatheroma.

particularly in coronary vessels, is the TCFA. As previously described, the thickness of the cap is far below the threshold of the ultrasound beam. IVUS diagnoses TCFA when the necrotic core component is in direct contact with the lumen, representing a fibrous cap thinner than 200 μm. Different lesion types are defined by IVUS-VH (Fig. 7.4b), each with its own corresponding sensitivity and specificity. Of note is the high specificity of this technique for TCFA (Table 7.2).

In this setting, the goal of the PROSPECT study has been to prospectively identify in patients with different types of acute coronary syndromes (ACSs) the distinctive characteristics of coronary lesions that in turn may be responsible for the onset of a new ACS. This study enrolled 697 patients who underwent percutaenous coronary intervention (PCI) for STEMI (30%), NSTEMI (66%), or unstable angina (4%). Those patients were submitted to intracoronary imaging (IVUS)

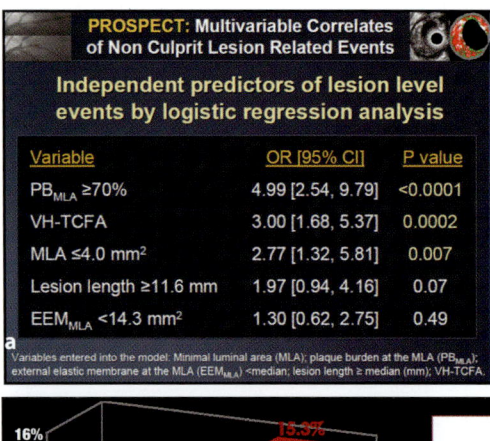

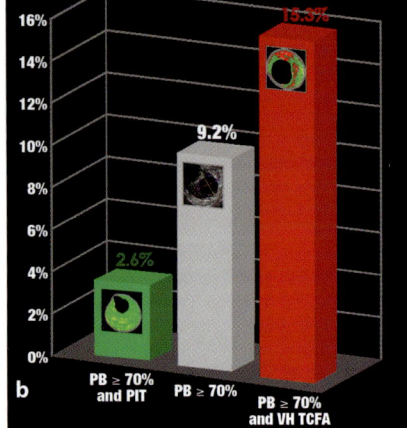

Fig. 7.5 a In the PROSPECT study minimal lumen cross-sectional area (MLA) ≤4.0 mm² and plaque burden ≥70% predict risk better than IVUS MLA alone. **b** In the PROSPECT study, the same lesions by gray-scale IVUS (plaque burden ≥70%, *MLA* <4 mm²) have dramatically different risk profiles when assessed with VH. However only a minority of those plaques caused a new acute coronary syndrome during a mean follow-up of 3.4 years. *PIT* pathological intimal thickening, *EEM* external elastic membrane

and intracoronary tissue characterization (IVUS-VH) of the proximal 6–8 cm of the three epicardial coronary arteries. During a mean follow-up of 3.4 years, new major cardiac events (MACE) occurred in 20.4% of cases (149 events in 135 patients). Of those, 12.9% were related to the culprit lesion treated by stenting during the index procedure (891 stents over 928 culprit lesions), and 11.6% to non-treated lesions. However, only 31 patients (4.9%) experienced irreversible events (death, cardiac arrest, myocardial infarction) related to the culprit lesion treated during the index procedure, while in a minority the irreversible events were related to disease progression on non-treated lesions and the rest were non-attributable. Of the lesions necessitating re-hospitalization for unstable angina, 74 (11.5%) were related to the treated lesion and 69 (10.8%) to other pre-existing lesions. The mean percentage stenosisi of the latter at the beginning of the study was 32%, which progressed to a mean of 66% at the time of re-hospitalization. The number of lesions with a >30% stenosis was 1814 as determined by angiography and 3100 as determined by IVUS, suggesting that the latter imaging technique is more sensitive for the assessment of atherosclerotic disease. Of the lesions causing an event, only 50% consisted of a plaque with a lipid pool and TCFA vulnerable lesions and those accounted for 4.9% out of 595 plaques with similar characteristics. With specific regard to TCFAs with a lumen ≤4 mm² and a plaque burden ≥70%, only 18.2% in 3 years caused a coronary event, while 81.8% did not. Thus, the conclusion of this study is that with current imaging modalities and pathogenetic knowledge the capability to predict an acute coronary syndrome is completely inadequate. In addition, it is important to note that there is an enormous discrepancy between the high number of complex plaques in the coronary tree and their predictive function with respect to a future coronary event.

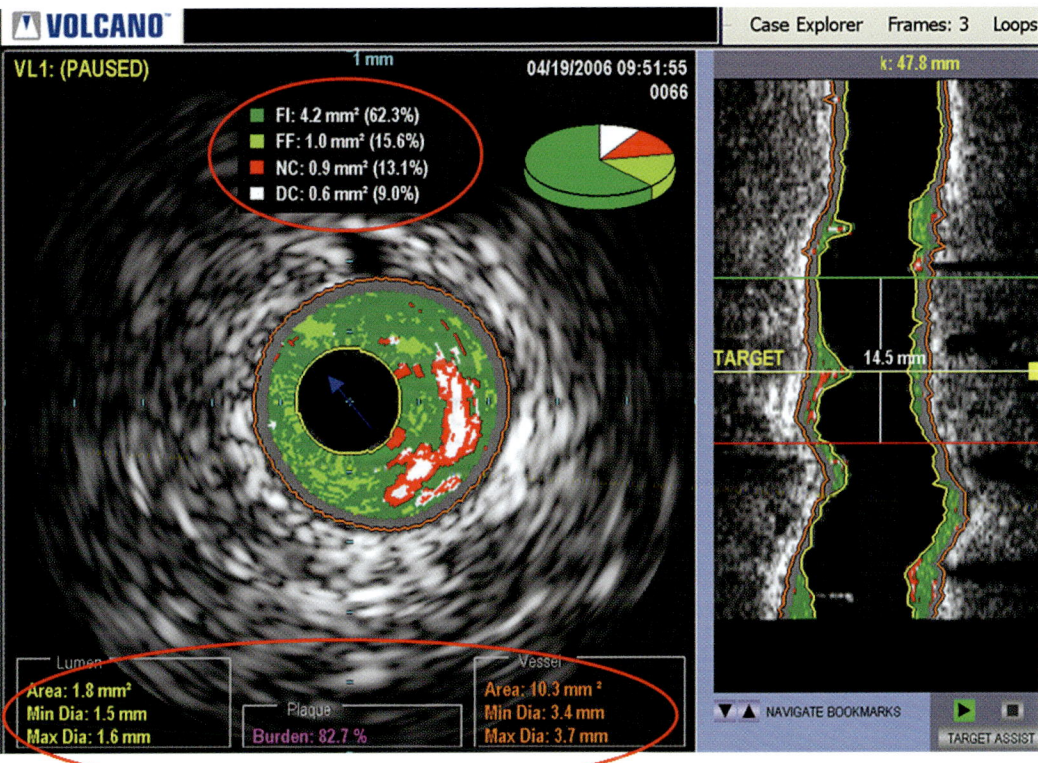

Fig. 7.6 The image displays the VH monitor view after a run acquisition. *Left* One section of the vessel, with the area of the plaque analyzed. In addition, the three panels display, from left to right, lumen area and diameters, plaque burden, and area and diameters of the external elastic lamina. Above, the different plaque components are presented as volume occupied by the different components and as percentage of the entire region of interest. *Right* a longitudinal section of the vessel. This plaque is classified as a calcific fibroatheroma

Multivariate analysis of the 152 variables evaluated showed that the simultaneous presence of a TCFA, a lumen ≤ 4 mm^2, and a plaque burden $\geq 70\%$, were the most important predictors of a coronary event (Fig. 7.5). This constellation of findings was related to an increased risk of a coronary events about 18 times higher than that associated with plaques without these three morphologic characteristics. These data are not surprising considering that two of the variables, i.e., lumen ≤ 4 mm^2 and plaque burden $\geq 70\%$, but not the plaque vulnerability, that is, the presence of TCFA, are the most important expression of atherosclerotic disease severity. If we analyze the different components for MACE development, it should be noted that the IVUS variable represented by plaque stenosis percentage has a relative risk of 5.0 compared to relative risk of 3.0 for the presence of a thin fibrous cap. However, these data need to be "adjusted" for the fact that: (1) all patients enrolled in the PROSPECT study were treated with optimal and maximized medical therapy and (2) the correlation between the event and the lesion was due to stent thrombosis in the same lesion treated during the index procedure.

7.4 IVUS-VH Console and Image Interpretation: Tips and Tricks

Figure 7.6 shows a typical screenshot from an IVUS-VH S5 consol. The current software version features automatic, real-time, border detection that

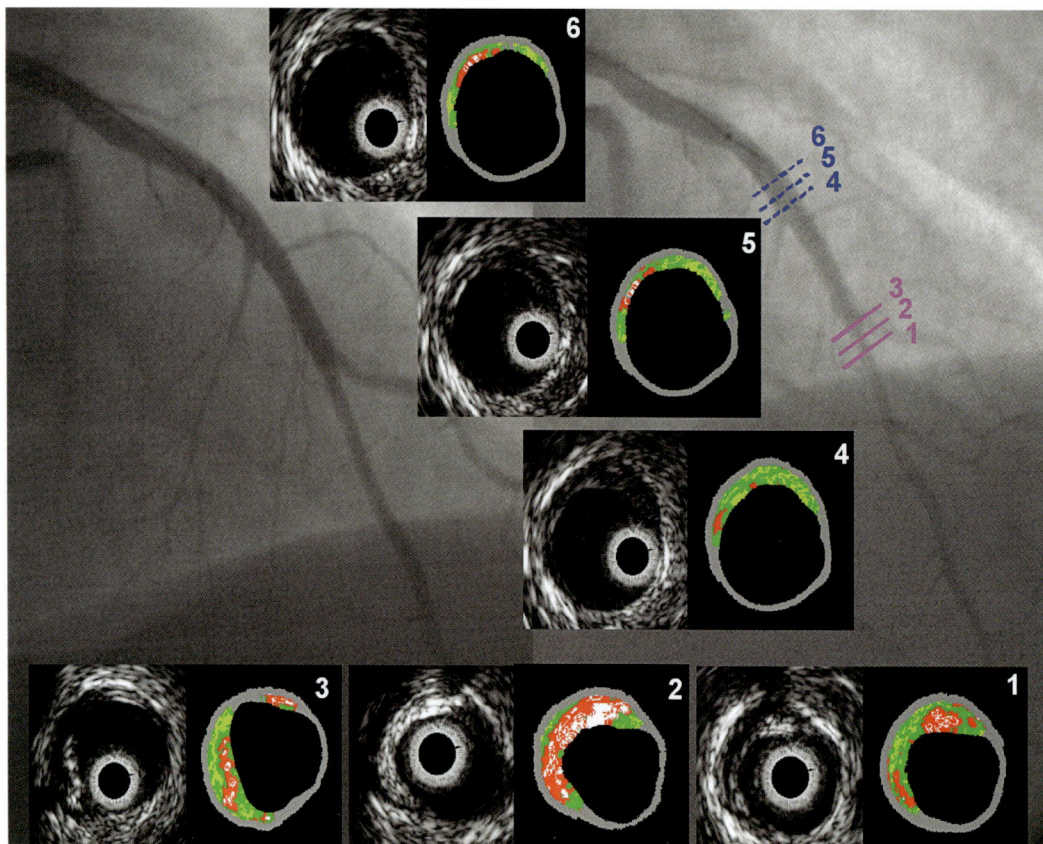

Fig. 7.7 Comparison between angiography, gray-scale IVUS, and IVUS-VH. Note that the left anterior descending artery appears normal along its entire length, according to angiography. The numbers indicate the different coronary segments corresponding to the images acquired by IVUS. A small fibrotic plaque is present in *segments 4, 5, and 6*. Conversely, a fibrocalcific plaque (*segments 2 and 3*) and a vulnerable plaque (*segment 1*) are identified by the lipidic content, close to the lumen (in the VH image shown as a red region), with the IVUS-VH technique

is extremely reliable. VH analysis is available only with 20-Mhz probes, which means less spatial resolution than obtained with the recently introduced 40-Mhz mechanical probes. The advantage of the electronic 20-Mhz probe is its lower crossing profile, which allows even more calcific and compact lesions to be easily crossed. Furthermore, the electronic probe is very flexible and can be more easily pushed than mechanical ones. Unfortunately, in the absence of an external layer, during pullback the probe may become entrapped in the plaque, slowing the speed of the maneuver. This is manifested as a less than perfect reading of the longitudinal axis. Also, unlike in gray-scale imaging, the need for ECG synchronization prohibits a constant frame-rate to speed ratio. This means that the slice number per length segment varies in every single acquisition, depending on the patient's heart rate; this is a major drawback in longitudinal studies evaluating, for example, plaque regression.

7.5 Conclusion

Despite the opportunity to identify and treat any critical stenosis directly in the catheterization laboratory, most of the acute events in patients with coronary artery disease cannot be prevented. Conversely, the identification of a vulnerable plaque (often not stenotic, Fig. 7.7), and even of a vulnerable patient (bearing multiple vulnerable asymptomatic plaques in his or her coronary tree) may help target interventions to those plaques most likely to become disrupted and to the prevention of related complications. Refined coronary imaging techniques will eventually corroborate autopsy studies demonstrating the heterogeneity of coronary atherosclerotic lesions, as stratified by individual patient risk-factor profile. The gap is still large and only prospective observations have reliably identified plaques that are prone to rupture, forcing a change in our approach to the treatment of coronary atherosclerotic disease. However, several prospective studies (SPECIAL, IBIS-2, PROSPECT) are currently ongoing. and their results, together with further advances in imaging modalities such as IVUS-VH, can be expected to bring new and life-saving treatments for patients with coronary artery disease.

Suggested Reading

König A, Klauss V (2007) Virtual histology. Heart 93:977-982

Maehara A, Cristea E, Mintz GS et al (2012) Definitions and methodology for the grayscale and radiofrequency intravascular ultrasound and coronary angiographic analyses. JACC Cardiovasc Imaging 5:S1-S9

Pu J, Mintz GS, Brilakis ES et al (2012) In vivo characterization of coronary plaques: novel findings from comparing greyscale and virtual histology intravascular ultrasound and near-infrared spectroscopy. Eur Heart J 33:372-383

Sangiorgi GM, Clementi F, Cola C, Biondi-Zoccai G (2007) Plaque vulnerability and related coronary event prediction by intravascular ultrasound with virtual histology: "It's a long way to Tipperary"? Catheter Cardiovasc Interv 70:203-210. Review

Stone GW, Maehara A, Lansky AJ et al (2011) A prospective natural-history study of coronary atherosclerosis. N Engl J Med 364:226-235

Identification and Characterization of the Atherosclerotic Plaque Using Coronary CT Angiography

Paolo Pavone, David A. Dowe and Roberto Leo

Coronary CT angiography (CTA) is the first diagnostic modality that allows simultaneous evaluation of the lumen and wall of these small, rapidly pulsating arteries. Catheter coronary angiography, by contrast, only evaluates the internal, patent lumen of these vessels, without providing direct information on the vessel wall or the extent of vascular parietal involvement by atherosclerosis. While it identifies areas of stenosis or obstruction, it does not show details of the plaque itself, unless heavy calcifications make the atherosclerotic plaque evident on the X-ray image. Intravascular ultrasonography (IVUS) is an excellent method to obtain high-resolution images of the vascular wall, with identification of the different layers and proper characterization of the atherosclerotic plaque; however, it is an invasive procedure, performed in the course of catheter coronary angiography, and does not simultaneously evaluate the vessel lumen. Coronary CTA is therefore the first non-invasive imaging technique that allows evaluation of the lumen and walls of the coronary arteries, a particular advantage in determining the atherosclerotic burden in these arteries. Since atherosclerosis is a disease of the vessel wall, obtaining proper and direct evidence of a coronary plaque is an important new diagnostic possibility. The technique provides morphological information and CT density measurements, with important prognostic and therapeutic implications.

8.1 Normal Vascular Wall

Coronary CTA creates an image during dynamic passage of a bolus of contrast agent in the coronary arteries. Thus, in images acquired using three-dimensional analysis, the vessel lumen has a high CT density and is therefore very bright. The vessel wall is not enhanced by contrast agent so that it is hypodense on CT. The normal vessel wall is too thin to be clearly defined in CT images, unless newer systems, which their very high spatial resolution (<0.3 mm), are employed, although experience with the most recent technology is still preliminary. The inability to identify the normal parietal vascular wall is not a negative factor in coronary CTA (Fig. 8.1), as non-visibility reflects a normal status and a lack of atherosclerotic involvement.

Identification of the vascular wall should always be performed using bi-dimensional reconstruction techniques (planimetric imaging, see Chap. 4). Only this type of image clearly displays the course of the vessel, with evidence of the hyperdense internal aspect of the patent lumen and the hypodense parietal layers. Care must be taken, as discussed previously, to evaluate the vessels in their longitudinal course and in the transverse, axial plane, in order to obtain a complete and detailed definition of the vascular wall.

P. Pavone (✉)
Radiology Department
Casa di Cura Mater Dei
Rome, Italy
e-mail: paolo.pavone@materdei.it

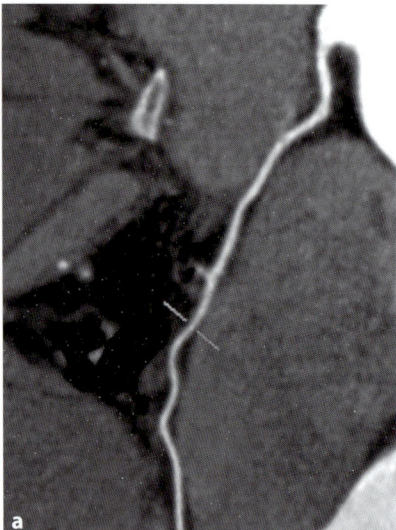 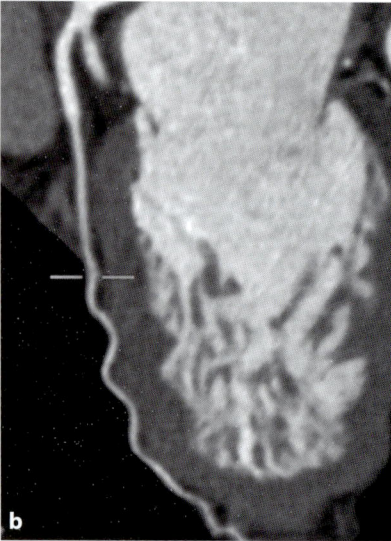

Fig. 8.1 Normal coronary arteries evaluated using a bi-dimensional technique. **a** Left circumflex coronary artery. **b** Left anterior descending coronary artery. The vessel wall is difficult to evaluate due to its normal thickness. The vessels themselves are well-evident, as they are surrounded by very hypodense epicardial fat tissue

8.2 Identification of Atherosclerotic Plaques in Coronary CT Angiography

The atherosclerotic plaque must always be identified by three-dimensional imaging reconstruction (volume rendering) in combination with bi-dimensional techniques. In the latter images, due to simultaneous visualization of the lumen and wall, atherosclerotic plaques are well-evidenced as areas of focal thickening. Images evaluated in the different orthogonal planes allow clear definition of the relationship between the atherosclerotic plaque and the lumen, and thus proper delineation of the extent of vascular stenosis.

8.3 CT Density Values and Plaque Characterization: Fibrolipidic and Calcific Plaques

In addition to its ability to identify atherosclerotic plaque, an intrinsic feature of CT is that the different components of the atherosclerotic plaque have different densities: (a) lipidic plaques, with very low density values (<0 HU); (b) fibrotic plaques, with intermediate tissue density (20–30 HU); and (c) calcific components of the plaque, which because of their high density (500–1000 HU) are always well evident in coronary CTA. Differentiation among these three plaque components is readily obtained by analysis and evaluation of the bi-dimensional images. In the examples shown in Fig. 8.2, the low-density plaque can be easily distinguished from the calcific high-density plaque, and different plaques in the same artery are distinctly visualized.

Plaques with a predominantly lipidic component cannot always be discriminated from those that are mostly fibrotic when clinically evaluated by CT. Therefore, during image evaluation and in the report, radiologists refer mostly to a "fibrolipidic" plaque, thereby indicating the absence of calcific components (Fig. 8.3). The difference between fibrolipidic and calcific plaque is always seen by coronary CTA.

Calcific plaques are strongly hyperdense and almost always well-evident in three-dimensional and in bi-dimensional images; whereas hypodense, non-calcific, fibrolipidic plaques are less obvious in appearance and require an experienced radiologist, who must carefully evaluate the targeted artery segment by segment (Fig. 8.4). The accuracy in the identification of non-calcific vs. calcific atherosclerotic plaque may be lower, especially in the more distal segments of the coronary arteries. For proximal segments, there is no difference since

8 Identification and Characterization of the Atherosclerotic Plaque Using Coronary CT Angiography

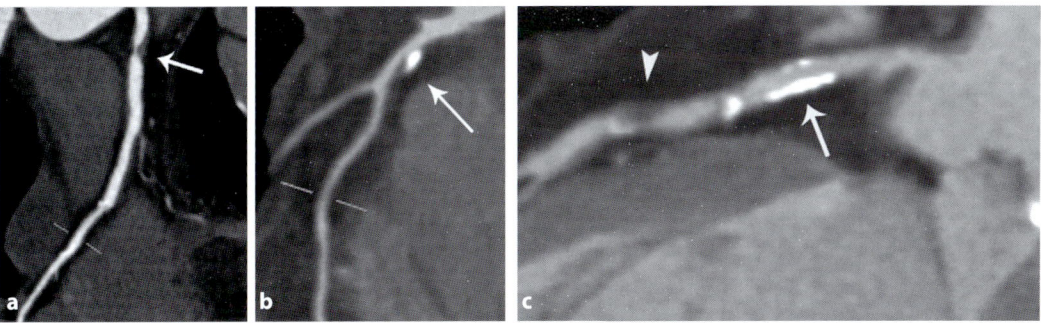

Fig. 8.2 Marginal plaques Evaluation of wall thickening, which is evident due to the difference in density compared to the lumen of the coronary artery, when opacified by contrast agent. **a** Fibrolipidic hypodense plaque (*arrow*). **b** Mixed plaque, partially calcified (*arrow*). **c** Soft fibrolipidic (*arrowhead*) and calcified plaques (*arrow*) on the same artery

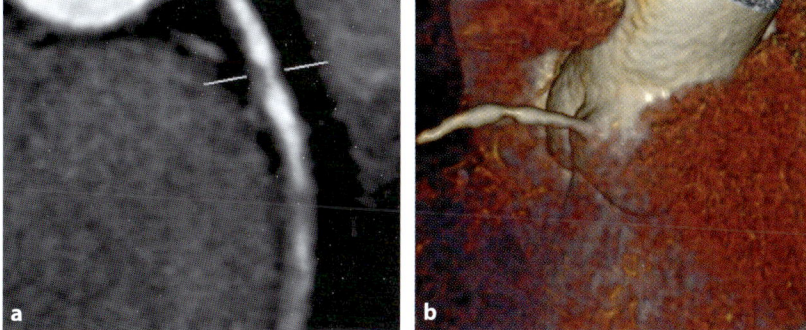

Fig. 8.3 Fibrolipidic marginal soft plaque of the right coronary artery evaluated with **a** bi-dimensional and **b** three-dimensional image reconstruction techniques

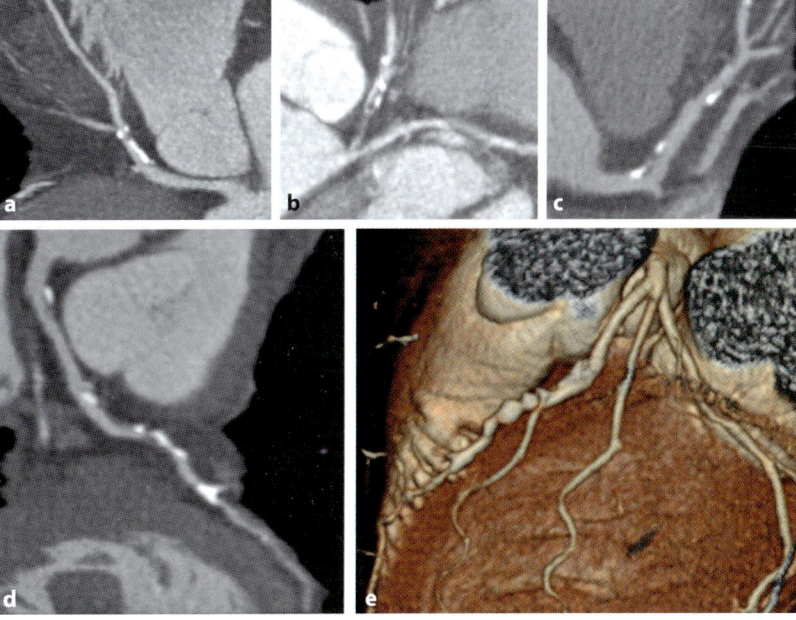

Fig. 8.4 Marginal calcific and mixed plaques. **a-d** Bi-dimensional image; **e** three-dimensional reconstructed image

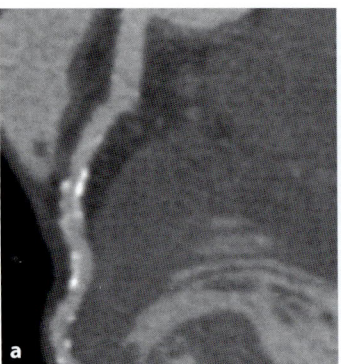
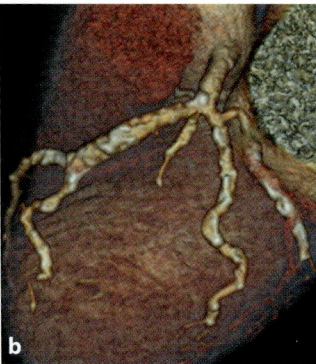

Fig. 8.5 a, b Diffuse atherosclerotic involvement of the *left* anterior descending and circumflex coronary arteries

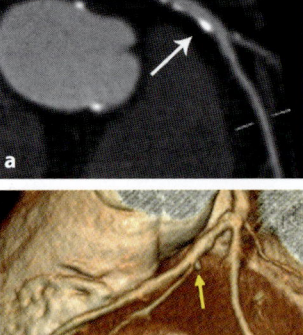
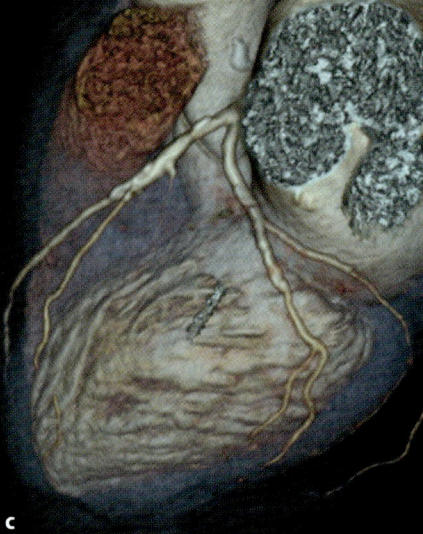

Fig. 8.6 Small marginal calcific plaque (*arrow*) of the left anterior descending coronary artery evaluated in **a** orthogonal bi-dimensional planes and **b** three-dimensional. **c** Image reconstruction technique

both calcific and non-calcific are correctly identified and characterized. The main goal of coronary CT examination is, in fact, to identify plaque burden, mostly in the proximal segments, while the definition of smaller, more distal, branches is limited. However, for disease prognosis, clinical involvement of the proximal and intermediate segments of the coronary arteries is more important than the involvement of distal segments.

8.4 Atherosclerotic Plaque and Disease Evolution

Atherosclerotic disease has a temporal course, with an evolution similar to that of inflammation. In this view, calcification may be considered as the end stage of pathological vascular involvement. With coronary CTA, eccentric calcific plaques, almost always in an extraluminal location, are frequently encountered. These represent areas of the vessel wall with limited and focal atherosclerotic involvement that have reached a final and stable pathological condition, without causing stenosis. Completely calcified plaques have to be considered as "safe" plaques since the atherosclerotic process has terminated. Of course, in the process, the plaque, although calcified and stable, may have caused significant stenosis, as is discussed in the next chapter.

Identification of a non-calcific fibrolipidic plaque – also when there is eccentric involvement of the vessel wall – that has not caused significant reduction of the lumen diameter (Figs. 8.5, 8.6)

8 Identification and Characterization of the Atherosclerotic Plaque Using Coronary CT Angiography

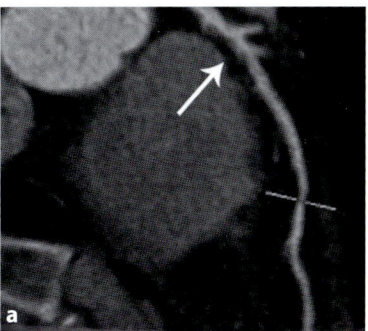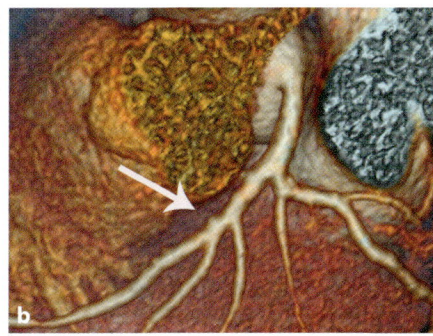

Fig. 8.7 a, b Ulcerated plaque (*arrow*) of the distal part of the left anterior descending coronary artery

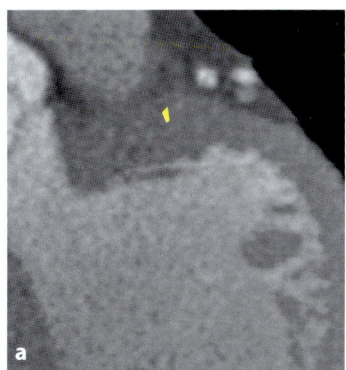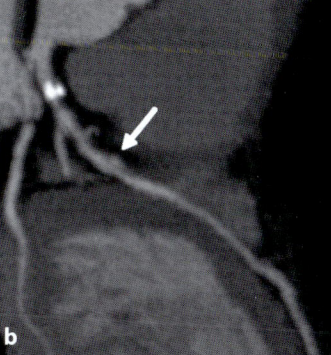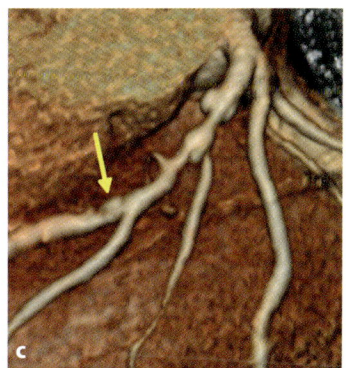

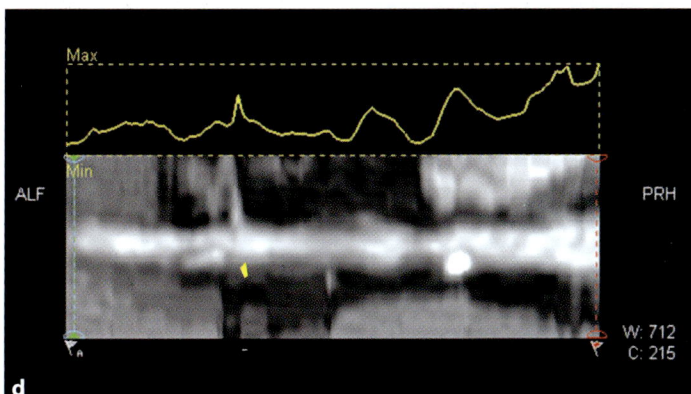

Fig. 8.8 Plaque dissection (*arrow*) of the left anterior descending coronary artery. **a** Axial image shows the intimal flap; the central component of the plaque is filled with contrast agent (**b, c**). The patient suffered acute clinical symptoms a few hours before CT. **d** Bi-dimensional reconstructed image also shows the intimal flap. There is also a mild reduction in the caliber of the vessel in the proximal segment and a second fibrolipidic plaque (*arrows*)

indicates to the cardiologist that the atherosclerotic process is still active and that other events may occur, leading to further progression of the disease and to worsening of the patient's clinical condition. These plaques (vulnerable plaques) may also create acute anatomo-pathological changes that lead to a sudden cardiac event and to infarction. In fact, vulnerable plaques may undergo different types of complications: (a) a further increase in size, with progressive reduction of the vessel lumen; (b) internal hemorrhage, leading to an immediate increase in plaque volume and sudden vascular occlusion, with acute infarction; (c) ulceration, with dispersion into the vessel lumen of atherosclerotic material, resulting in vascular occlusion or turbulent flow in the vascular ulcer, with subsequent development of thrombi; (d) intimal dissection at the plaque level, leading to immediate vascular occlusion (Figs. 8.7, 8.8). These potential complications, well-known mostly to

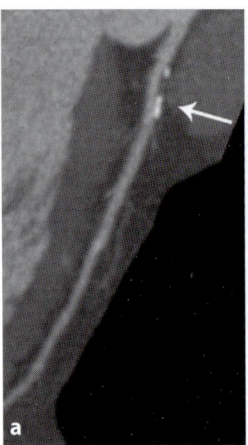 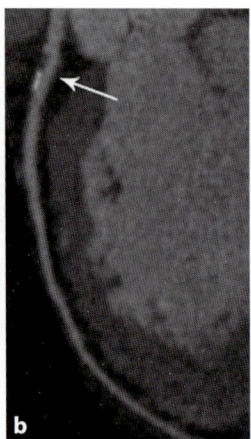 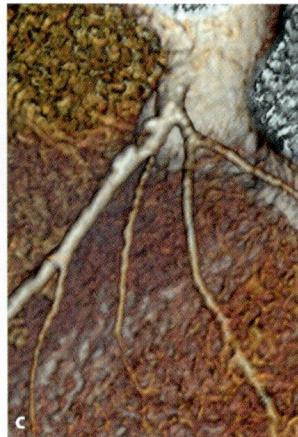

Fig. 8.9 Mixed calcific and fibrolipidic plaques (*arrows*). **a, b** Bi-dimensional images; **c** three-dimensional image

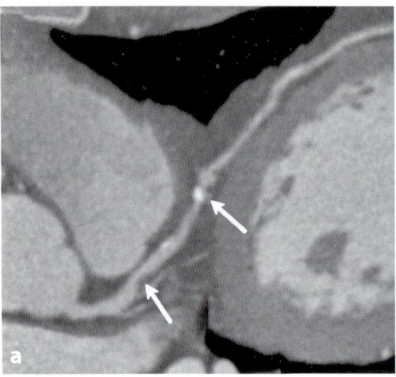 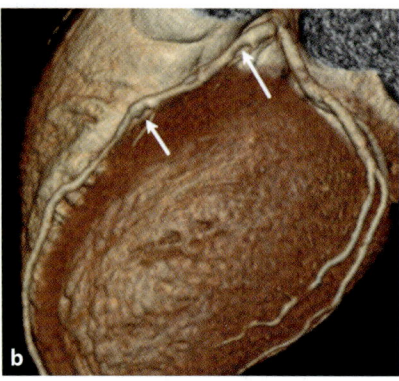

Fig. 8.10 Mixed plaque involving the proximal segment of the left anterior descending artery and a calcific plaque of the middle third of the same vessel (*arrows*). The bi-dimensional (**a**) and three-dimensional (**b**) images are displayed

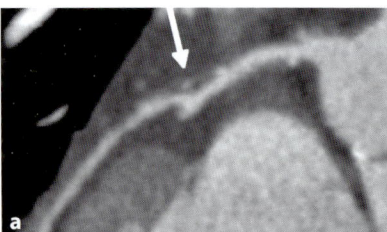 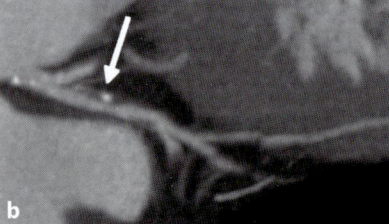

Fig. 8.11 a Mixed plaque (*arrow*) with **b** a central hyperdense calcific core and a peripheral fibrolipidic cap. The plaque is eccentric, with non-significant reduction of the vessel lumen

pathologists, must always be considered by both the radiologist and the cardiologist carrying out a coronary CTA examination. Knowledge of the morphology and characteristics of the atherosclerotic plaque provide a better and more defined prognostic and therapeutic approach to atherosclerotic disease of the coronary arteries. While in a non-stenosing calcific plaque the diagnosis is always "stabilized atherosclerotic disease", in the presence of a non-stenosing fibrolipidic plaque the cardiologist may recommend support therapies, i.e., drugs or lifestyle changes, that limit disease progression while at the same time reducing the possibility of an acute event, which may lead to a further reduction in the diameter of the vessel lumen and to vascular occlusion.

Mixed plaques may be encountered as well; these have to be considered as at-risk, vulnerable plaques if the fibrolipidic component is prevalent, with only small internal, central calcifications (Figs. 8.9–8.11).

8 Identification and Characterization of the Atherosclerotic Plaque Using Coronary CT Angiography   69

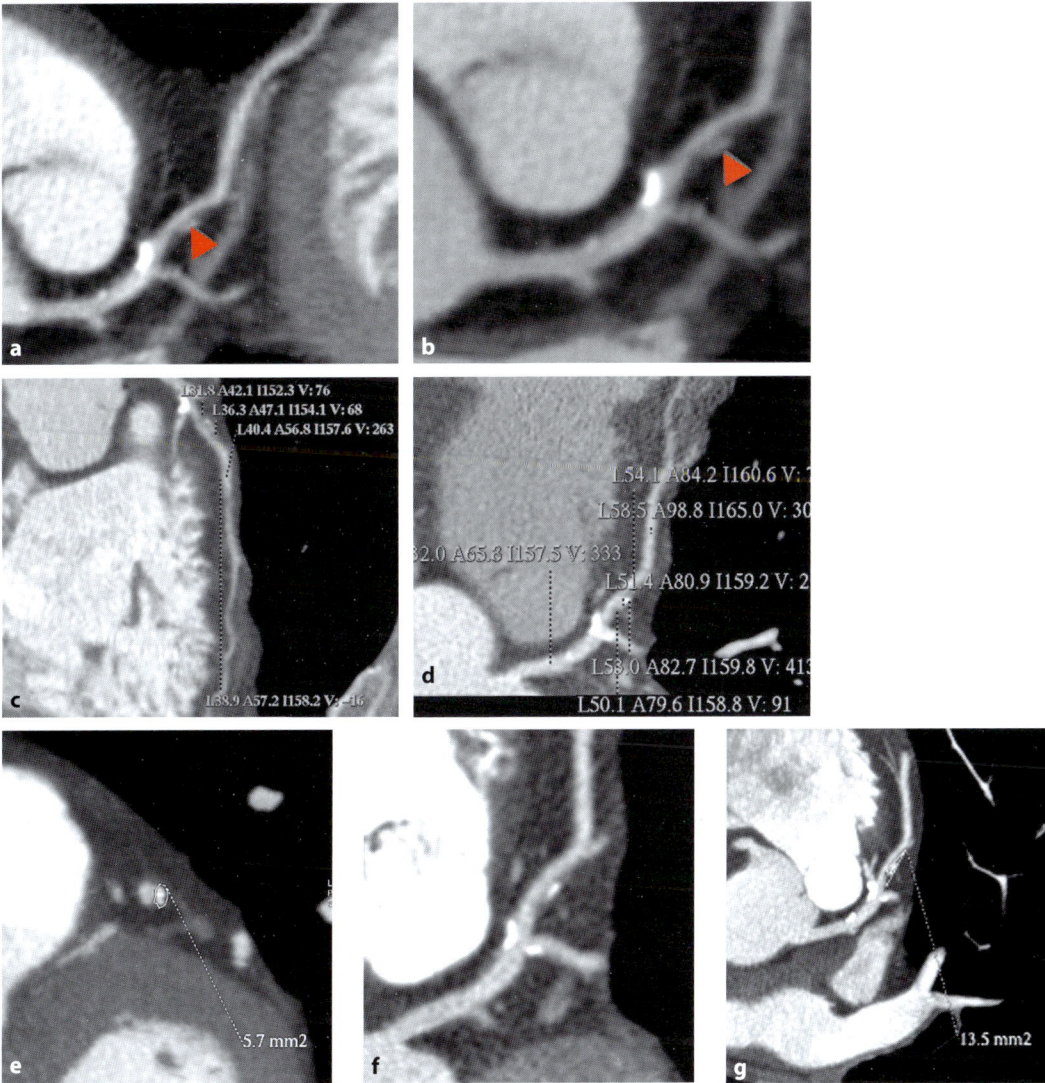

Fig. 8.12 Reduction of the volume of an atherosclerotic plaque (*arrowheads*). **a** Follow-up controls after statin therapy. **b** 03-04-02, **c**, **d** 09-06-03, **e-g** 26-06-04

8.5 Diagnostic Evaluation of Coronary Disease During Medical Therapy

The development and widespread clinical use of drugs aimed at significantly decreasing serum cholesterol levels may lead to a reduction in the size of the atherosclerotic plaques of most patients with coronary artery disease. This, of course, applies only to fibrolipidic plaques, as in the calcific plaque complete stabilization of the atherosclerotic process has been already achieved and the plaque burden of the vessel wall can no longer be reduced.

CT is not only able to identify and characterize the fibrolipidic component of the plaque, but, as a non-invasive procedure, it allows the clinician to monitor plaque evolution over time. For example, the three-dimensional images acquired with CT can show the effect of statins on plaque size (Fig. 8.12, Table 8.1).

The clinical relevance of CT in patients with atherosclerosis of the coronary arteries is that non-calcific, non-stenosing fibrolipidic plaques, which do not require interventional procedures, can be accurately identified. These patients can be started on a therapeutic approach with drugs (statins) that target both plaque volume and the overall atherosclerotic burden on the vessels. At the very least, statins are able to reduce further growth of the plaque, therefore limiting the possibility that it will undergo sudden anatomic changes (see above). A few years after the start of therapy, plaque volume can be monitored in follow-up controls with coronary CTA.

These concepts are new and not completely accepted by clinicians. Moreover cost-benefit effects must be considered. Today, statins are recommended for all at-risk patients with high serum cholesterol levels. Imaging of the coronary arteries prior to the beginning of therapy would screen for patients with non-calcific fibrolipidic plaques who may benefit from this type of therapy, distinguishing them from patients with only calcified plaques or with normal arteries, neither of whom would benefit from statins. In addition, long-term monitoring may indicate the proper time to terminate medical therapy and thus lead to important savings in drug and medical care costs.

Table 8.1 Atherosclerotic involvement and volume change of the atherosclerotic plaque over the course of statin therapy

Date	Panels[a]	Plaque length (mm)	Plaque area (mm^2)
03.04.2002	b	13.6	19.8
09.06.2003	c, d	13.2	13.7
26.06.2004	e-g	13.2	10.8

[a] See Fig. 8.12.

Suggested Reading

Budoff MJ, Shaw LJ, Liu ST et al (2007) Long-term prognosis associated with coronary calcification: observations from a registry of 25,253 patients. J Am Coll Cardiol 49:1860-1870

Ehara S, Kobayashi Y, Yoshiyama M et al (2004) Spotty calcification typifies the culprit plaque in patients with acute myocardial infarction. An intravascular ultrasound study. Circulation 110:3424-3429

Hendel RC, Patel MR, Kramer CM et al (2006) ACCF/ACR/SCCT/SCMR/ASNC/NASCI/SCAI/SIR 2006 appropriateness criteria for cardiac computed tomography and cardiac magnetic resonance imaging. J Am Coll Cardiol 48:1475-97

Leber AW, Knez A, von Ziegler F et al (2005) Quantification of obstructive and nonobstructive coronary lesions by 64-slice computed tomography. A comparative study with quantitative coronary angiography and intravascular ultrasound. J Am Coll Cardiol 46:147-154

Redberg R (2006) Computed tomographic angiography. More than just a pretty picture? J Am Coll Cardiol 49:1827-1829

Coronary CT Angiography: Evaluation of Stenosis and Occlusion

Paolo Pavone and Roberto Leo

Once an atherosclerotic plaque has been identified and properly characterized by means of coronary CT angiography (CTA), the next step is to define the extent of atherosclerotic involvement, i.e., significant reduction of the lumen by stenosis or complete occlusion of the vessel. A reduction in the caliber of the vessel lumen is associated with a reduction in blood flow and may have significant hemodynamic consequences; however, an important and clearly evident parietal atherosclerotic plaque may be present without significantly reducing lumen caliber. Thus, an exact definition of the extent of lumen reduction by means of coronary CTA is very important from a clinical point of view. In most cases, this diagnostic procedure is employed in not highly symptomatic patients (in patients in whom there is strong clinical suspicion of coronary disease, catheter angiography is directly performed); then, depending on the results of the clinical examination, a decision is made as to whether a more invasive approach (catheter angiography) is required. This decision depends at least in part on the significance of the vessel stenosis. Both the aim and the key role of coronary CTA are to differentiate patients with normal coronary vessels from those with limited atherosclerotic involvement without evidence of stenosis (who may benefit from supportive drug therapy) and from those with significant stenosis. In this latter group, catheter coronary angiography may confirm the significance of the disease and define the therapeutic approach.

The direct evidence of arterial stenosis provided by coronary CTA yields additional information. For example, a stenosis > 70% causes a significant hemodynamic reduction of vascular flow. Completely asymptomatic patients, with negative treadmill tests, may present with important and significant stenosis of one or more coronary arteries but with an overall reduction in flow that is less than the 70% threshold.

In clinical practice, a stenosis is considered significant when the vessel caliber is reduced by > 50%. Thus, the goal is to interpret coronary CTA images such that the level of stenotic vascular involvement is precisely determined.

9.1 Non-significant Moderate Stenosis

As discussed in the previous chapter, marginal atherosclerotic plaques not causing a significant reduction of the lumen caliber are frequently encountered in coronary CTA images. Once a plaque has been identified, it must be properly analyzed. This requires that the vessel be evaluated in the orthogonal and axial planes, in order to define the influence of this marginal plaque on lumen caliber, using qualitative as well as semi-automated quantitative approaches (Figs. 9.1, 9.2). If the non-significance of the lumen reduction is established, no further procedure is necessary, as coronary CTA is by itself diagnostic, allowing identification and

P. Pavone (✉)
Radiology Department
Casa di Cura Mater Dei
Rome, Italy
e-mail: paolo.pavone@materdei.it

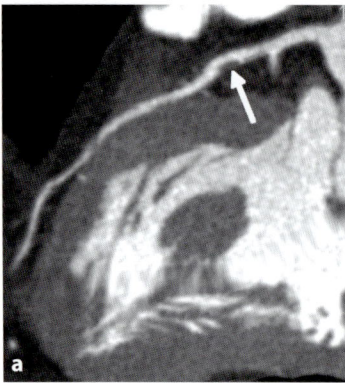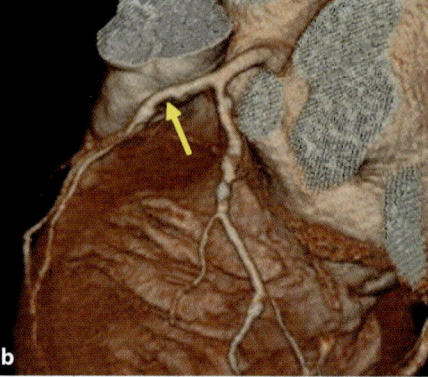

Fig. 9.1 Marginal fibrolipidic plaque (*arrows*) of the middle third of the left anterior descending artery (LAD), without significant caliber reduction. **a** Bi-dimensional image and **b** three-dimensional volume-rendered image

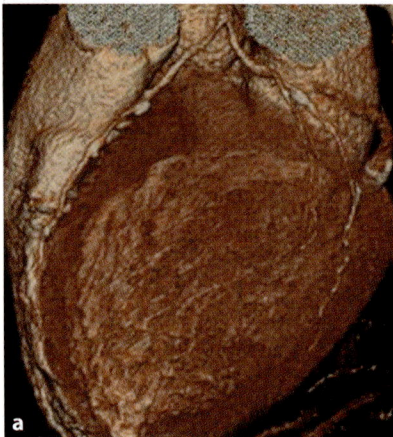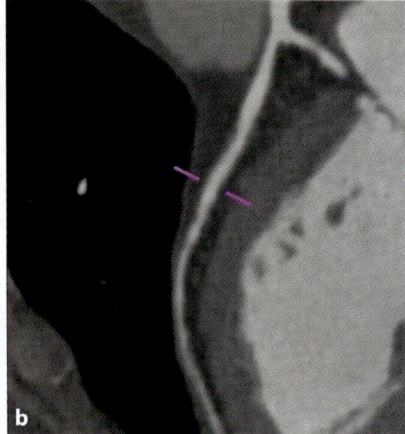

Fig. 9.2 Mild stenosis of the LAD. **a** Three-dimensional image and **b** bi-dimensional image showing mild reduction in the caliber of the middle segment of the artery

characterization of the plaque as well as definition of the extent of lumen reduction.

The semi-automated approach to analyzing lumen reduction is a fascinating and important alternative to the qualitative, operator-dependent, method. Specific software analyzes the vessel in a bi-dimensional planimetric image and displays axial, transverse images simultaneous with the longitudinal vascular exploration. The software is able to evaluate the caliber of normal-sized vessels and the area of the lumen in the segment involved by atherosclerotic plaque, providing an estimate of the degree of stenosis. However, while definitely useful, the semi-automated approach is usually combined with a more personalized approach; that is, qualitative definition by the radiologist of the influence exerted by the parietal plaque on the vessel lumen, thus differentiating significant from non-significant stenosis.

9.2 Calcified Plaques: Problems in Defining Vascular Stenosis

In a vessel with atherosclerotic calcified plaque involvement, the challenge to the clinician is to define and properly specify the degree of vessel reduction. However, densely calcified plaques create a "blooming" effect on CTA, i.e., in both three- and bi-dimensional reconstructed images, the volume of the calcified plaque appears much larger than it is in reality (Fig. 9.3). This CT artifact is similar to that observed when metal objects are present in the area being imaged (for instance, the metallic wires of pacemakers). In the blooming effect, there are large bright streaks and lines surrounding the object, both of which limit the definition of its contours. Calcified plaques create a larger volume, thereby impeding

9 Coronary CT Angiography: Evaluation of Stenosis and Occlusion

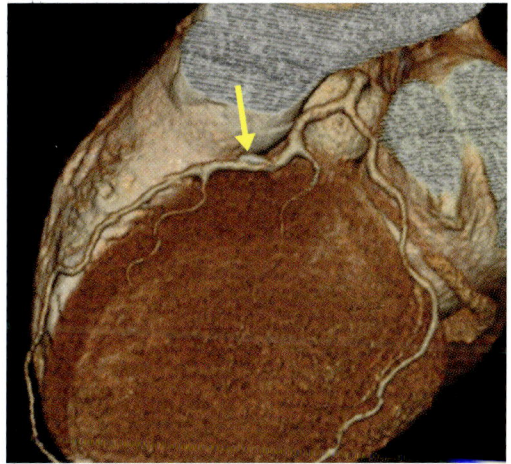

Fig. 9.3 Short segmental isolated plaque of the LAD. Blooming artifacts create a false external expansion of the plaque out of the vessel lumen (*arrow*)

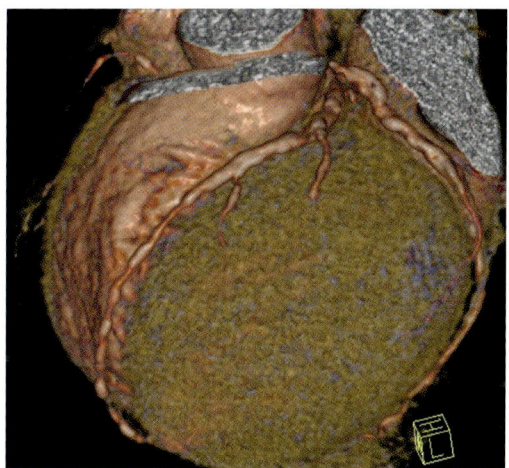

Fig. 9.4 Diffuse atherosclerotic involvement with densely calcified plaques; an artifactual blooming effect is present

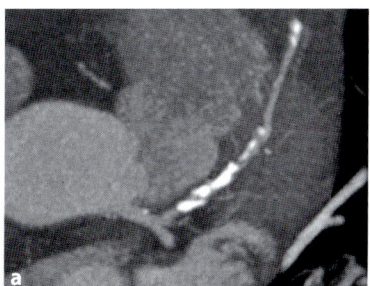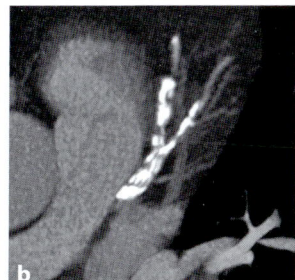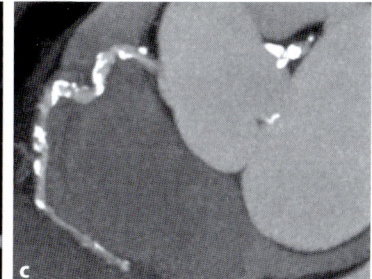

Fig. 9.5 Bi-dimensional images of densely calcified plaques with artifactual blooming effect. **a**, **b** Extensive plaques of the left descending coronary artery. **c** Calcified plaque of the circumflex arteries

Fig. 9.6 Diffuse calcified plaques of the LAD. **a** A normal filter (value 30) shows the strong blooming effect, with plaques appearing larger then they actually are. **b** The blooming effect is reduced with a 46-value filter. Calcified parietal plaques with moderate stenosis are shown

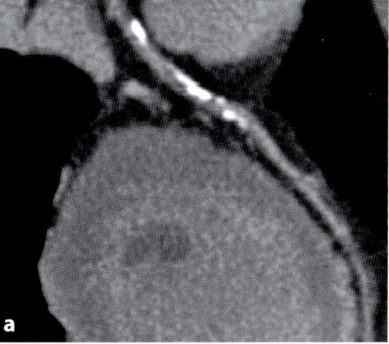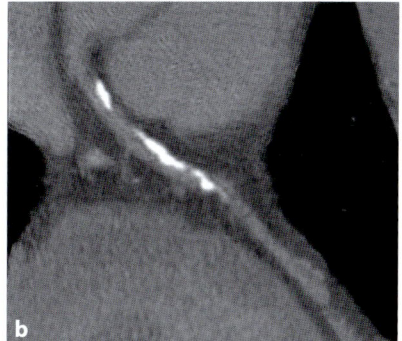

the radiologist's efforts to understand the effective influence of the plaque on the vessel lumen (Figs. 9.4, 9.5). It is then difficult to clearly estimate (even with automated software) the significance of the stenosis. Thus, in the evaluation of calcified plaques, care must be taken in image analysis and reconstruction. Proper reconstruction protocols that limit the blooming effect have to be employed. In the evaluation of stents, better results are obtained using reconstruction filters of intermediate value (usually a value of 46 is indicated) (Fig. 9.6). Moreover, in bi-dimensional

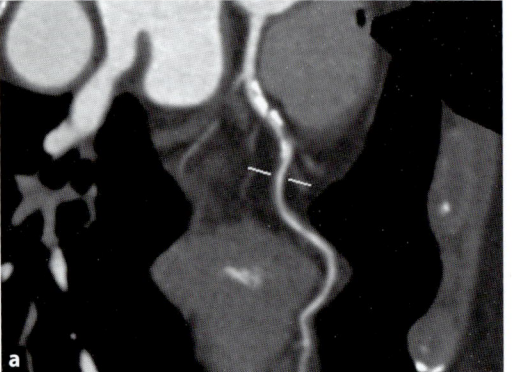
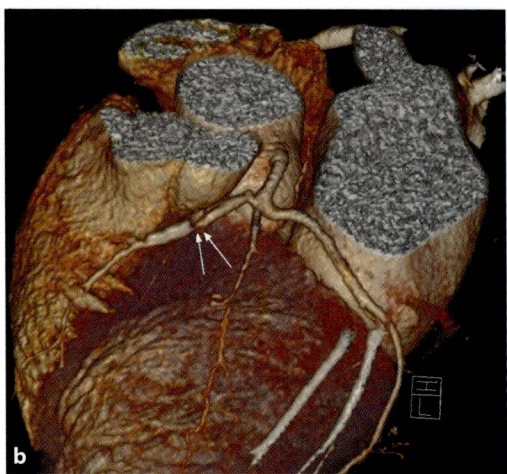

Fig. 9.7 Significant stenosis caused by a mixed plaque with a central calcific core (*arrows*), as seen using **a** bi-dimensional and **b** three-dimensional techniques

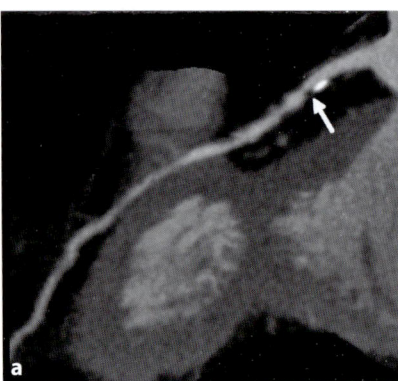
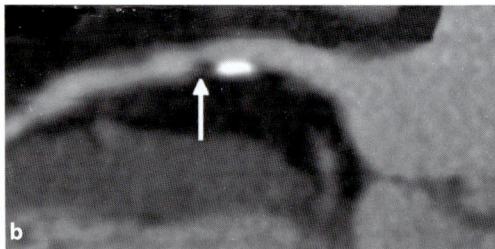

Fig. 9.8 Bi-dimensional images show **a** both a marginal calcific plaque and a second, non-calcific fibrolipidic plaque, with 50% vessel stenosis (*arrow*). **b** A third, non-calcific plaque is also present (*arrowhead*)

image reconstruction and analysis, images of the vessels must be reviewed in the three orthogonal planes; for images in the longitudinal axis, the plane located in the most central position of the vessel has to be selected, while avoiding the so-called partial volume effects (well-known to radiologists) that may further lead to overestimation of the stenosis.

Despite these considerations, atherosclerotic calcified plaques remain difficult to evaluate. The real degree of stenosis is frequently overestimated in current clinical practice, leading to the unnecessary use of catheter coronary angiography. Experience with CTA and the development of newer software (using image subtraction) will further improve our diagnostic confidence in this field.

9.3 Significant Stenosis

Atherosclerotic plaques that cause significant stenosis may be eccentric, marginally located, or concentric. Coronary CTA images are able to define the influence of the plaque on lumen caliber and to identify patients with significant stenotic involvement. Stenosing plaques may be calcific or fibrolipidic, and proper characterization of the atherosclerotic plaques will result in a more appropriate therapeutic approach (Figs. 9.7–9.9). In the evaluation of three-dimensional images acquired by CT, a complete analysis on three planes has to be performed, as discussed previously, in order to better define the degree of stenosis. Manual reconstruction methods provide qualitative measurement of the

Fig. 9.9 Severe stenosis caused by a concentric plaque of the proximal segment of the right coronary artery. **a** Axial image shows the plaque involvement and allows analysis of the reduced vessel lumen. **b** Bi-dimensional reconstructed image shows evidence of the stenosis, but with good distal vascular opacification

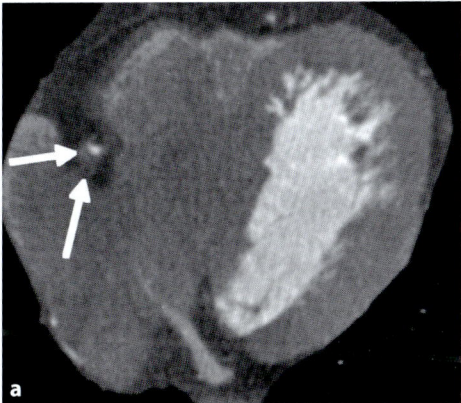 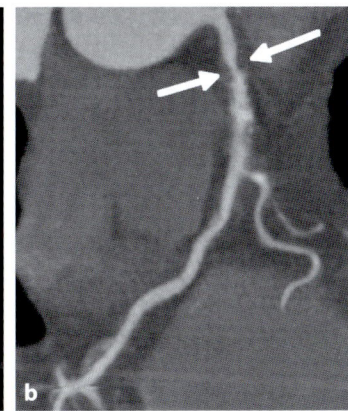

Fig. 9.10 a, b Anomalous origin of three vessels from the same left coronary sinus. A stenosis of the middle segment of the circumflex artery is also present (*arrow*)

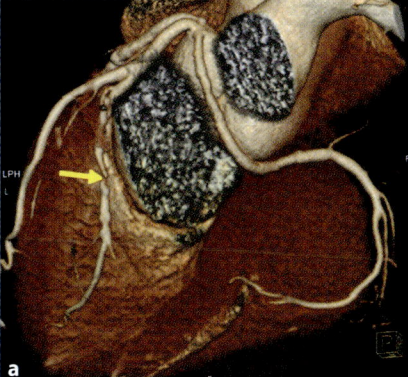 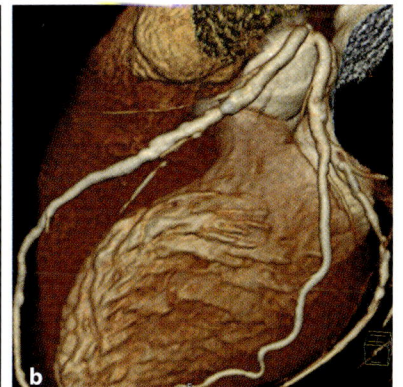

Fig. 9.11 a, b Significant stenosis of the right coronary artery just proximal to the crux (vascular bifurcation). The stenosis is evident both in **a** three-dimensional and **b** bi-dimensional images

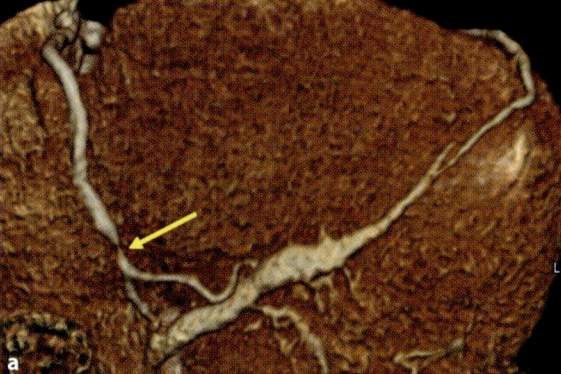 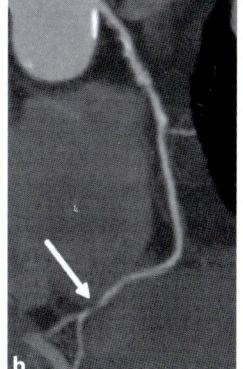

degree of stenosis, whereas semi-automated procedures generate quantitative information.

The extension of the atherosclerotic burden on the coronary bed has to be properly assessed and defined in CTA images, specifically, whether one, two, or three coronary vessels are involved, since multi-vessel involvement influences clinical outcome and the course of coronary atherosclerotic disease (Figs. 9.10–9.12). In addition, patient survival is directly related to the extent of atherosclerotic involvement; being high for non-significant stenosis, low in the presence of significant

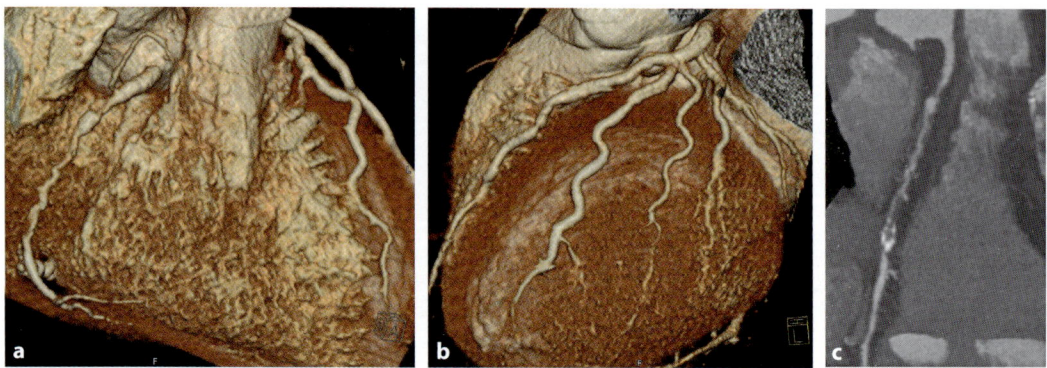

Fig. 9.12 a-c The right coronary artery is involved in multiple plaques, with focally significant reduction in the caliber of the arterial lumen. Strong compensatory hypertrophy of the vessels of the left vascular anatomy is well evident in three-dimensional volume-rendering images (**a**, **b**)

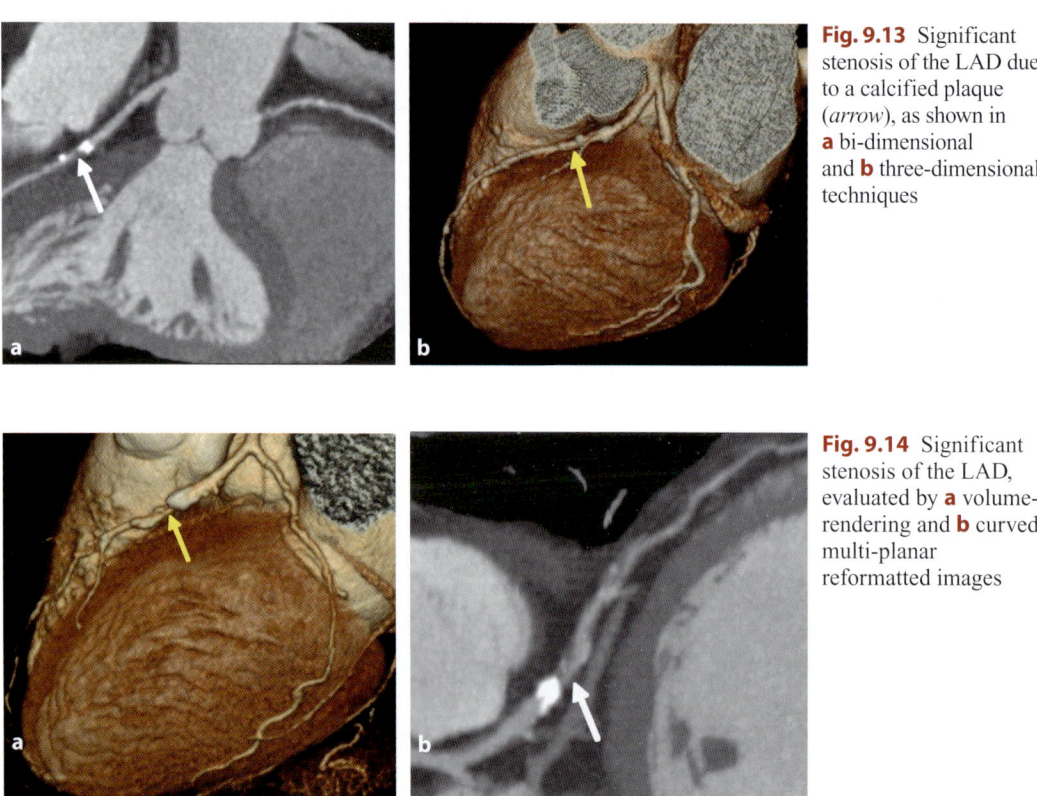

Fig. 9.13 Significant stenosis of the LAD due to a calcified plaque (*arrow*), as shown in **a** bi-dimensional and **b** three-dimensional techniques

Fig. 9.14 Significant stenosis of the LAD, evaluated by **a** volume-rendering and **b** curved multi-planar reformatted images

stenosis of a single vessel (Figs. 9.13–9.15), and even lower when three-vessel disease is evident.

Stenosing atherosclerotic disease of the coronary arteries has to be correlated with the anatomic configuration of the coronary bed. If congenital hypertrophy of one coronary vessel is present (see Chapter 1), stenosis of that single vessel will cause more significant pathological findings, whereas stenosis of a congenitally hypoplastic vessel may have less influence on myocardial perfusion. The same applies to coronary occlusion, which may be compatible with life only if a hypoplastic or non-dominant vessel is involved.

9 Coronary CT Angiography: Evaluation of Stenosis and Occlusion 77

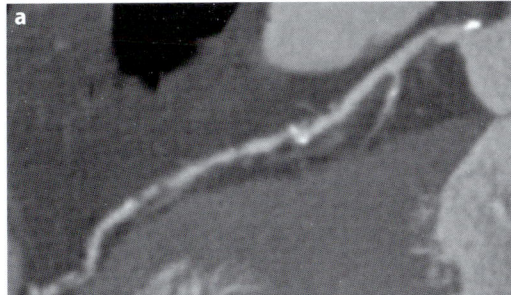
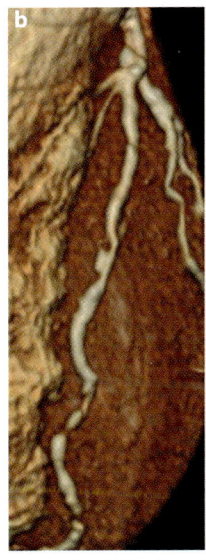

Fig. 9.15 Diffuse atherosclerotic involvement of the LAD, evaluated on **a** bi-dimensional and **b** three-dimensional images

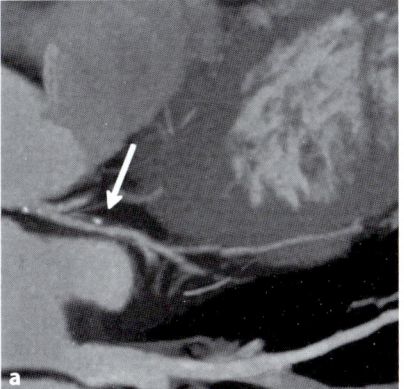
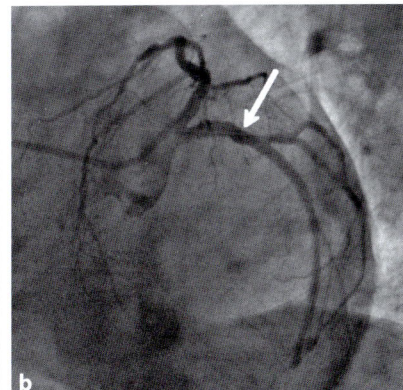

Fig. 9.16 Vascular remodeling. **a** The CT image evidences a thick peripheral marginal and eccentric coronary plaque (*arrow*) of the circumflex coronary artery. **b** Catheter coronary angiography does not show any significant area of lumen reduction, due to vascular remodeling

9.4 Remodeling

The presence of an atherosclerotic plaque is not always paralleled by vessel stenosis. Coronary arteries are rapidly pulsating vessels with consistent elasticity; significant remodeling of the vessel lumen may reduce the effect of a parietal plaque on vessel caliber and lumen. It is possible to have an important marginal plaque, e.g., 2 mm thick, that does not significantly influence the vessel lumen. This is exclusively found in coronary arteries and does not apply to other vessels in the body. Progression of an atherosclerotic plaque of the carotid arteries will be paralleled by a reduction of the lumen, with an increase of the plaque volume. In the coronary arteries, however, if the vessels retain their elasticity, the volume increase induced by a parietal, eccentric atherosclerotic plaque will lead to distension of the contralateral vessel wall, with deformity of the vessel course but also an increase in the vessel lumen and thus a lack of stenosis. This phenomenon is called vascular remodeling and is often well-evidenced in coronary CTA images (Fig. 9.16). In these cases, coronary CTA may be even more accurate than catheter angiography. In case of remodeling, the caliber of the vessel, as shown by catheter angiography, may be completely normal. Only coronary CTA will correctly demonstrate and characterize the important, eccentric

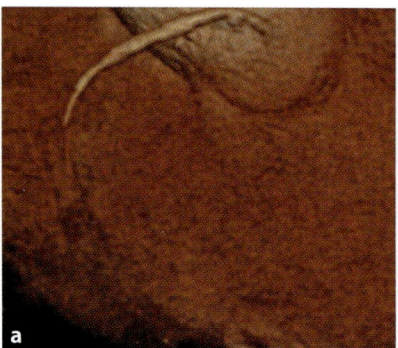 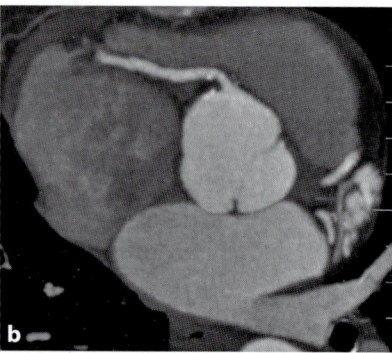

Fig. 9.17 Occlusion of the right coronary artery without distal revascularization and without collateral vessels. **a** Three-dimensional image and **b** the bi-dimensional reconstructed image

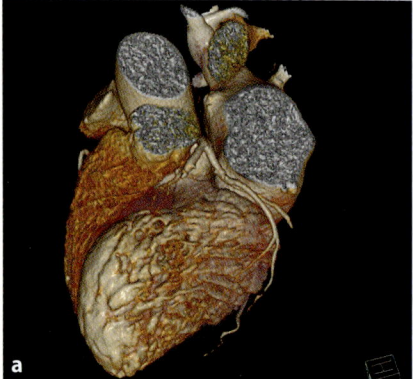 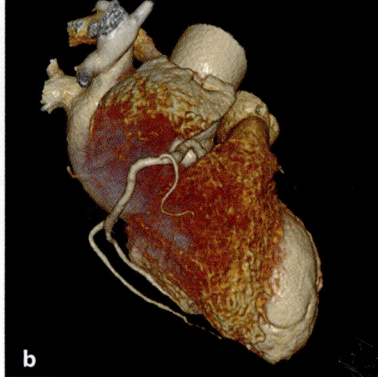

Fig. 9.18 Complete occlusion of the LAD. **a** Aneurysmal dilatation of the lateral part and the apex of the left ventricle. **b** Hypertrophy of the right coronary artery and the circumflex artery, thereby vascularizing the remaining part of the left ventricular wall

plaque. These findings have important prognostic value; in fact, only CTA is able to show that such patients have coronary artery disease (mostly in the presence of fibrolipidic atherosclerotic plaque) and require treatment to limit the possibility of atherosclerotic progress and to reduce the risks of complications of soft plaques (ulceration, hemorrhage), especially the development of acute coronary syndrome.

9.5 Occlusion of the Coronary Arteries and the Development of Collateral Circulation

Coronary artery occlusions can be easily evaluated with coronary CTA, due to the fact that distal to an atherosclerotic plaque the lack of visualization of a coronary vessel is diagnostic for coronary occlusion (Fig. 9.17). While complete occlusion of the main left artery is never diagnosed, because it is a fatal condition, it is not rare to find occlusions of the right coronary artery or of a relatively hypoplastic left coronary branch, without concomitant significant clinical findings. In fact, the anatomic configuration (dominant vessels, congenitally hyperplastic arteries) may greatly reduce the influence of vascular occlusion, at least regarding the clinical aspect.

The coronary arterial bed is considered a "terminal" vascular bed in that distal arteries, once occluded, cannot be revascularized by other, contiguous vessels. This is true only for acute coronary occlusions; myocardial infarction will develop if an occlusion occurs acutely, such that contiguous vessels are unable to compensate for the reduced perfusion. However, atherosclerosis is more frequently a slowly progressing, chronic disease and there is sufficient time for the development of coronary collateral circulation. Collaterals are very thin, peripheral intramyocardial vessels with an inverted vascular flow that allows revascularization distal to the vascular occlusions (Figs. 9.18–9.20). They are usually too small for their proper and direct

9 Coronary CT Angiography: Evaluation of Stenosis and Occlusion

Fig. 9.19 Occlusion of the right coronary artery, with evidence of collateral circulation providing flow distal to the occluded segment (collateral circulation is not directly evident in acquired CT images). **a** Bi-dimensional and **b** three-dimensional images

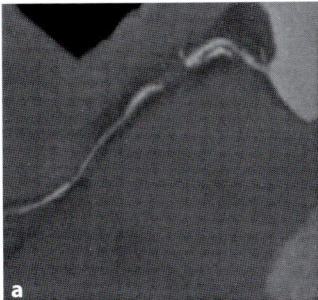
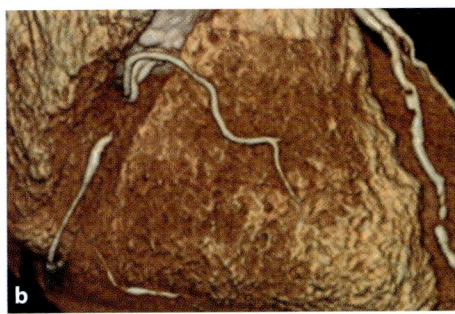

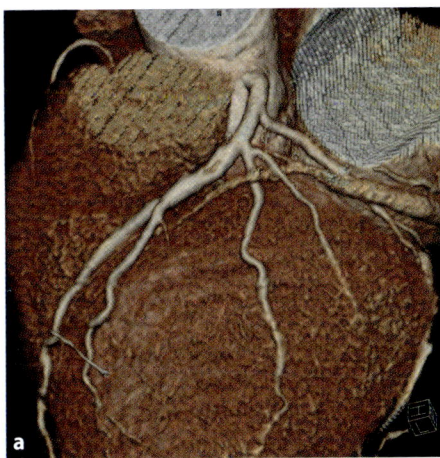
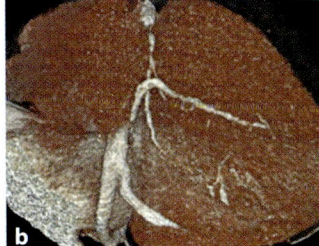
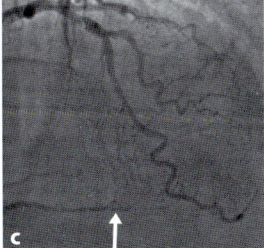

Fig. 9.20 Collateral circulation from the LAD shows revascularization distal to the occlusion of the right coronary artery. **a**, **b** Three-dimensional images acquired with CT. **c** Catheter coronary CT angiography shows small collateral vessels and revascularization of the distal right coronary vessel

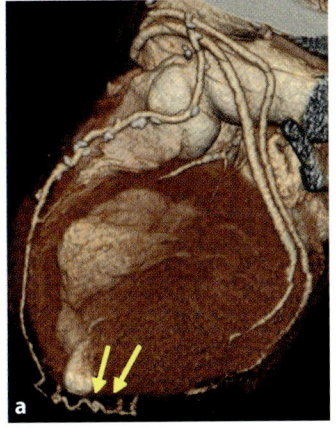
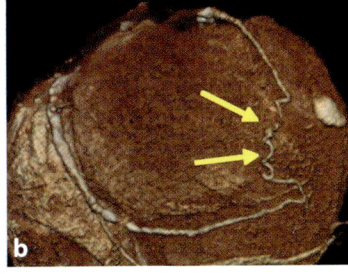
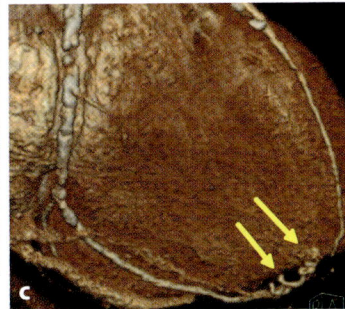

Fig. 9.21 a-c Volume-rendering images obtained from a patient who underwent a coronary artery bypass graft (CABG) procedure. The LAD provides collateral circulation, with large and tortuous vessels (*arrows*), to the occluded right coronary artery

demonstration by coronary CTA and may be opacified only at catheter angiography. CTA instead provides indirect evidence of their presence. In complete vascular occlusion, with distal re-filling of the involved vessel, a diagnosis of collateral circulation can be made, thus also providing information on the vessel that is contributing the inverted flow for revascularization. Only in a few instances is it possible to directly evaluate collateral circulation, based on evidence of hypertrophic superficial epicardial vessels or the "corkscrew" appearance of the vessels (Fig. 9.21). In addition, collateral circulation may develop in the same coronary vessel (homocoronary collateral circulation) (Fig. 9.22).

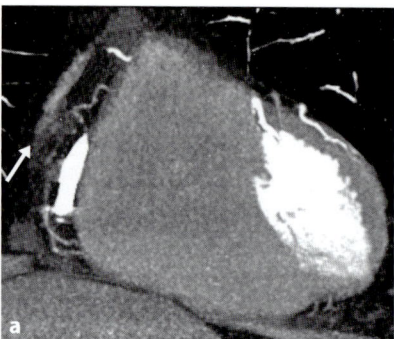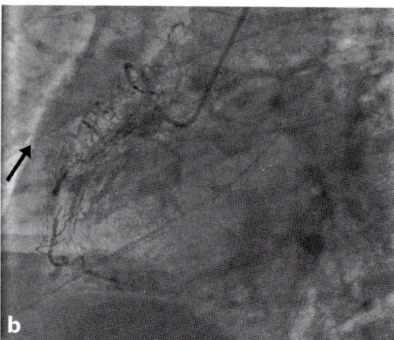

Fig. 9.22 Ipsilateral collateral circulation. The right coronary artery is occluded (stent occlusion). The small tortuous vessels providing revascularization of the distal right coronary artery (*arrow*) are readily seen on **a** CT and **b** catheter coronary angiography

9.6 Evaluation of Coronary Artery Stenosis: A Review of the Literature

Coronary CTA exhibits a high sensitivity and specificity in the definition of coronary artery stenosis. The sensitivity in defining significant stenosis (> 50% caliber reduction) is 93% for the evaluation of single vessels and even higher on a per patient basis, as shown in a recent meta-analysis of literature data. Not surprisingly, the sensitivity with 64-slice systems is much higher than that obtained with 16-slice systems (83 vs. 93%), a difference that may also be related to methodological improvements (more concentrated contrast agent, better injection protocol) or to the faster rotational speed of the X-ray tube and advances in detector characteristics. Further improvements are expected with technical advances, such as larger and more sensitive detector arrays and even faster rotation times, leading to reduced acquisition times of coronary images.

As far as specificity is concerned, the current overall value is high, in the range of 96%. Another important issue is related to the negative predictive value, which is 97–98%. The significance of the latter is very important from a clinical point of view; in fact, it defines the ability of coronary CTA to determine whether the vessels are normal, i.e., free of atherosclerotic involvement. Accordingly, if the arteries are normal with respect to the CTA findings, then there is a 98% certainty that the patient does not have coronary atherosclerosis. This stresses the important role that CTA plays – in symptomatic as well as in asymptomatic at-risk patients – in screening patients without or with atherosclerotic involvement. The first group consists of patients with normal coronary arteries, in whom no further diagnostic evaluation is needed. In the second group are patients with coronary artery disease, which needs to be further characterize and staged by CTA, either alone or, in the presence of clearly significant stenosis, by means of catheter angiography. It is estimated that at least 30% of the catheter angiography examinations currently performed identify a normal coronary bed; thus, a large number of these procedures could be avoided. At the same time, once significant coronary disease has been diagnosed at CTA, it is not crucial whether the same method is able to properly address the exact degree of stenosis; rather, further definition and characterization of the atherosclerotic vascular involvement are left to catheter angiography.

9.7 Saving Lives

Radiologists, especially those who have only recently gained experience in the field of cardiology, should be well aware of the fact that there are a number of truly asymptomatic patients who would have never undergone catheter angiography, due to a lack of clinical indications. In this group, only the use of coronary CTA is able to show the presence of important coronary disease. These patients can thus be regarded as lives saved by CTA.

By being alert to such patients, we hope to overcome the indifference with which some clinicians still regard coronary CTA. In fact, several developments advocate its increased use: (1) the problem of high radiation exposure has been solved (80% reduction with newer equipment, i.e., much less than the exposure associated with nuclear-medicine procedures); (2) the technology is no longer primitive and the procedures have become standard; and (3) the image quality is consistent, facilitating good professional collaboration between cardiologists and radiologists and thus better-informed clinical diagnoses. The frequency and ease with which CTA can be used should reassure the properly informed patient that he or she is undergoing a standard, routine clinical procedure, not a dangerous examination. CTA is, in this aspect, no different than, e.g., a CT scan of the kidneys for the evaluation of kidney stones (which has made intravenous pyelography almost completely obsolete) or magnetic resonance of the brain (which has totally replaced the very invasive procedures used by neuroradiologists until the 1970s). Indeed, "seeing" the coronary arteries, as is possible with CTA, is the best approach to directly determine whether a patient has coronary artery disease. Every other diagnostic procedure provides only indirect information.

In the following three representative cases, the patients had highly significant CTA findings but either absent or limited clinical findings and a negative treadmill test.

Case 1

A 40-year-old patient with mild symptoms, related to the epigastric area. Negative endoscopy, negative treadmill test. Stenting of the stenotic lesion was performed (Figs. 9.23, 9.24).

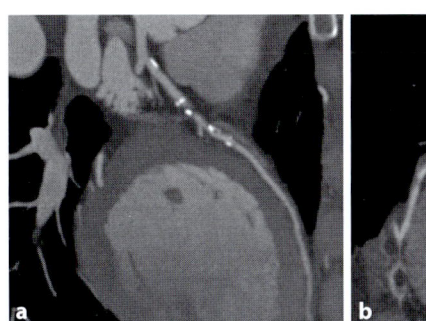
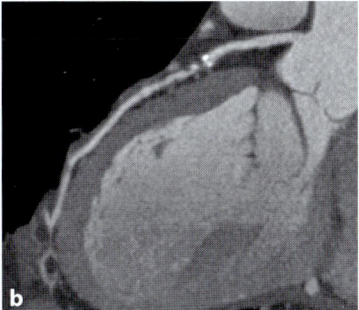
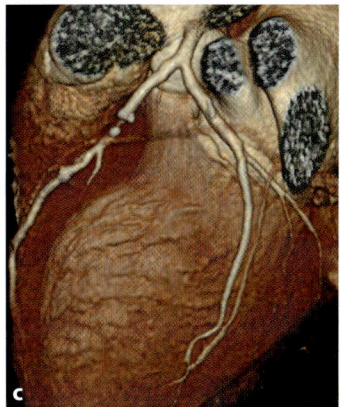

Fig. 9.23 a, b Bi-dimensional MPR images and **c** 3D images show a severe stenosis of the middle segment of the LAD due to a calcified plaque

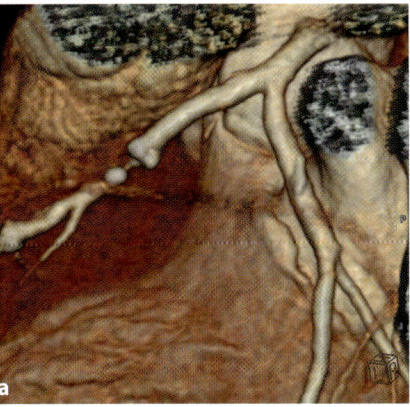
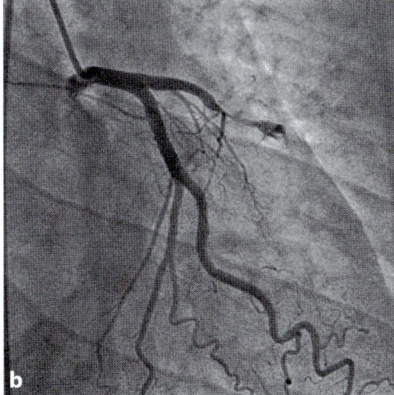

Fig. 9.24 a Three-dimensional image of the stenosis. **b** Catheter coronary angiography confirms the diagnosis and the absence of vascular flow distal to the diseased segment

Case 2

A 70-year-old patient with no symptoms and a negative treadmill test. The only indication for CTA was the fact that his son had died of an acute cardiac arrest while playing football. The patient underwent stenting of a stenotic lesion (Fig. 9.25).

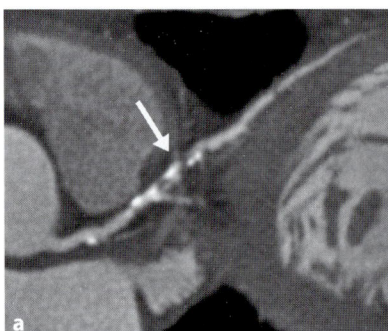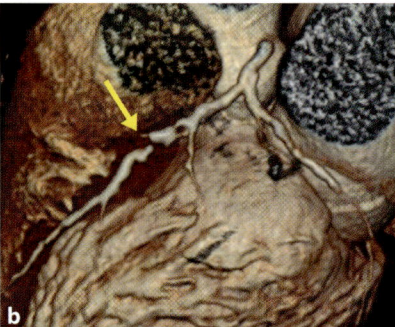

Fig. 9.25 Severe stenosis of the LAD evaluated on **a** bi-dimensional and **b** three-dimensional images

Case 3

A 68-year-old asymptomatic patient with a negative treadmill test who requested CTA after learning of the procedure in the media. A coronary artery bypass graft was performed after coronary angiography (Figs. 9.26–9.28).

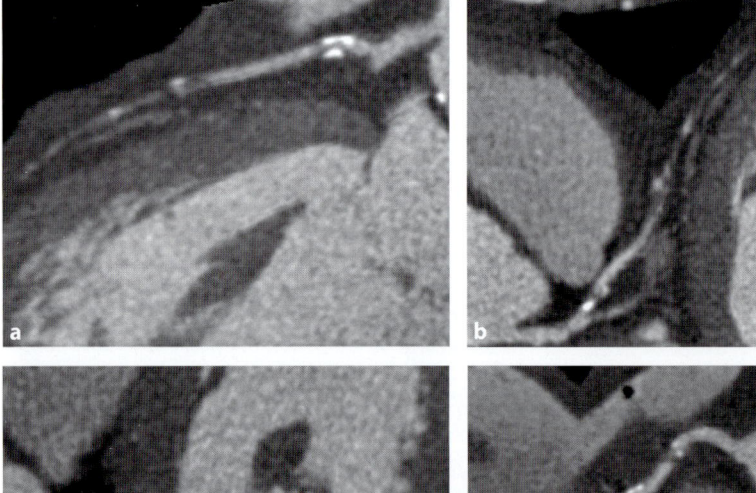

Fig. 9.26 a-d Bi-dimensional images show occlusion of both the right coronary artery and the LAD. There is also a marginal plaque in the middle segment of the cirumflex artery, with significant stenosis (*arrow*)

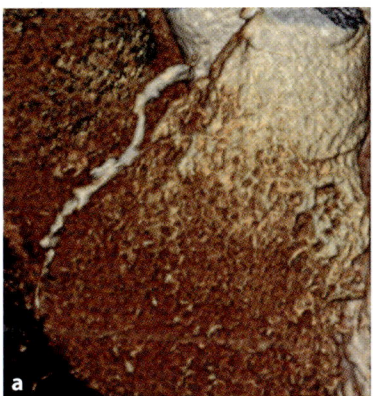 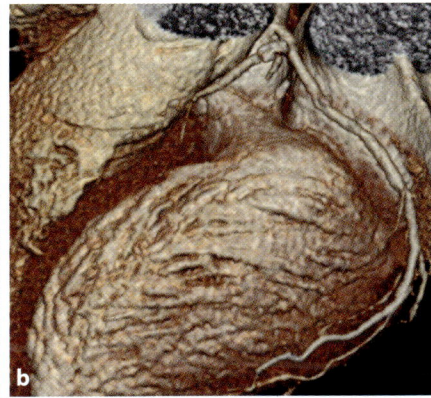

Fig. 9.27 Three-dimensional volume-rendering images show occlusion of **a** the middle third of the right coronary artery and **b** the LAD. The circumflex artery is hypertrophic

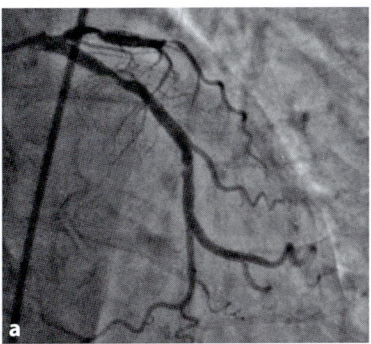 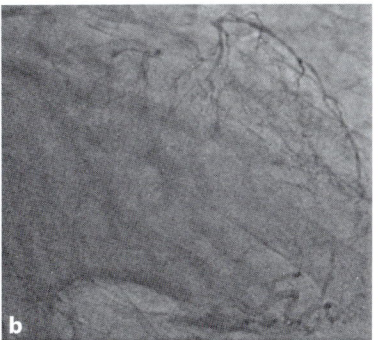 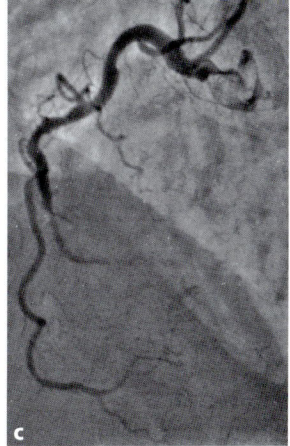

Fig. 9.28 Catheter coronary angiography shows occlusion of the LAD and stenosis of the circumflex artery. **a** In late angiographic phase, there is re-vascularization of the distal LAD through collateral circulation. **b** The right coronary artery is occluded (**c**) and the acute marginal artery is hypertrophic

Suggested Reading

Kerl JM, Schoepf UJ, Zwerner PL, Bauer RW, Abro JA, Thilo C, Vogl TJ, Herzog C. Accuracy of coronary artery stenosis detection with CT versus conventional coronary angiography compared with composite findings from both tests as an enhanced reference standard. Eur Radiol. 2011 Sep;21(9):1895-903. Epub 2011 May 1. PubMed PMID: 21533864

Min JK, Koo BK, Erglis A, Doh JH, Daniels DV, Jegere S, Kim HS, Dunning AM, Defrance T, Lansky A, Leipsic J. Usefulness of Noninvasive Fractional Flow Reserve Computed from Coronary Computed Tomographic Angiograms for Intermediate Stenoses Confirmed by Quantitative Coronary Angiography. Am J Cardiol. 2012 Jun 28. [Epub ahead of print] PubMed PMID: 22749390

Shmilovich H, Cheng VY, Tamarappoo BK, Dey D, Nakazato R, Gransar H, Thomson LE, Hayes SW, Friedman JD, Germano G, Slomka PJ, Berman DS. Vulnerable plaque features on coronary CT angiography as markers of inducible regional myocardial hypoperfusion from severe coronary artery stenoses. Atherosclerosis. 2011 Dec;219(2):588-95. Epub 2011 Aug 7. PubMed PMID: 21862017; PubMed Central PMCID: PMC3226846

Vavere AL, Arbab-Zadeh A, Rochitte CE, Dewey M, Niinuma H, Gottlieb I, Clouse ME, Bush DE, Hoe JW, de Roos A, Cox C, Lima JA, Miller JM. Coronary artery stenoses: accuracy of 64-detector row CT angiography in segments with mild, moderate, or severe calcification--a subanalysis of the CORE-64 trial. Radiology. 2011 Oct;261(1):100-8. Epub 2011 Aug 9. PubMed PMID: 21828192; PubMed Central PMCID: PMC3176425

Current Strategies in Cardiac Surgery

10

Andrea Montalto and Francesco Musumeci

10.1 Introduction

Atherosclerotic coronary artery disease (CAD) may cause narrowing of the coronary arteries due to the thickening and loss of elasticity of their walls. The arterial narrowing, when significant, will reduce blood flow to the myocardium during exercise and, in the presence of severe coronary artery disease, even at rest. Revascularization by coronary artery bypass grafting (CABG) surgery has been shown to offer symptomatic and prognostic benefits [1].

10.2 Indications for Surgery

The indications for CABG are based on the comparative benefits of surgery relative to medical treatment or coronary angioplasty percutaneous interventions [2]. According to the most recent clinical evidence, based on over 40 years of clinical experience in the management of CAD, surgery is the best treatment option in the presence of lumen narrowing ≥50% in the left main coronary artery, either as an isolated lesion or in combination with narrowing in other

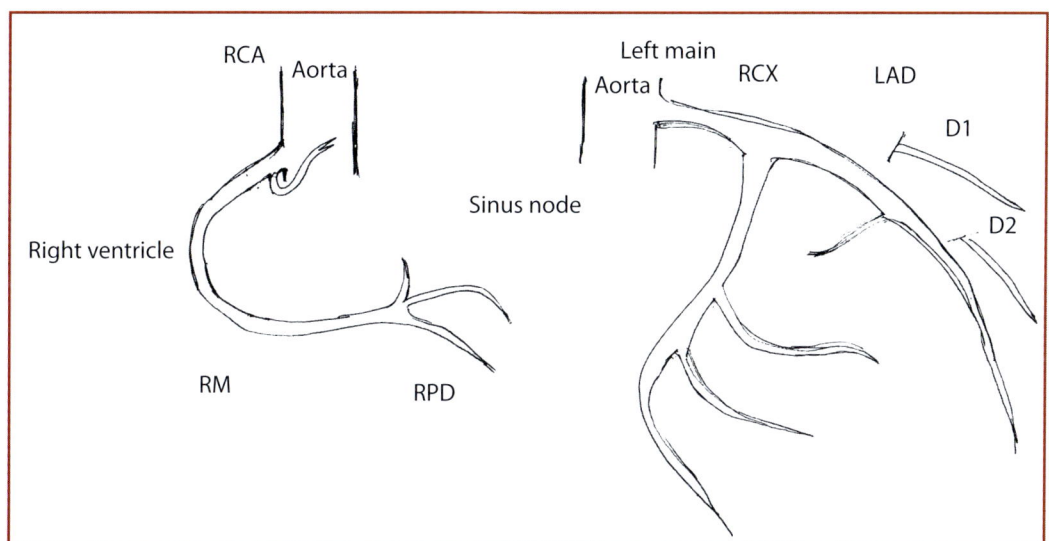

Fig. 10.1 *RCA* right coronary artery, *RM* right marginal, *RPD* right posterior descending, *LAD* left anterior descending, *D1* first diagonal, *D2* second diagonal

F. Musumeci (✉)
Department of Cardiac Surgery and Transplantation
San Camillo Hospital, Rome, Italy
e-mail: fr.musumeci@libero.it

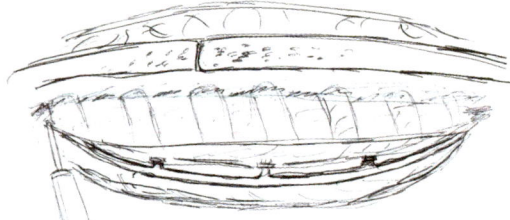

Fig. 10.2 Preparation of the internal thoracic artery

coronary arteries. Surgery provides better outcome also in the presence of three-vessel CAD, particularly in diabetic patients. Surgery is also indicated in patients with one- or two-vessel CAD if there is critical proximal narrowing of the left anterior descending coronary artery (LAD). Finally, surgery has the best prognostic impact compared to alternative treatments in patients with multi-vessel CAD and impaired LV function [3] (Fig. 10.1).

10.3 Conduits Used in Coronary Surgery

10.3.1 Arterial Grafts

10.3.1.1 Internal Thoracic Artery

The use of the left internal thoracic artery (ITA) as a bypass graft for the LAD has been demonstrated to provide superior early and late survival and better event-free survival after CABG surgery. The histological and biological characteristics of the ITA result in better clinical outcomes than achieved with venous conduits, making the ITA the conduit of first choice for myocardial revascularization. The ITA is usually mobilized immediately after the sternum has been opened, before heparin is administered. The artery can either be dissected from the chest wall within a pedicle with the internal thoracic veins, fat, muscle and pleura or it may be skeletonized (Fig. 10.2). The remarkable remodeling capacities of the ITA allows it to adapt its diameter and flow to the demand for blood of the supplied myocardium. In fact, the ITA increases its flow in the same way as normal coronary arteries, i.e., through an increase in velocity and caliber mediated by the endothelium [4].

10.3.1.2 Radial Artery

The use of the radial artery (RA) as a conduit for CABG surgery was originally described by Carpentier in the early 1970s. The initial results were disappointing, with 32% of grafts occluded at 2 years. Acar and colleagues postulated that harvest injury was responsible for the graft occlusion. Encouraging mid- and long-term results have been demonstrated with the RA harvested as a pedicle together with the surrounding tissues. RA harvesting is performed through an incision made in the forearm beginning over the radial pulse at the wrist. It is then extended proximally over the belly of the brachioradialis for the necessary length.

10.3.1.3 Right Gastroepiploic Artery

The gastroepiploic artery (GEA) may be used in re-operation for myocardial revascularization in the absence of other suitable conduits, or as a second- or third-choice arterial conduit to provide a total arterial revascularization. To expose the right GEA, the midline incision over the sternum is extended over the upper abdomen. Dissection extends from the pylorus along the greater curvature of the stomach until a sufficient length is obtained.

10.3.2 Venous Grafts

The saphenous vein continues to be the most commonly used conduit in CABG. The greater saphenous vein is, in fact, easy to harvest, readily available, and versatile. If the saphenous vein from the lower leg is to be used, the initial skin incision is located anterior to the medial malleolus. If the upper portion of the vein is used, then the skin incision is performed in the groin. In either case, a continuous incision over the length of the vein is made. After the vein has been exposed, the proximal end is isolated and divided between ligatures (Fig. 10.3).

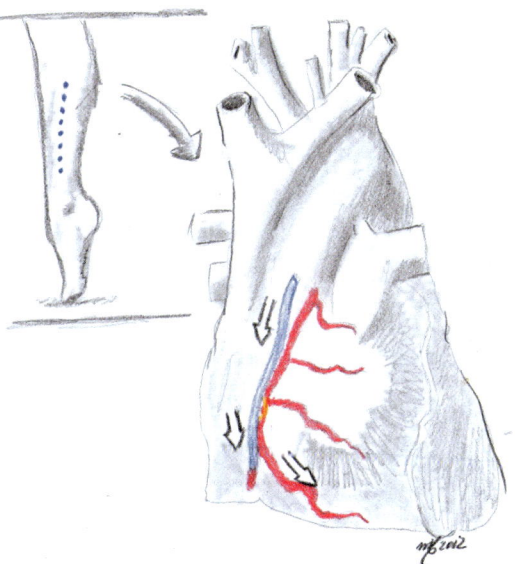

Fig. 10.3 Example of aorto-coronary bypass grafting using the saphenous vein

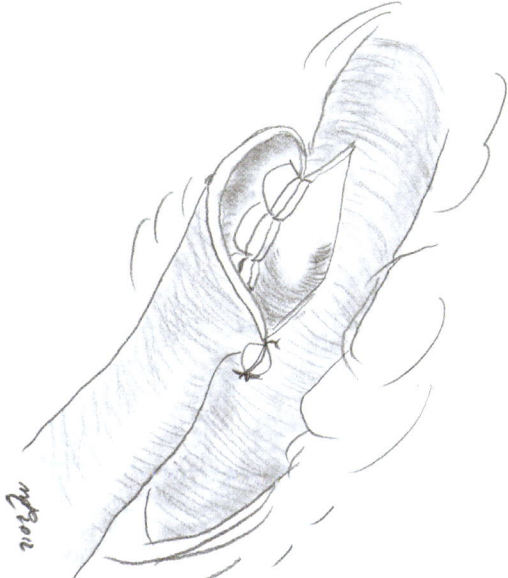

Fig. 10.4 Standard end-to-side anastomosis

Branches may be ligated with fine sutures and divided, or divided between hemostatic clips.

10.4 Surgical Strategy

The objective of CABG is to obtain complete myocardial revascularization by bypassing all critical coronary-artery narrowings in vessels having a diameter ≥1 mm (Fig. 10.4). The most widely used strategy in CABG involves routine grafting of the left ITA to the LAD and segments of the saphenous vein to the remaining diseased coronary arteries. Vein graft can be used in different combinations. The vein can be anastomosed end-to-side to a coronary artery, providing blood supply only to the myocardial segment supplied by that coronary branch. If additional coronary branches need to be bypassed, sequential grafting can be performed by connecting one venous segment to two or more coronary arteries using side-to-side anastomoses. This technique is usually employed for the circumflex coronary artery when there is more than one obtuse marginal branch, each with proximal narrowing. In this setting, the grafted vein is anastomosed side-to-side to one or more proximal marginal branches and end-to-side to most distal marginal branches. Sequential grafts to the circumflex system can be extended to include the postero-lateral branch or the posterior descending branch of the right coronary artery (RCA).

The left ITA is most often used to bypass the LAD. Sequential grafting using the left ITA may include a diagonal branch of the LAD. In a bypass of the RCA, the right ITA can be used either alone or in combination with a left ITA graft to the LAD system. Alternatively, the right ITA can be passed through the transverse sinus and anastomosed to one or more marginal branches of the left circumflex coronary artery (Fig. 10.5).

The right GEA may be used to bypass branches of the RCA and the circumflex coronary arteries in combination with an ITA graft to the LAD circulation (Fig. 10.6).

A graft of the RA may be used as a sequential graft to bypass arteries on the lateral and posterior surfaces of the left ventricle. Proximally, the radial artery can be anastomosed to the left ITA or directly to the ascending aorta. The RA may be used to extend the right ITA to allow revascularization of the arteries of the postero-lateral wall of the left ventricle [5-9] (Fig. 10.7).

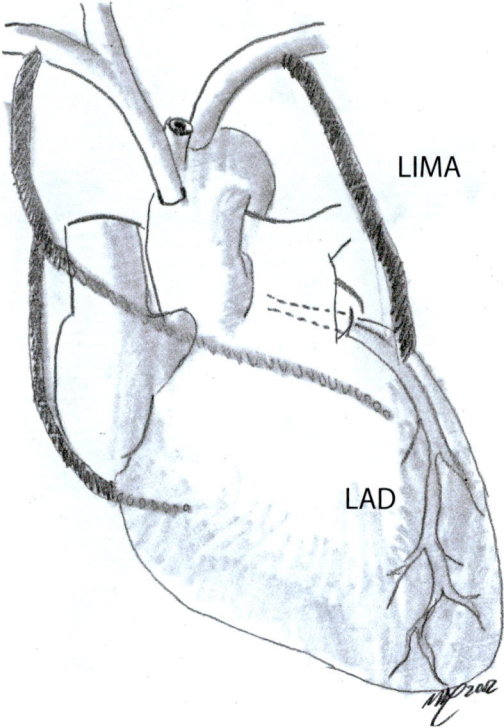

Fig. 10.5 *LIMA* left internal mammary artery, *LAD* left anterior descending artery

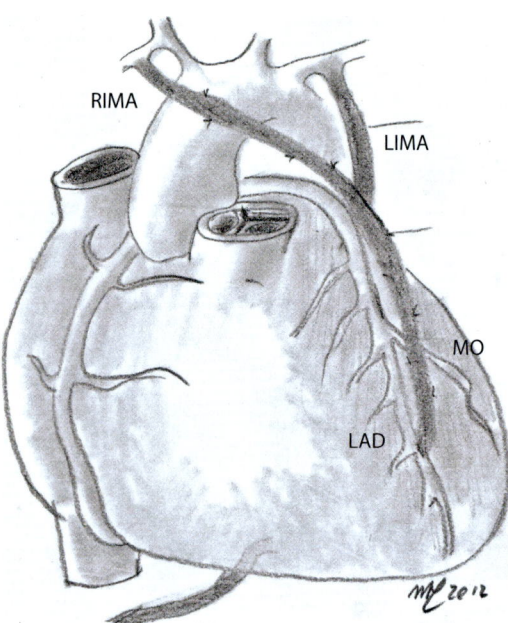

Fig. 10.6 *LIMA* left internal mammary artery, *LAD* Left anterior descending artery, *RIMA* right internal mammary artery, *MO* obtuse marginal

10.4.1 On-Pump Myocardial Revascularization

A medial sternotomy is made and at the same time a segment of the saphenous vein is harvested. Heparin is administered after dissection of the ITA is completed. Purse-string sutures are then placed at the cannulation sites in the ascending aorta and right atrial wall. Cardiopulmonary bypass is established using a single venous cannula. The aorta is clamped and the cardioplegic solution infused.

10.4.2 Off-Pump Myocardial Revascularization

Off-pump coronary artery bypass gafting (OPCABG) is a recognized valuable alternative to conventional CABG on a cardiopulmonary bypass. Despite ongoing controversy over its relative benefits, OPCABG has been shown to reduce mortality in numerous prospective randomized trials and in retrospective comparisons. With the development of stabilization devices that permit adequate and safe exposure of all surfaces of the left ventricle in the beating heart, OPCABG can be performed also in patients with three-vessel disease and with left main coronary artery disease [10] (Fig. 10.8).

10.5 Results

At 15 years post-operatively, a grafted left ITA provides higher cumulative survival ($p<0.01$), less early recurrence of angina ($p<0.01$), fewer recurrences of myocardial infarction ($p<0.02$), fewer re-operations ($p<0.001$), and better cumulative event-free survival ($p<0.01$) than a saphenous vein graft [11, 12]. Even better long-term results can be achieved if both ITAs are used.

Fig. 10.7 a-e *LIMA* left internal mammary artery, *LAD* left anterior descending, *RIMA* right internal mammary artery *MO* obtuse marginal, *RA* radial artery, *RITA* right internal thoracic artery, *LITA* left internal thoracic artery

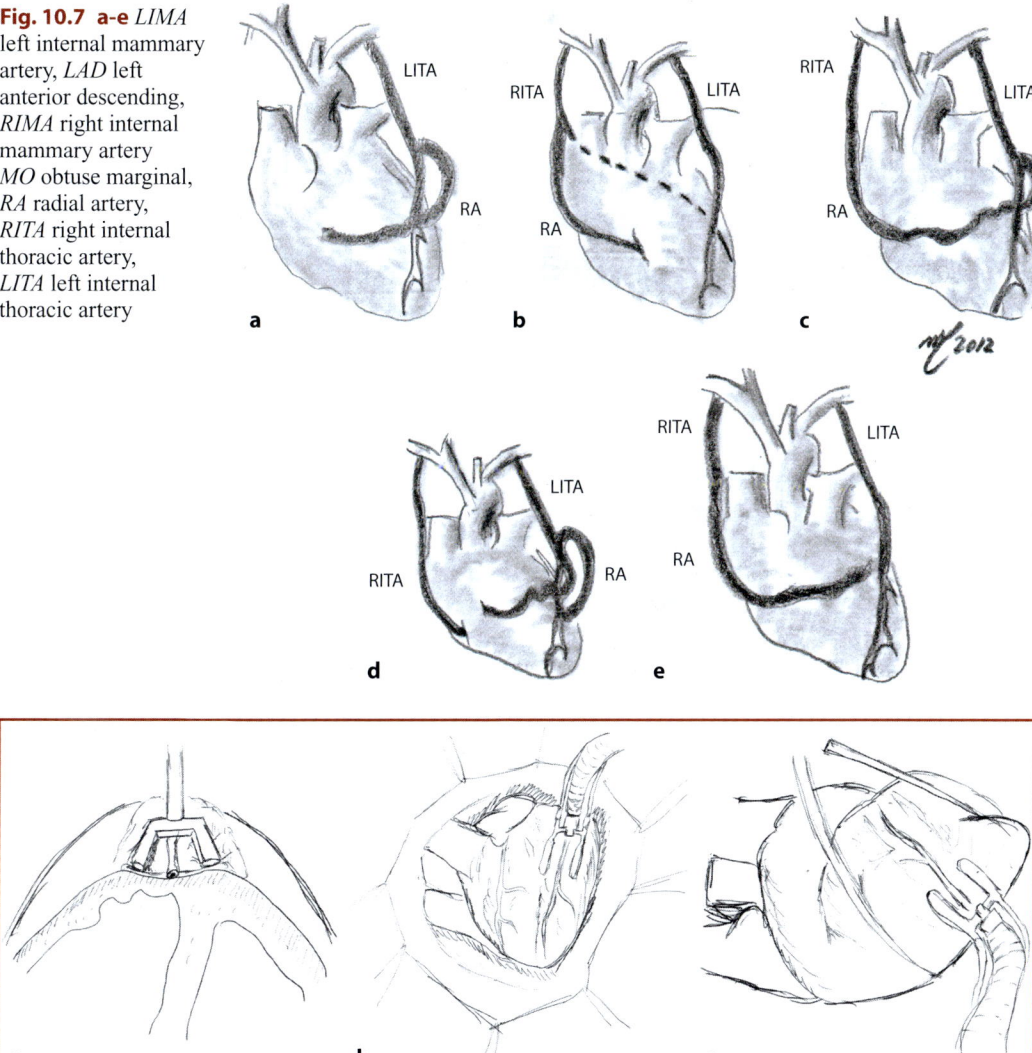

Fig. 10.8 a-c Example of coronary stabilization during off-pump procedure

10.6 Conclusion

The left ITA to the LAD should be the graft of choice in all patients undergoing surgical myocardial revascularization. The use of both ITAs is recommended to provide total arterial revascularization of the left heart, in addition to being the preferred strategy of myocardial revascularization in all patients up to 70 years of age.

Acknowledgement The drawings in this chapter were made by Marco Montalto.

References

1. Abramov D, Tamariz MG, Fremes SE et al (2000) Trends in coronary artery bypass surgery results: a recent, 9-year study. Ann Thorac Surg 70:84
2. Califf RM, Harrell FE Jr, Lee KL et al (1989) The evolution of medical and surgical therapy for coronary artery disease. A 15-years perspective. JAMA 261:2077
3. Eagle KA, Guyton RA, Davidoff R et al American College of Cardiology; American Heart Association (2004) ACC/AHA 2004

guideline update for coronary artery bypass graft surgery: a report of the American College of Cardiology/American Heart Association Task Force on Practice Guidelines. Circulation 110:e340-e347
4. Eagle Formica F, Ferro O, Greco P et al (2004) Long-term follow-up of total arterial myocardial revascularization using exclusively pedicle bilateral internal thoracic artery and right gastroepiploic artery. Eur J Cardiothorac Surg 26:1141-1148
5. Henriquez-Pino JA, Gomes WJ, Prates JC, Buffolo E (1997) Surgical anatomy of the internal thoracic artery. Ann Thorac Surg 64:1041-1045
6. Pevni D, Mohr R, Lev-Ran O et al (2003) Technical aspects of composite arterial grafting with double skeletonized internal thoracic arteries. Chest 123:1348-1354
7. Kobayashi J, Tagusari O, Bando K et al (2002) Total arterial off-pump coronary revascularization with only internal thoracic artery and composite radial artery grafts. Heart Surg Forum 6:30-37
8. Wendler O, Hennen B, Demertzis S et al (2000) Complete arterial revascularization in multivessel coronary artery disease with 2 conduits (skeletonized grafts and T grafts). Circulation 102 (19 Suppl 3):III,79-83
9. Bonacchi M, Prifti E, Battaglia F et al (2003) In situ retrocaval skeletonized right internal thoracic artery anastomosed to the circumflex system via transverse sinus: technical aspects and postoperative outcome. J Thorac Cardiovasc Surg 126:1302-1313
10. Puskas JD, Williams WH, Duke PG (2003) Off-pump coronary artery bypass grafting provides complete revascularization with reduced myocardial injury, transfusion requirements, and length of stay: a prospective randomized comparison of two hundred unselected patients undergoing off-pump versus conventional coronary artery bypass grafing. J Thorac Cardiovasc Surg 125:797-808
11. Cameron A, Davis KB, Green G, Schaff HV (1996) Coronary bypass surgery with internal-thoracic-artery grafts-effects on survival over a 15-year period. N Engl J Med 334:216-219
12. Fiore AC, Naunheim KS, Dean P et al (1990) Results of internal thoracic artery grafting over 15 years: single versus double grafts. Ann Thorac Surg 49:202-208

Coronary CT Angiography: Evaluation of Coronary Artery Bypass Grafts

Carlo Nicola De Cecco, Gorka Bastarrika and Marco Rengo

11.1 Introduction

Coronary revascularization, comprising coronary artery bypass graft (CABG) surgery and percutaneous coronary intervention (PCI), is among the most common major medical procedures provided by the US health care system, with more than 1 million procedures performed annually [1, 2]. Several innovations in coronary revascularization, such as drug-eluting stents, minimally invasive CABG surgery, and "off-pump" CABG surgery, have been adopted widely in the past decade, with the promise of improved clinical outcomes compared with older revascularization technologies and techniques [3, 4]. However, with the advent of PCI and the increased efficacy of medical therapy, a constant decrease in the number of CABG procedures has been steadily observed in the USA. Nonetheless, the results of the recent SYNTAX trial indicated that CABG surgery remains the better choice for coronary revascularization among patients with previously untreated three-vessel or left main coronary artery disease [5-7].

Multi-detector computed tomography (MDCT) coronary angiography is well-established as an excellent imaging technique in the evaluation of graft patency after CABG. The improved accuracy and safety of MDCT has reduced the need for catheter-based coronary angiography; in fact, an increasing number of patients undergo annual CABG patency assessment with this non-invasive imaging technique [8]. The avoidance of unnecessary coronary angiography through the use of MDCT is expected to result in overall cost savings along the diagnostic pathway.

11.2 CABG Indications and Clinical History

Indications for CABG surgery include triple-vessel disease, one- or two-vessel disease involving the left anterior descending artery, and main trunk disease. The rate of graft patency at 10 years is 50–60% for venous grafts and 80–90% for arterial grafts [6, 7]. The arterialization of venous grafts over time following exposure to systemic blood increases the risk of stenosis and graft occlusion, due to intimal hyperplasia. Recurrent cardiac ischemia after CABG surgery occurs in a significant proportion of patients, demanding further investigations and re-intervention. Early graft failure is the result of technical factors including graft kinking or stretching, suboptimal conduit quality, competitive flow in the native artery, or poor runoff distal to the anastomosis. Diabetes, renal failure, and poor left ventricular function are predictors of poor outcome in graft patency.

C.N. De Cecco (✉)
Department of Radiological Sciences
Oncology and Pathology, University of Rome
"La Sapienza" Polo Pontino, Latina, Italy
e-mail: carlodececco@gmail.com

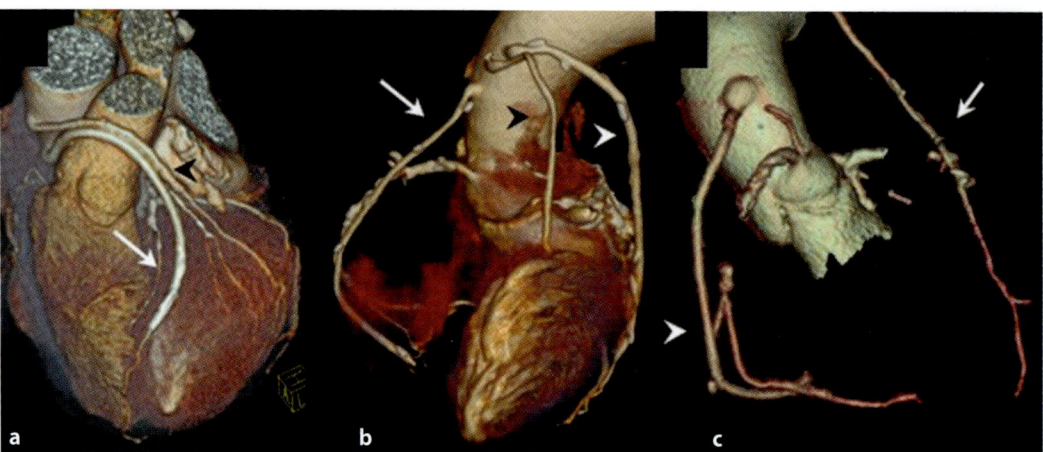

Fig. 11.1 Different types of CABG. **a** Venous grafts on the LAD (*arrow*) and the marginal vessel (*black arrowhead*). **b** Venous grafts on the RCA (*arrow*), diagonal (*black arrowhead*) and marginal vessels (*white arrowhead*). **c** LIMA graft on the LAD (*arrow*) and a venous graft the on RCA (*arrowhead*)

11.3 CABG Classification

In CABG surgery, either venous or arterial grafts can be used. The choice of graft type and anastomosis depends on several factors, such as conduit availability and target-vessel position.

Venous grafts are harvested from the saphenous vein as free grafts and are then anastomosed proximally to the aorta and distally to the target vessel.

Arterial grafts can be in situ grafts, usually from the left internal mammary artery (LIMA) but less frequently from the right internal mammary artery (RIMA), or free conduits harvested from other arteries. LIMA grafts are used to revascularize the left anterior descending (LAD) artery, while the RIMA is used to target the right coronary artery (RCA). The right gastroepiploic artery less frequently serves as the graft vessel, i.e., only in case of redo surgery when no other conduits are available. A LIMA graft is the procedure of choice for LAD revascularization based on the anatomical and biological characteristics of this artery (Fig. 11.1).

In sequential grafts, a proximal anastomosis is established with one vessel followed by a distal anastomosis with adjacent vessels in order to revascularize multiple coronary branches using only one conduit.

Two bypass conduits can be used to form a Y (or T) graft to revascularize different vessels. In most cases, a LIMA graft on the LAD is used with a second venous graft that is laterally anastomosed to a diagonal or marginal vessel [9, 10].

11.4 Current Indications for CABG Imaging with MDCT

The most recent document establishing appropriateness criteria for the use of non-invasive cardiac imaging with CT is that of the American College of Cardiology Foundation [11]. In their report, a technical panel scored each indication on a numerical scale of 1 to 9, considering scores between 7 and 9 as appropriate (imaging is generally acceptable and is a reasonable approach for the indication), scores between 4 and 6 as uncertain (imaging may be generally acceptable and a reasonable approach for the indication, but more research and/or patient information is needed to definitively classify the indication), and scores between 1 and 3 as inappropriate (imaging is not generally acceptable and is not a reasonable approach for the indication).

According to this document (Table 11.1), MDCT in CABG evaluation is considered appropriate in symptomatic patients in order to demonstrate con-

Table 11.1 Summary of the criteria for the appropriate use of cardiac multidetector computed tomography (MDCT) imaging in patients with CABG. Modified from [11]

	Clinical scenario	Appropriate use score (1-9)	
Symptomatic (ischemic equivalent)	Evaluation of graft patency	A (8)	
	Time of prior CABG surgery	< 5 years	≥ 5 years
Asymptomatic	Evaluation of graft patency	I (2)	U (5)

A appropriate, *I* inappropriate, *U* uncertain.

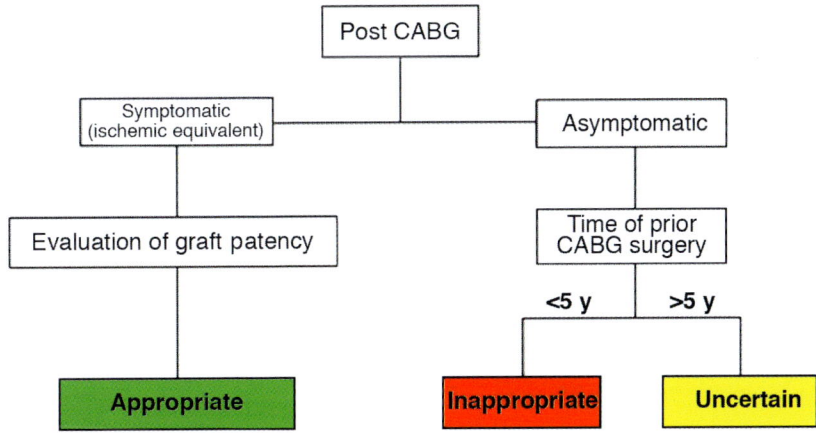

Fig. 11.2 Criteria for the appropriate use of cardiac MDCT imaging in patients with CABG. Modified from [11]

Table 11.2 Accuracy of 64- and 320-row MDCT in the assessment of graft patency compared with conventional coronary angiography

					Occlusion				Stenosis			
Author	Pts	N	Arterial	Venous	Sens	Spec	PPV	NPV	Sens	Spec	PPV	NPV
Malagutti [12]	52	109	45	64	-	-	-	-	100	98.3	98	100
Pache [13]	31	93	22	71	-	-	-	-	97.8	89.3	90	97.7
Ropers [14]	50	138	37	101	100	100	-	-	100	94	92	100
Dikkers [15]	34	69	52	17	100	100	100	100	100	98.7	75	100
Jabara [16]	50	147	47	100	100	100	100	100	100	100	100	100
Feuchtner [17]	41	70	46	24	100	100	100	100	85	95	80	97
Meyer [18]	138	397	144	253	-	-	-	-	97	97	93	99
Nazeri [19]	89	287	89	198	-	-	-	-	98	97	95.5	99
Weustink [20]	52	111	48	63	-	-	-	-	100	100	100	100
Lee [21]	44	137	31	108	100	100	100	100	94.1	97.6	88.9	98.8
De Graaf [22][a]	40	89	28	61	100	94	85	100	96	92	83	98

[a] 320-row

duit stenosis or occlusion. In clinical practice, the detection of a chronic occlusion in a patient with chest pain of sudden onset can avoid the need for percutaneous graft recanalization attempts.

In asymptomatic patients evaluated for CABG patency at least 5 years after surgery, MDCT is considered uncertain; although there is increasing evidence supporting the role of MDCT in this setting, especially given the increasing availability of new-generation scanners, in which radiation exposure has been significantly reduced. In asymptomatic patients who underwent CABG surgery less than 5 years previously, MDCT imaging is considered inappropriate (Fig. 11.2).

As reported in Table 11.2, MDCT demonstrates high accuracy in the assessment of graft occlusion

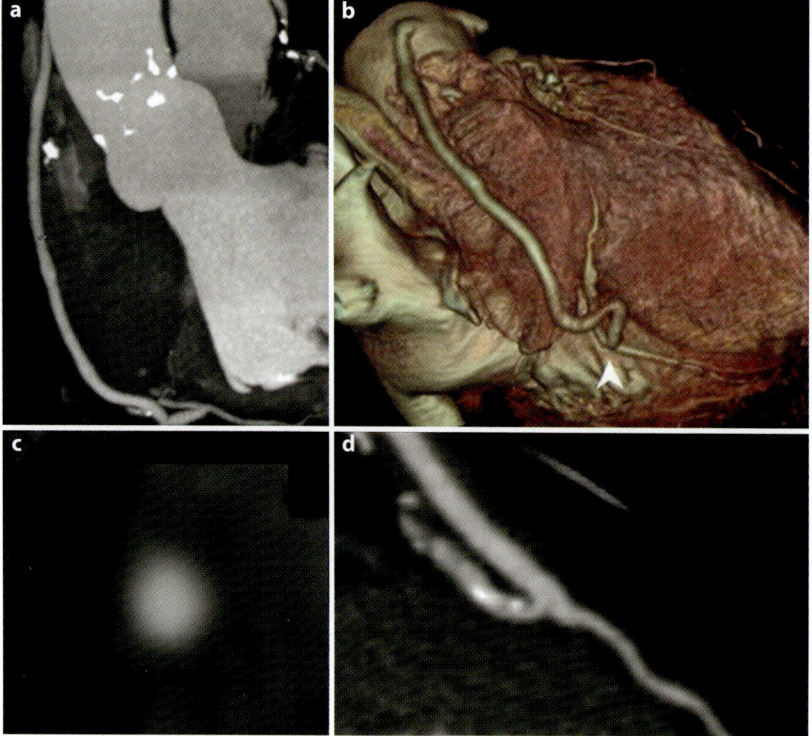

Fig. 11.3 Asymptomatic patient 5 years after the CABG intervention. **a** Right coronary artery CABG patency. **b-d** The distal anastomosis is well-depicted (*arrowhead*). **c** Lumen analysis shows no evidence of intimal hyperplasia

or stenosis [12-22]. In a recent meta-analysis [23], 64-row MDCT enabled the assessment of graft obstruction (> 50% stenosis or occlusion) with a sensitivity of 99%, a specificity of 96%, a positive predictive value of 93%, and a negative predictive value of 99% (Figs. 11.3–11.5). No significant difference was reported for 16- vs. 64-row MDCT, due to the low heart rate of CABG patients, the large size of the conduit, the relative immobility of the vessel, and the absence of calcifications. However, the 64-row scanner is able to assess a greater number of coronary artery segments [24, 25].

Chest pain in post-CABG patients may be caused by disease progression in native coronary arteries or in non-grafted or distal runoff vessels. Disease progression in non-grafted vessels was determined in up to 40% of patients examined 5–10 years post-CABG [26]. Although accurate for detecting bypass graft disease, MDCT has significant limitations in the evaluation of native arteries because of the typically severe vessel calcifications and the small diameter of post-anastomotic segments [27, 28] (Fig. 11.6). In patients with suspected disease progression, the assessment of CABG patency with MDCT should be followed by a stress test or coronary angiography.

Coronary CT analysis of unprotected coronary territories is also of prognostic value in CABG patients, adding to the overall clinical picture [29].

MDCT angiography can additionally be used as a preoperative diagnostic tool for identifying target vessels for CABG surgery and for choosing the best site for anastomosis, particularly when severely calcified vessels are observed [30]. It is also of interest in evaluating the length of the required conduit.

MDCT imaging plays an important role in redo intervention, assessing the relationship between the grafts, the aorta, the right ventricle, and the thoracic wall [31]. Post-operative changes and fibrosis can involve vascular structures in close proximity with the sternum, which, in turn, increases the risk of severe vascular injury during sternotomy (Fig. 11.7). When performed before redo surgery, MDCT can modify the surgical approach and its use is associated with shorter

11 Coronary CT Angiography: Evaluation of Coronary Artery Bypass Grafts

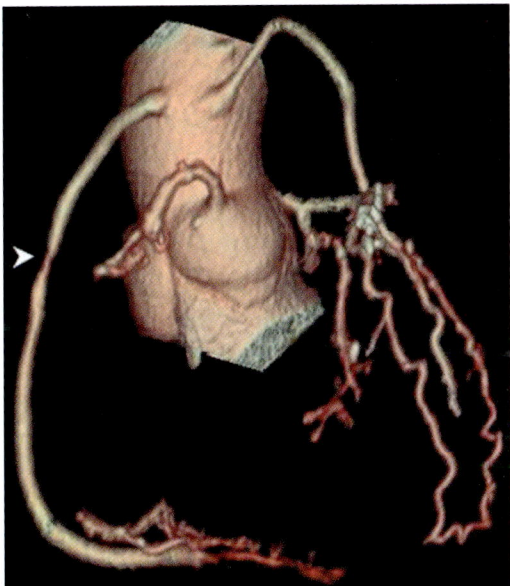

Fig. 11.4 Symptomatic patient 3 years after CABG intervention. Severe right coronary artery graft stenosis (*arrowhead*)

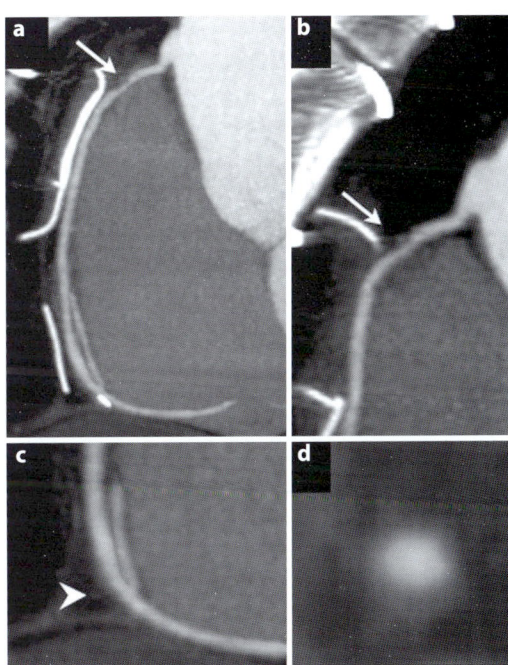

Fig. 11.5 Asymptomatic patients 7 years after CABG intervention. **a, b, d** Mild stenosis of the proximal graft segment on the RCA (*arrow*). **c** The distal anastomosis is well visualized (*arrowhead*)

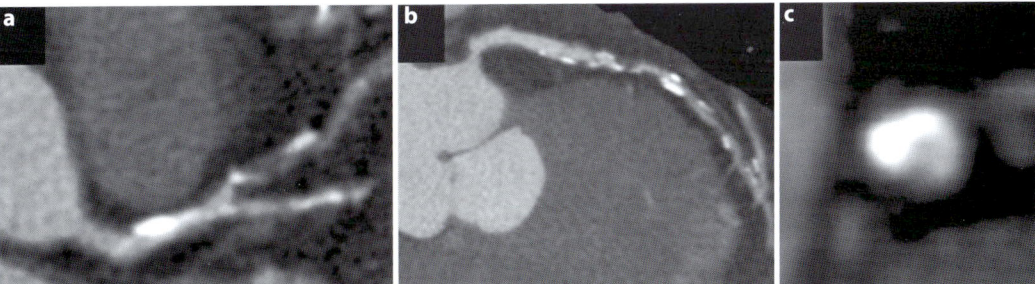

Fig. 11.6 Evaluation of the native arteries in a CABG patient. **a-c** Severe calcified stenosis on the LAD artery hampered the analysis of disease progression

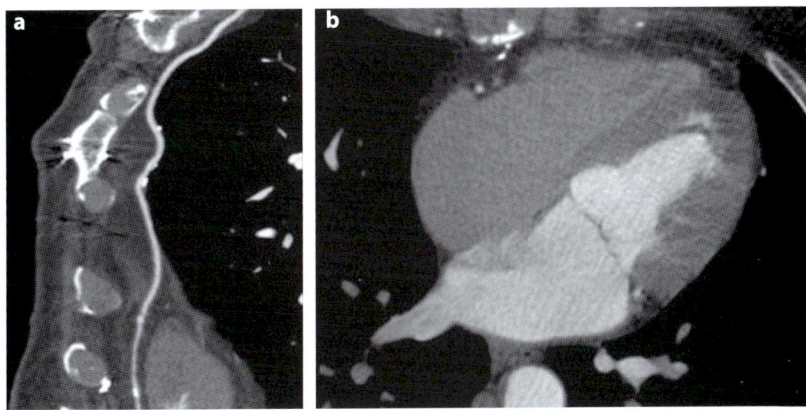

Fig. 11.7 MDCT in redo intervention planning. Close relationships between the LIMA (**a**), the right ventricle (**b**), and the sternum

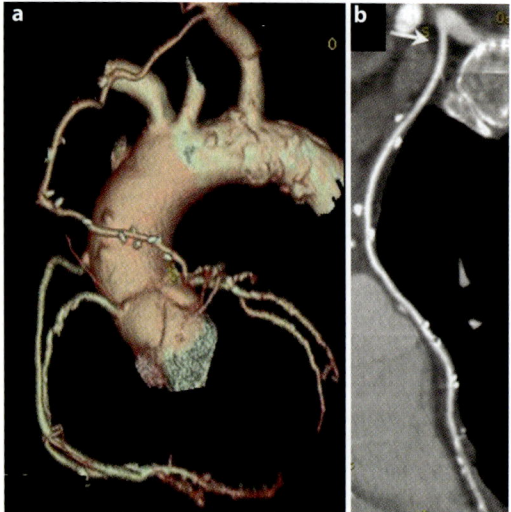

Fig. 11.8 Coronary CT in a patient with LIMA and venous CABG. **a, b** The upper limit of the examination should include the origin of the LIMA (*arrow*) to allow a complete evaluation

perfusion and cross-clamp times, shorter ICU stays, and less frequent perioperative myocardial infarct [32, 33]. The increasing acceptance of minimally invasive surgery further establishes the need for preoperative imaging assessment.

11.5 Coronary CT Acquisition Protocols for CABG

In CABG evaluation, the MDCT acquisition volume is larger than during analyses of the native coronary arteries. The upper limit of the examination in patients with an arterial graft should be the subclavian arteries, to allow complete evaluation of the origin of the mammary arteries (Fig. 11.8). In case of isolated venous graft, the acquisition should nonetheless include the entire ascending aorta and the aortic arch. In patients with an arterial bypass in which the right gastroepiploic artery was used, the imaging volume must include the upper abdomen.

In addition, if conventional MDCT systems are used for coronary CT in the context of CABG assessment, a heart rate of less than 65 beats per minute is usually recommended [34-36]. However, dual-source CT allows CABG evaluation in patients with a faster heart rate, yielding images of good quality [37-39]. In patients who have undergone revascularization, pre-medication is not usually required as beta-blocker therapy, and thus a low heart rate, is routine in this group.

For the evaluation of severely calcified native vessels or a LIMA with numerous metallic clips, a high-convolution kernel (B46f) will reduce beam-hardening artifacts [40].

Contrast material should be administered continuously through a right antecubital vein at a high injection flow rate (4–6 ml/s) followed by a saline chaser. Administration of contrast via the left arm is not recommended because the resulting high concentration in the innominate vein could hamper evaluation of the LIMA origin and cause streak artifacts. As a general rule, the volume of contrast medium for a coronary CT angiography examination is calculated as follows: volume of contrast (ml) = scan time (s) × flow (ml/s) [41].

11.6 CABG Image Analysis

For stenosis assessment, each graft can be considered as consisting of three segments: the proximal and distal anastomoses and the main body.

Radiologists should be aware of the surgical technique used and the characteristics of the bypass in order to be able to assess all relevant features. Otherwise, for example, a chronically occluded bypass can be easily missed.

Axial image analysis is important to obtain an overall visualization of graft number and patency as well as other significant characteristics, such as conduit course and relationships between the graft and adjacent structures, especially if redo surgery has been planned.

Curved multiplanar reformations (cMPR) are fundamental to assess and quantify graft stenosis. Particular attention should be paid to the vascular anastomoses, which should be accurately visualized in order to confirm graft patency (Fig. 11.9). Caution is required in case of contrast opacification of the distal target vessel without direct assessment of the graft anastomosis, as collateral-vessel reflow can be mistaken for graft patency.

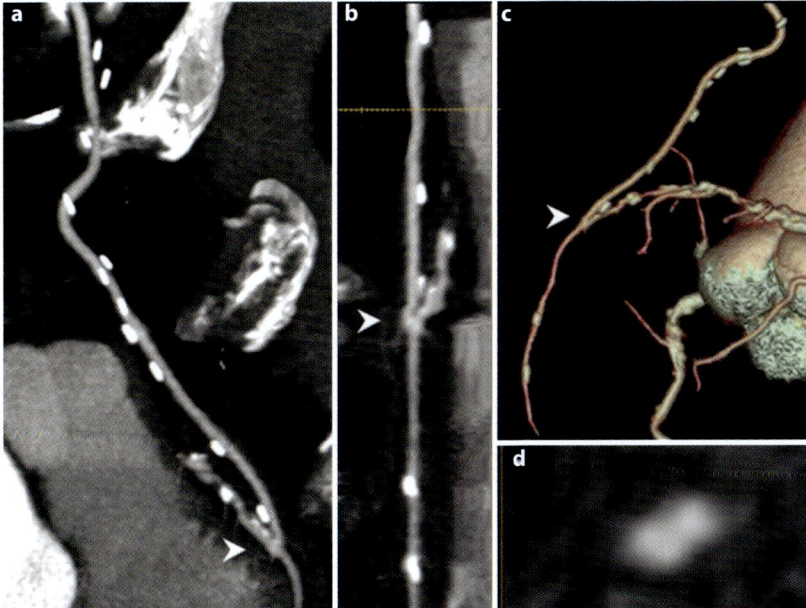

Fig. 11.9 LIMA graft on the LAD. **a-c** Distal anastomosis (*arrowheads*). **d** Anastomosis patency evaluated on a cross-sectional image

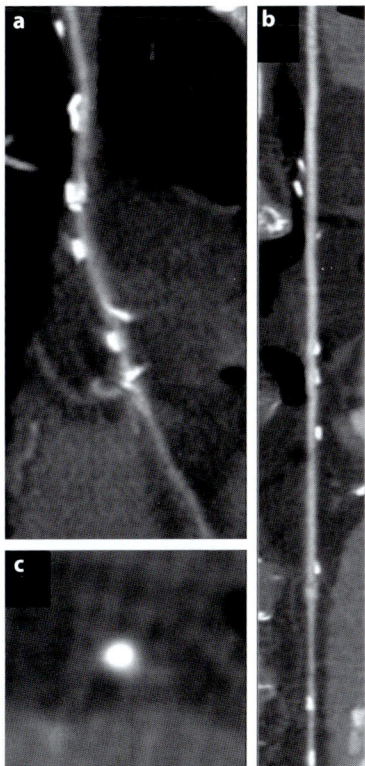

Fig. 11.10 Surgical clips on the LIMA can impair vessel analysis. **a, b** Severe metallic artifacts hamper CABG evaluation. **c** LIMA with less extensive metallic artifacts, allowing lumen visualization

Venous conduits usually are of good caliber, without the need for significant metallic clips, hence allowing their easier evaluation than arterial grafts. Surgical clips used during the harvesting of arterial vessels are normally present along the graft and may be responsible for heavy streak artifacts, which can impair vessel analysis (Fig. 11.10).

The evaluation of native arteries is challenging but essential in determinations of disease progression, especially in non-grafted vessels. Since the occlusion of side-branch vessels can explain the onset of new symptoms, the radiologist should accurately evaluate any changes compared to the previous coronary angiography or MDCT. In case of dubious findings, a stress test or coronary angiography is recommended.

In CABG patients, evaluation of the cardiac function index and cardiac volumes is particularly important in assessing the development or progression of cardiac failure. Cardiac CT allows an accurate evaluation of cardiac volumes and systolic function and in these respects is comparable with cardiac MRI [42, 43] (Figs. 11.11, 11.12). With the latest-generation CT technology, morphological and functional information can be obtained simultaneously in a "one-stop-shopping" acquisition in which myocardial perfusion is assessed during

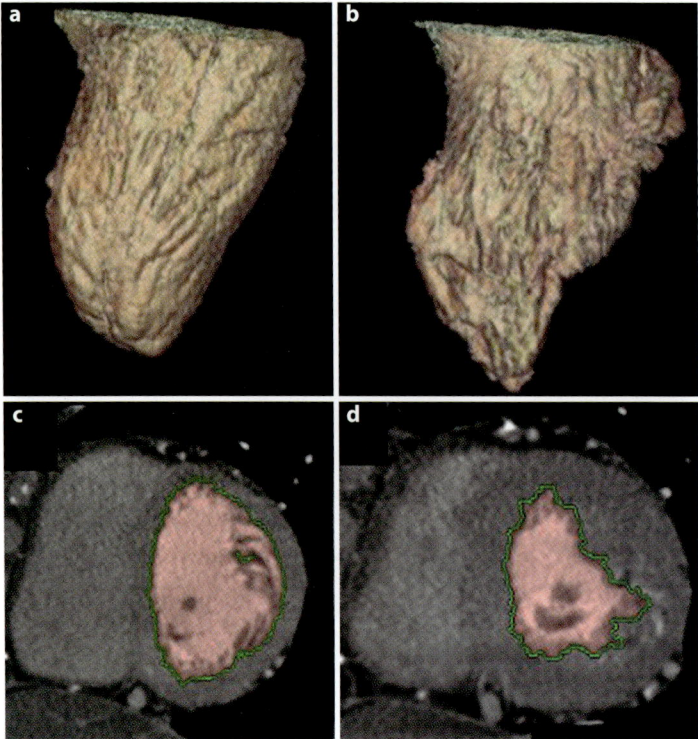

Fig. 11.11 Left ventricle function analysis. **a, c** Diastolic phase; **b, d** systolic phase

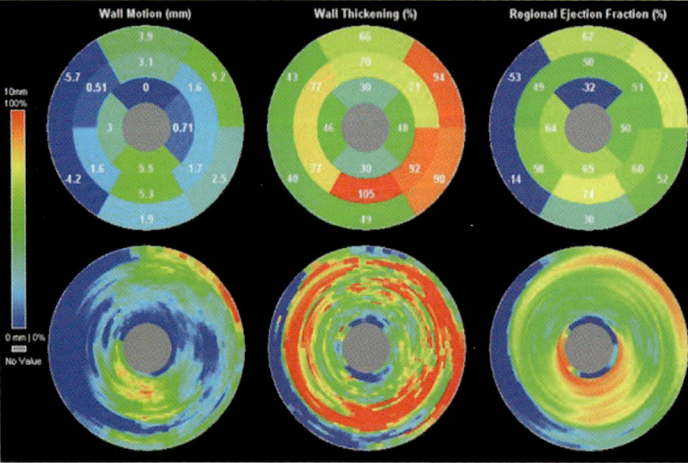

Fig. 11.12 Bulls-eye plots of wall motion, thickening, and regional ejection fraction

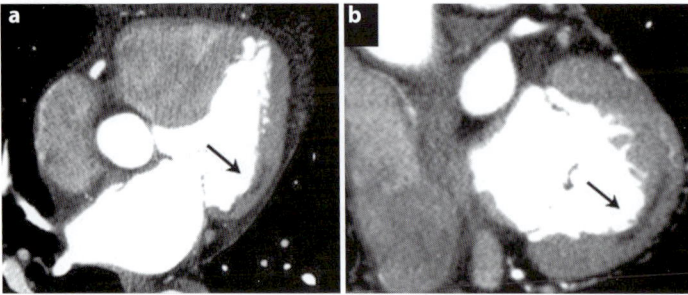

Fig. 11.13 a, b Left ventricle: chronic infarct of the basal postero-lateral wall (*arrows*)

pharmacological stress testing [44]. Areas of chronic myocardial infarction are also detectable as subendocardial hypodense streaking (Fig. 11.13).

Finally, volume-rendering images play a fundamental role in the reporting process because of their relevance for the cardiac surgeon or interventional cardiologist in choosing the best surgical approach.

References

1. DeFrances CJ, Lucas CA, Vuie VC, Golosinskiy A (2008) 2006 National Hospital Discharge Survey. Hyattsville, MD: National Center for Health Statistics
2. Epstein AJ, Polsky D, Yang F et al (2011) Coronary revascularization trends in the united state, 2001-2008. JAMA 305:1769-1776
3. Serruys PW, Morice MC, Kappetein AP et al (2009) Percutaneous coronary intervention versus coronary- artery bypass grafting for severe coronary artery disease. N Engl J Med 360(10):961-972
4. Patel MR, Dehmer GJ, Hirshfeld JW et al (2009) ACCF/SCAI/STS/AATS/AHA/ASNC 2009 Appropriateness Criteria for Coronary Revascularization J Am Coll Cardiol 53:530-553
5. Hannan EL, Racz MJ, Walford G et al (2005) Long-term outcomes of coronary-artery bypass grafting versus stent implantation. N Engl J Med 352:2174-2183
6. Myers WO, Blackstone EH, Davis K et al (1999) CASS Registry long-term surgical survival. Coronary artery surgery study. J Am Coll Cardiol 33:488-498
7. Goldman S, Zadina K, Moritz T et al (2004) Long-term patency of saphenous vein and left internal mammary artery grafts after coronary artery by-pass surgery: results from a Department of Veterans Affairs Cooperative Study. J Am Coll Cardiol 44:2149-2156
8. Jones CM, Chin KY, Yang GZ et al. Coronary artery bypass graft imaging with 64-slice multislice computed tomography: literature review. Semin Ultrasound CT MRI 2008;29:204-213
9. Marano R, Liguori C, Rinaldi P et al (2007) Coronary artery bypass grats and MDCT imaging: what to know and what to look for. Eur Radiol 17:3166-3178
10. Calafiore AM, Di Giammarco G, Teodori G et al (1996) Left anterior descending coronary artery grafting via left anterior small thoracotomy without cardiopulmonary bypass. Ann Thorac Surg 61:1658-1663
11. Taylor AJ, Cerqueira M, Hodgson JM et al (2010) ACCF/SCCT/ACR/AHA/ASE/ASNC/ NASCI/SCAI/SCMR 2010 Appropriate Use Criteria for Cardiac Computed Tomography. J Am Coll Cardiol 56:1864-1894
12. Malagutti P, Nieman K, Meijboom WB et al (2007) Use of 64-slice CT in symptomatic patients after coronary bypass surgery: evaluation of grafts and coronary arteries. Eur Heart J 28:1879-1885
13. Pache G, Saueressig U, Frydrychowicz A et al (2006) Initial experience with 64-slice cardiac CT: non-invasive visualization of coronary artery bypass grafts. Eur Heart J 27:976-980
14. Ropers D, Pohle FK, Kuettner A et al (2006) Diagnostic accuracy of noninvasive coronary angiography in patients after bypass surgery using 64-slice spiral computed tomography with 330-ms gantry rotation. Circulation 114:2334-2341
15. Dikkers R, Willems TP, Tio RA et al (2006) The benefit of 64-MDCT prior to invasive coronary angiography in symptomatic post-CABG patients. Int J Cardiovasc Imaging 23:369-377
16. Jabara R, Chronos N, Klein L et al (2007) Comparison of multidetector 64-slice computed tomographic angiography to coronary angiography to assess the patency of coronary artery bypass grafts. Am J Cardiol 99:1529-1534
17. Feuchtner GM, Schachner T, Bonatti J, Friedrich GJ et al (2007) Diagnostic performance of 64-slice computed tomography in evaluation of coronary artery bypass grafts. Am J Roentgenol 189:574-580
18. Meyer TS, Martinoff S, Hadamitzky M et al (2007) Improved non-invasive assessment of coronary artery bypass grafts with 64-slice computed tomographic angiography in an unselected patient population. J Am Coll Cardiol 49:946-950
19. Nazeri I, Shahabi P, Tehrai M, Sharif-Kashani et al (2009) Assessment of patients after coronary artery bypass grafting using 64-slice computed tomography. Am J Cardiol 103:667-673
20. Weustink AC, Nieman K, Pugliese F, Mollet NR et al (2009) Diagnostic accuracy of computed tomography angiography in patients after bypass grafting. JACC Cardiovasc Imaging 2:816-24
21. Lee JH, Chun EJ, Choi SI et al (2011) Prospective versus retrospective ECG-gated 64-detector coronary CT angiography for evaluation of coronary artery bypass graft patency: comparison of image quality, radiation dose and diagnostic accuracy. Int J Cardiovasc Imaging 27:657-667

22. de Graaf FR, van Velzen JE, Witkowska AJ, Schuijf JD et al (2011) Diagnostic performance of 320-slice multidetector computed tomography coronary angiography in patients after coronary artery bypass grafting. Eur Radiol 21:2285-2296
23. Mowatt G, Cummins E, Waugh N, Walker S et al (2008) Systematic review of the clinical effectiveness and cost-effectiveness of 64-slice or higher computed tomography angiography as an alternative to invasive coronary angiography in the investigation of coronary artery disease. Health Technology Assessment 17
24. Hamon M, Lepage O, Malagutti P, Riddel J et al (2008) Diagnostic Performance of 16- and 64-Section Spiral CT for Coronary Artery Bypass Graft Assessment: Meta-Analysis. Radiology 247:679-686
25. Khan R, Rawal S, Eisenberg MJ (2009) Transitioning from 16-slice multidetector computed tomography for the assessment of coronary artery disease: are we really making progress? Can J Cardiol 9:533-542
26. Dunlay SM, Rihal CS, Sundt TM et al (2009) Current trends in coronary revascularization. Curr Treat Options Cardiovasc Med 11:61-70
27. Türkvatan A, Biyikoglu, Büyükbayraktar FG, Cumhur T et al (2009) Noninvasive evaluation of coronary artery bypass graft and native coronary arteries: is 16-slice multidetector CT useful? Diagn Interv Radiol 15:43-50
28. Andreini D, Pontone G, Ballerini G, Bertella E et al (2007) Bypass graft and native postanastomotic coronary artery patency: assessment with computed tomography. Ann Thorac Surg 83:1672-1678
29. Chow BJW, Ahmed O, Small G et al (2011) Prognostic value of CT angiography in coronary bypass patients. JACC Cardiovasc Imaging 5:496-502
30. Bedi HS, Gill JAS, Bakshi SS (2008) Can we perform coronary artery bypass grafting on the basis of computed tomography angiography alone? A comparison with conventional coronary angiography. Eur J Cardiothorac Surg 33:633-638
31. Maluenda G, Goldstein MA, Lemesle G, Weissman G et al (2010) Perioperative outcomes in reoperative cardiac surgery guided by cardiac multidetector computed tomography angiography. Am Heart J 159:301-306
32. Gasparovic H, Rybicki FJ, Millstine J et al (2005) Three-dimensional computed tomography imaging in planning the surgical approach for redo cardiac surgery after coronary revascularization. Eur J Cardiothorac Surg 28:244-249
33. Kamdar AR, Meadows TA, Rosselli EE et al (2008) Multidetector computed tomography angiography in planning of reoperative cardiothoracic surgery. Ann Thorac Surg 85:1239-1245
34. Leschka S, Alkadhi H, Plass A et al (2006) Accuracy of MSCT coronary angiography with 64-slice technology: first experience. Eur Heart J 26:1482-1487
35. Wintersperger BJ, Nikolaou K, von Ziegler F et al (2006) Image quality, motion artifacts, and reconstruction timing of 64-slice coronary computed tomography angiography with 0.33-second rotation speed. Invest Radiol 41:436-442
36. Leschka S, Wildermuth S, Boehm T et al (2006) Noninvasive coronary angiography with 64-section CT: effect of average heart rate and heart rate variability on image quality. Radiology 241:378-385
37. Achenbach S, Ropers D, Kuettner A et al (2006) Contrast-enhanced coronary artery visualization by dual-source computed tomography-initial experience. Eur J Radiol 57:331-335
38. Bastarrika G, De Cecco CN, Arraiza M et al (2008) Dual-source CT for visualization of the coronary arteries in heart transplant patients with high heart rates. Am J Roentgenol 191:448-454
39. Scheffel H, Alkadhi H, Plass A et al (2006) Accuracy of dual-source CT coronary angiography: First experience in a high pre-test probability population without heart rate control. Eur Radiol 16:2739-2747
40. Seifarth H, Raupach R, Schaller S et al (2005) Assessment of coronary artery stents using 16-slice MDCT angiography: evaluation of a dedicated reconstruction kernel and a noise reduction filter. Eur Radiol 15:721-726
41. Schoepf UJ, Zwerner PL, Savino G et al (2007) Coronary CT angiography. Radiology 244:48-63
42. Busch S, Johnson TR, Wintersperger BJ et al (2008) Quantitative assessment of left ventricular function with dual-source CT in comparison to cardiac magnetic resonance imaging: initial findings. Eur Radiol 18:570-575
43. Thilo C, Hanley M, Bastarrika G et al (2010) Integrative computed tomographic imaging of cardiac structure, function, perfusion, and viability. Cardiol Rev 18:219-229
44. Bastarrika G, Ramos-Duran L, Rosenblum MA et al (2010) Adenosine-stress dynamic myocardial CT perfusion imaging: initial clinical experience. Invest Radiol 45:306-313

Coronary Stents

12

Enrica Mariano, Giuseppe M. Sangiorgi
and Massimo Fioranelli

12.1 Introduction

Coronary stent technology is a crucial part of most interventional procedures for percutaneous revascularization. Previously, vessel-wall injury and plaque fracture were the usual sequelae in response to the mechanical effect of balloon angioplasty. Nowadays, a sophisticated engineering tool serves not only as a scaffolding platform but also as an advanced vector for local antiproliferative drug delivery to the arterial wall. The wide acceptance of coronary stenting is based on the results of pioneering trials such as the BENESTENT and STRESS trials, which showed the superiority of stenting over balloon angioplasty in terms of a reduction in angiographic re-stenosis and the need for repeated intervention. Since then, the growing use of stents in ever more complex lesions and patients has stimulated the introduction of a rapidly increasing number of different stent designs. These have been proposed in order to address physiological concerns; indeed, a primary aim of stent development is to reduce device profiles and increase flexibility, thus facilitating safe delivery of the stent.

Percutaneous coronary stent implantation frequently results in significant three-dimensional changes in the geometry of native coronary arteries. These changes may increase the risk of in-stent re-stenosis due to altered vessel-wall compliance and subsequent alterations in shear stress. Additionally, the implantation of a stiff stent within the coronary arteries may result in flexion or hinge points due to the abrupt changes in vessel-wall rigidity at the ends of the stent. These hinge points have been associated with increased rates of re-stenosis and may increase the risk of edge dissection and the need for additional stent implantation. Other significant issues are lesion coverage, to avoid plaque prolapse, and radial support, to prevent elastic recoil of the artery. Furthermore, the ability to easily access arterial side branches through the struts of a deployed stent in bifurcation lesions has progressively gained importance. Finally, radiological visibility during angiography is another crucial element in optimizing the clinical benefits of a stent, especially during placement, while the attenuation index must be considered if, for example, a computed tomography study will be obtained in the follow-up after the procedure.

This chapter summarizes the components of stent design that are important in terms of both the biological response of the arterial wall and clinical outcome. In addition, new stent platforms, mainly represented by the biodegradable stent, are reviewed since they are expected to provide a more "physiological" answer to stent implantation, reducing vascular injury and accelerating vessel healing with consequent improvement in clinical outcome.

12.1.1 Types of Stents

In clinical practice, the international cardiologist must decide which stent is most appropriate for the patient and, even more importantly, for the lesion to be treated. Although the "ideal" stent, i.e., one

E. Mariano (✉)
Interventional Cardiology Unit
"Tor Vergata" University, Rome, Italy
e-mail: enrica_mariano@hotmail.com

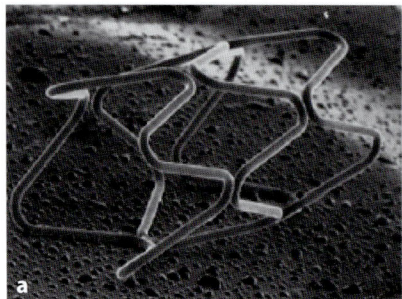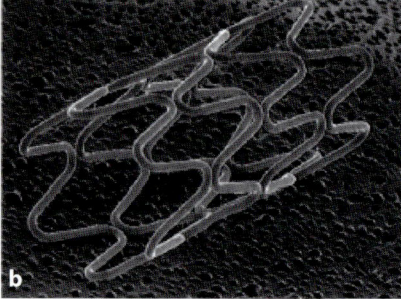

Fig. 12.1 Scanning electron micrographs showing stents of **a** 8-strut and **b** 12-strut design after balloon expansion

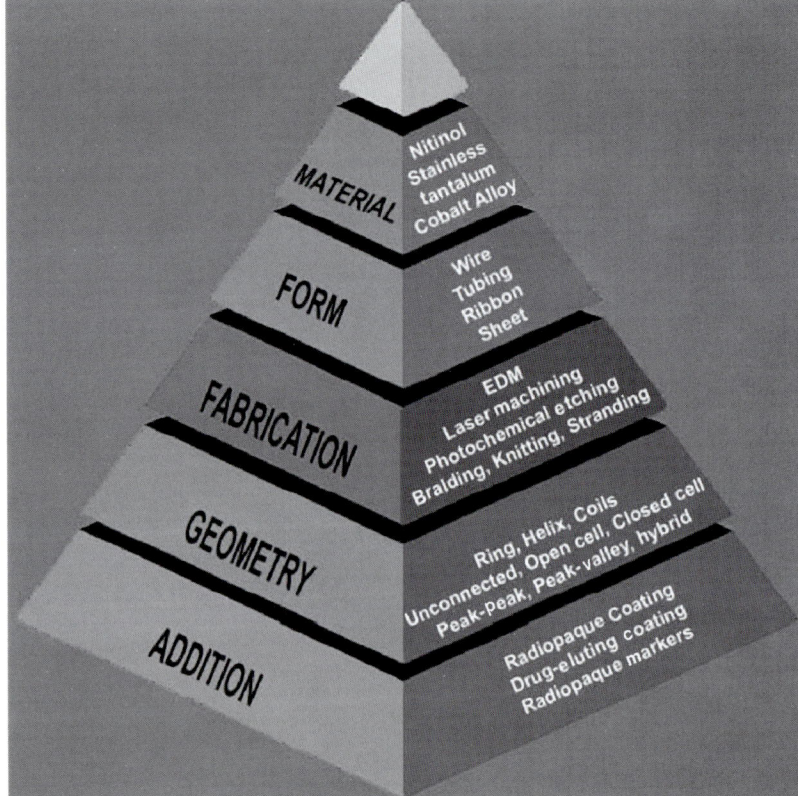

Fig. 12.2 Stent-design pyramid showing the different materials and construction characteristics

that is tailor-made to treat a given lesion or a particular subset of patients, does not exist, the general characteristics of the "perfect" stent can be summarize as follows:
- Flexible
- Trackable
- Low unconstrained profile
- Radio-opaque
- Thromboresistant
- Biocompatible
- Reliably expandable
- High radial strength
- Circumferential coverage
- Low surface area
- Hydrodynamic compatibility.

In general, stents can be classified according to several engineering variables that influence the characteristics and biocompatibility of the stent as well as patient outcome (Figs. 12.1, 12.2). These variables are:

- Mechanism of expansion (self-expanding or balloon-expandable)
- Materials (stainless steel, cobalt-based alloy, tantalum, nitinol, inert coating, active coating, or biodegradable)
- Forms (sheet, wire, or tube)
- Manufacturing methods (laser-cut, water-jet cutting, photo-etching, etc.)
- Geometrical configurations/design (mesh structure, coil, slotted tube, ring, multi-design, or custom design)
- Additions (grafts, radio-opaque markers, coatings, etc.).

12.1.2 Mechanism of Stent Expansion

Balloon-expandable stents are made from materials that can be plastically deformed through the inflation of a balloon; after the balloon is deflated, the stent remains in its expanded shape, except for a slight recoil caused by the elastic portion of the deformation. Self-expanding stents, by contrast, are manufactured in the expanded shape, then compressed and constrained in a delivery system. Upon their release from the delivery system they spring back, i.e., self-expand, to the pre-set diameter. Indeed, this characteristic of a self-expandable stent can be used when metallic struts are needed to cover a soft plaque, in which case a larger stent can be chosen that will not fully expand in the vessel but will remain compacted among the different cells, producing greater lesion coverage.

12.2 Materials

Materials for metallic balloon-expandable or self-expanding stents must exhibit excellent corrosion resistance and biocompatibility (Table 12.1); they should be adequately radio-opaque and create minimal artifacts during MRI. For balloon-expandable stents, the ideal material for construction should have a low yield stress (to make it deformable at manageable balloon pressures), a high elastic modulus (for minimal recoil), and be work hardened through expansion, and therefore of high strength. The most widely used material for balloon-expandable stents is stainless steel, typically 316L, a particularly easily deformable material of low carbon content and additions of molybdenum and niobium. Alternative materials for balloon-expandable stents are tantalum, platinum alloys, niobium alloys, and cobalt alloys. Their advantages are better radio-opacity, higher strength, improved corrosion resistance, and better MRI compatibility.

For self-expanding stents, the ideal material should have a low elastic modulus and a high yield stress for large elastic strains. Currently, the most widely used material is nitinol, a nickel-titanium alloy that can recover from an elastic deformation of up to 10%. This unusually wide elastic range, commonly known as super-elasticity, is the result of a thermo-elastic martensitic transformation.

12.2.1 Raw Material

Stents can be made from sheet, wire (round or flat), or tubing. The latter two account for a large majority of balloon-expandable and self-expanding stents. Stents made from sheet metal have to be rolled into a tubular configuration after the pattern has been created.

12.3 Fabrication Methods

The choice of fabrication method depends mainly on the form of the selected raw material. Wires can be formed into stents in various ways using conventional wire-forming techniques, such as coiling, braiding, or knitting. The simplest shape for a wire stent is a coil. All coil stents marketed today are balloon-expandable. The wire-mesh stent (such as the self-expanding Wallstent, Boston Scientific, Natick MA) and the coil stent (such as the older Gianturco-Roubin Flex/GR-II, Cook, Bloomington IN; and the Wiktor, Medtronic, Minneapolis MN) have been shown to have a high propensity for thrombosis and re-stenosis and are thus no longer used by cardiologists for coronary interventions.

The vast majority of coronary stents, and probably the majority of peripheral vascular stents, are produced by laser cutting from tubing, typically, Nd:YAG lasers. Balloon-expandable stents are cut

Table 12.1 Overview of the materials used in the manufacture of balloon-expandable and self-expandable stents, the different stent forms, stent fabrication, stent geometry, and stent additions

Materials	Balloon-expandable stents	Stainless steel 316L (vast majority) Tantalum Martensitic nitinol Platinum iridium Polymers Niobium alloy Cobalt alloy	
	Self-expanding stents	Super-elastic Nickel-titanium Nitinol (majority) Cobalt alloy) Full hard (stainless steel)	
Form	Wire	Wallstent (cobalt alloy) Bridge, S7, S660, (stainless steel, welded rings) Angiostent (platinum iridium) Strecker (tantalum) Expander (nitinol)	
	Tube	(Vast majority)	
	Sheet	NIR (stainless steel) ZR1 (stainless steel) GRII (stainless steel) Endotex (nitinol)	
	Ribbon	Horizon Prostatic (nitinol) EndoCoil, Esophacoil (nitinol)	
Fabrication	Laser-cutting Photochemical etching	(Vast majority) NIR Nitinol sheet Coiled nitinol framework, ePTFE covering	
	Brading	Wallstent (cobalt alloy)	
	Knitting	Streaker (tantalum)	
	Vapor deposition		
	Water jet	SCS, SCS-Z stent	
Stent geometry Slotted tube/coil	Helical spiral	Periodic peak-to-peak connections No/minimal connections Axial spine Integral with graft	
	Woven	Braided Knitted	
	Individual rings		
	Sequential rings	Open cells	Peak-to-peak connections Peak-to-valley connections Midstruts connections Hybrids Other
		Closed cells	Regular peak-to-peak connection Non-flex connector Flex connector Combined connector Hybrid
		Coil	
Additions	Covering	WallGraft; coiled nitinol framework, ePTFE covering	
	Radio-opaque markers	Tabs (tantalum end, gold end, platinum within strut) Sleeve (gold, platinum) Welded (tantalum)	
	Radio-opaque coating	Gold, silicone carbide over gold	
	Biocompatibility coatings	Tantal7m coating, phosphorylcholine, carbon coating, silicone carbide	
	Drug-eluting coating	Rapamycin, paclitaxel	

12 Coronary Stents

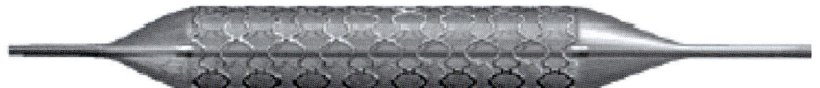

Fig. 12.3 The Skylor is a balloon-expandable cobalt-chromium stent characterized by a closed cell and thin struts pre-mounted on a rapid-exchange-type balloon catheter

in a crimped or near-crimped condition and only require post-cutting deburring and surface treatment, typically electropolishing.

Self-expanding nitinol stents can be cut either in the "small" configuration, requiring post-cutting expansion and shape-setting, or in the expanded condition. In either case, these stents have to be deburred and polished. A cutting method that does not produce a heat-affected zone is water-jet cutting, in which a focused jet of water and an abrasive additive are used instead of a laser beam to cut the pattern. Another interesting manufacturing method is photochemical etching.

12.3.1 Geometry

Early designs were generally classified as either slotted-tube geometries, such as the Palmaz stents, or coil geometries, such as the Gianturco-Roubin Flex stent. While the former had excellent radial strength, they lacked flexibility. The opposite was the case for coil designs. The subsequent evolution of stent design led to the development of a rich variety of stent geometries. These can be classified into five main categories: coil, helical spiral, woven, individual rings, and sequential rings.

12.3.2 Closed Cell

In sequential ring construction, all internal inflection points of the structural members are connected by bridging elements. This condition is typically only possible with regular peak-to-peak connections (Fig. 12.3). The primary advantages of closed-cell designs are optimal scaffolding and a uniform surface, regardless of the degree of bending. However, these advantages result in a structure that is typically less flexible than that conferred by a similar open-cell design.

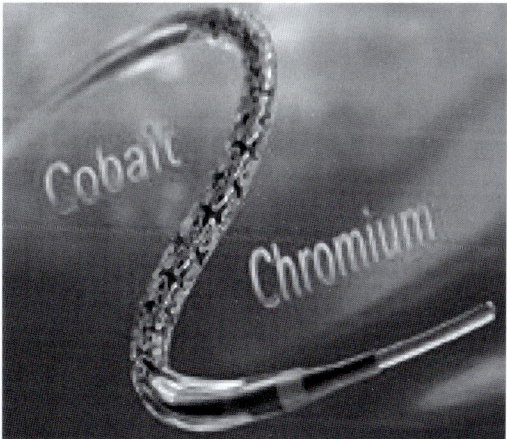

Fig. 12.4 Coroflex Blue™, with its open-cell design, represents a new-generation cobalt-chromium stent endowed with characteristics of high flexibility and thin struts (65 μm)

12.3.3 Open Cell

In this type of construction, some or all the internal inflection points of the structural members are not connected by bridging elements. The unconnected structural elements contribute to the longitudinal flexibility of the stent (Fig. 12.4). Periodically connected peak-to-peak designs are common among self-expanding stents, such as the SMART stent, and in balloon-expandable stents, such as the AVE S7.

12.3.4 Coatings

Several active compounds have been used to cover stents in order to increase their biocompatibility, thereby enhancing their safety and effectiveness. Among the different compounds tested, heparin was one of the first, based on its ability to reduce the coagulation cascade (and thus possibly the thrombogenic risk) following its release after stent deployment. Other coatings, such as phosphorylcholine and silicon carbide, have been used in order to reduce platelet activation and interaction, with the goal of limiting platelet adhesion to the struts of the stent during the acute phase of stent re-endothelialization.

Passive coverage also has been shown to be useful. Indeed, covered stents have been created in which a polytetrafluoroethylene (PTFE) layer was placed between two stents (Jostent graft, Jomed) or one stent was covered by an inner and an outer layer of PTFE (Symbiot, Boston Scientific). These devices have been assessed in the treatment of degenerated saphenous vein grafts containing a considerable amount of friable atherothrombotic material. Other useful indications for PTFE-covered stents are coronary aneurysm exclusion and coronary perforation. The MGuard coronary stent (Inspire-MD, Tel-Aviv, Israel) is designed to protect against a post-procedural embolic shower. This device presents a novel combination of a coronary stent and an embolic protection device. To date, the MGuard coronary stent has shown safety in human coronary and vein-graft indications.

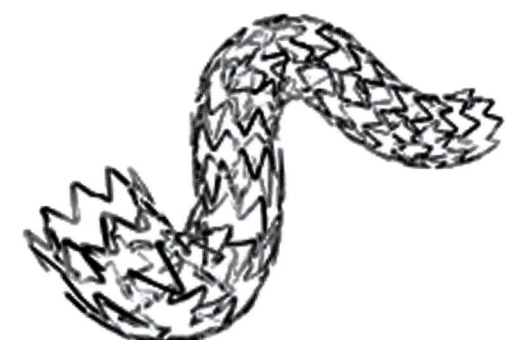

Fig. 12.5 The Taxus (paclitaxel-eluting) stent (Boston Scientific, Natick, MA)

12.4 Additions

12.4.1 Radio-opacity Enhancements

To improve the X-ray visibility of stents made from stainless steel or nitinol, gold, platinum, or tantalum markers are added to the stent struts. Electroplating (with gold) is another option.

12.4.2 Drugs

The combination of highly refined metallic-stent designs and polymer materials has been the standard approach in several drug-eluting stent (DES) initiatives. Stent-based drug delivery has been accomplished by three distinct mechanisms:
- Bio-absorbable polymeric stents can be loaded with a drug that is eluted slowly over time.
- Metal stents can have a drug either bound to their surfaces or embedded within macroscopic fenestrations or microscopic nanopores, thus providing more rapid drug delivery.
- Metal stents coated with an outer layer of polymer (bio-absorbable or non-bio-absorbable) can be drug-loaded, thus providing more controlled and sustained drug delivery and, consequently, more effective drug-tissue interactions.

In DESs in which the drugs have wide toxic-to-therapeutic ratios, such as those loaded with members of the sirolimus family (e.g., the sirolimus-eluting Cypher stent; Cordis, Johnson & Johnson, Miami Lakes, FL), the regularity of strut spacing might be less important and adequate drug doses can be applied to the stent surface so that, despite broad variability in the delivery location, an adequate dose is uniformly released.

For DESs containing drugs with narrower toxic-to-therapeutic ratios (e.g., the paclitaxel-eluting Taxus; Boston Scientific) (Fig. 12.5), inadequate dosing may occur at sites where the stent struts lie far apart, resulting in over-therapeutic or toxic dosing at sites where the struts bunch together, due to vessel curvature or asymmetric expansion. While the Cypher stent has a closed-cell-design, the tandem architecture of the Taxus stent features neither a closed- nor an open-cell design; instead, there are intervals with a shorter or longer axis to increase radial force. Both stents have inert and non-erodible polymeric coatings. The Endeavor stent (Medtronic, Minneapolis, MN) uses the non-erodible polymer phosphorylcholine to release the sirolimus analogue ABT-578; it is the first DES in which a non-stainless-steel alloy serves as the foundation for a polymer-coated DES, i.e., the thin-strut cobalt-

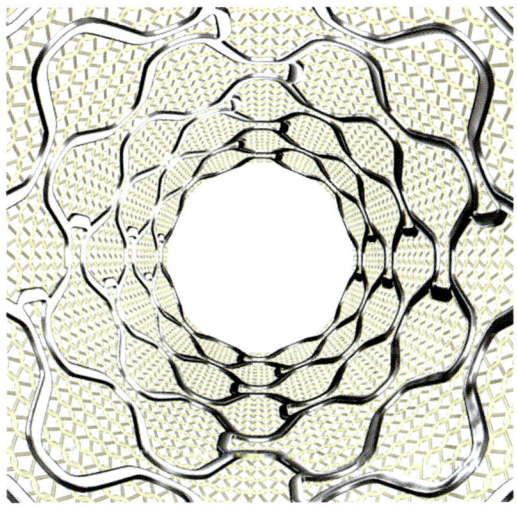

Fig. 12.6 A 3D view of the MGuard coronary stent (Inspire-MD, Tel-Aviv, Israel). Its ultra-thin PET sleeve is designed to provide embolic-shower protection during and after the procedure

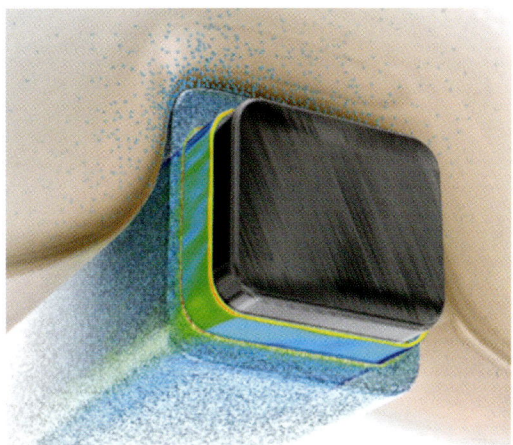

Fig. 12.7 Illustration of a hybrid design of the stent, showing a close-up of a stent strut implanted in a vessel. The strut is represented by the metallic object in the center. Here, the PROBIO passive coating is the very thin layer surrounding the surface of the stent, shown in blue, green, and gold. On top of the passive coating is the BIOlute active coating, shown as a translucent outer coating, that elutes drug and is absorbed over time

chromium alloy (Driver). The platform of the Xience V stent is a L-605 cobalt chromium (CoCr) balloon-expandable stent that is remarkably similar to its successful bare metal stent (BMS) equivalent, the Multi-Link Vision (Abbott Laboratories), whose main characteristics are low strut thickness, high flexibility and deliverability, an acceptable degree of compliance, recoil, and risk of plaque prolapse, and overall good radio-opacity. Everolimus (Certican, Novartis, Basel, Switzerland) is a sirolimus analogue and it has a useful role in the prevention of allograft rejection after organ transplantation. With its potent suppression of reactive neointimal ingrowth, this drug has been shown to significantly reduce neointimal proliferation. Specifically, 3-year data from the SPIRIT I, II, and III trials demonstrated no significant increase in major adverse cardiac events or late stent thrombosis in patients treated with the everolimus-eluting stent Xience V.

The Platinum trial compared the Promus with the Promus Element stent (stent platform Element, Boston Scientific, and the drug everolimus) while the Taxus Perseus trial evaluated the TAXUS Element (stent platform Element and the drug paclitaxel). In the Taxus Element, the polymer is SIBS (polymer translute) while in the Promus Element it is a fluorine copolymer (PVDF-HFP). The delivery system of the Element stent (Fig. 12.6) and its platinum-chromium steel composition improve the deliverability, flexibility, and radial force of the device, reducing elastic recoil and offering the thinnest strut profile among the various DESs (Fig. 12.13).

Recently, a new DES stent has been introduced into clinical practice. The ORSIRO (Biotronik) represents a unique solution for the treatment of de novo coronary stenosis (Figs. 12.7–12.10), with its combination of active and passive components. The passive component consists of the covered stent struts, which avoid contact between stent and tissue. The active component is a matrix of bioabsorbable polymer and the drug sirolimus. The Pro Kinetic Energy platform (strut thickness 60 μm) provides optimal deliverability for this hybrid device. The BIOlute polymer consists of polylactic acid (PLLA), a biodegradable polymer (with CO_2 and H_2O as the degradation products) used in many clinical applications and chosen for this device because of its high biocompatibility and controlled drug release. Clinical data on the safety and feasibility of the ORSIRO stent have been obtained from clinical studies such as the BIOFLOW-1, a first-in-humans (n=30 patients), prospective, multicentric single-arm study carried out for Certification Experts

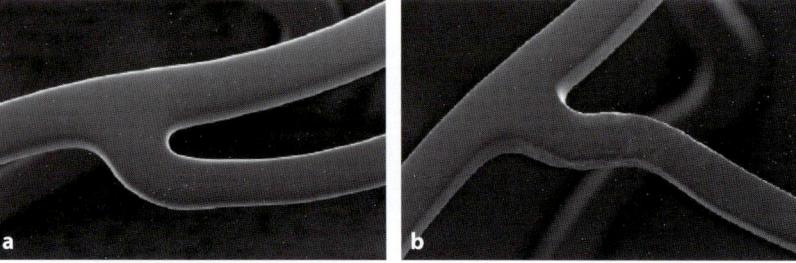

Fig. 12.8 a, b Non-dilated stent sections are covered by a uniform non-crystalline coating associated with a non-covalent mode to stent surface

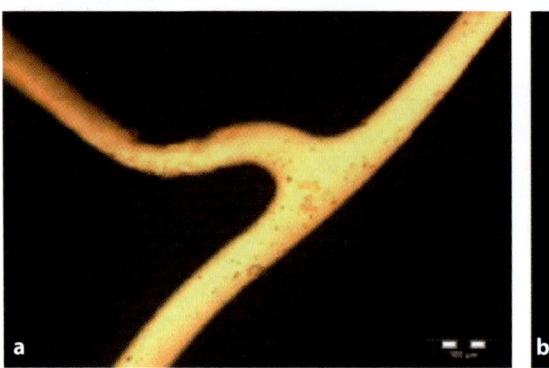
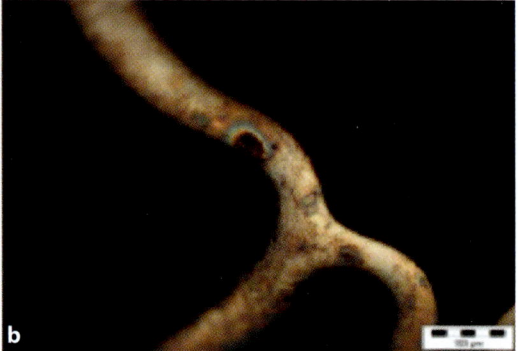

Fig. 12.9 a, b The ORSIRO stent reduces the incidence of allergic reactions to metal ions by the tissues. According to the literature, 10–12% of women and 6% of men suffer adverse reactions to nickel. The PROBIO coating avoids contact between electrolytes and struts of the stent, thus reducing the inflammatory response (**a**). Sirolimus is eluted over a period of 12–14 weeks, with a drug dosage of 1.4 µg/mm^2 of stent struts, with release kinetics similar to those of Cypher and Resolute. **b** ML-VISION without coating

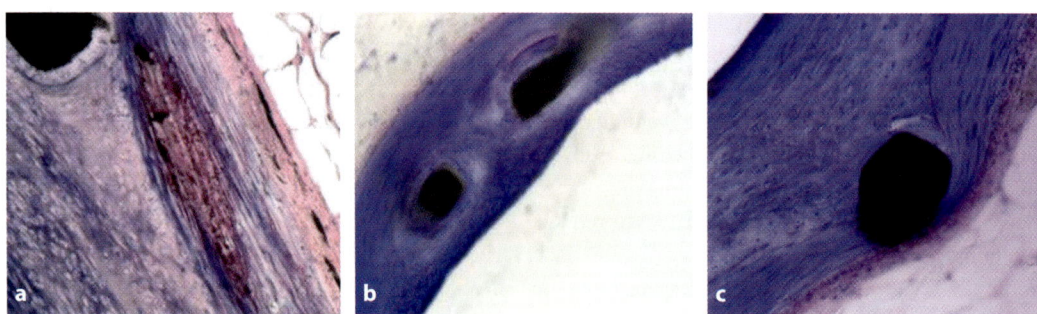

Fig. 12.10 The polymer coating as seen on histology at 12 months (**a**). Note that at 24 (**b**) and 36 months (**c**) the PLLA is completely degraded

(CE) approval; BIOFLOW INDIA (n=100 patients), a pivotal study for ORSIRO approval in India; BIOFLOW-2 a prospective, multicentric, randomized trial (n=400 patients) that concluded non-inferiority of ORSIRO vs. Xience V; and BIOFLOW-3 (n=1500 patients) a prospective multicentric study that evaluated the absence of major adverse cardiac events (MACE), post-marketing surveillance, and the long-term outcome of patients treated with ORSIRO stent implantation.

Another polymer-free DES recently introduced into clinical practice is the CRE8, an exclusive technology of the manufacturer (CID SpA) that couples abluminal reservoir technology, which allows controlled and directed drug

Fig. 12.11 CRE8: distinctive features

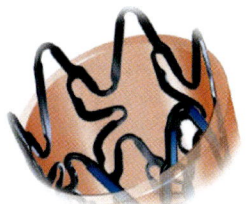
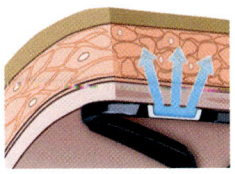
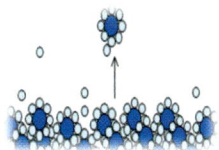
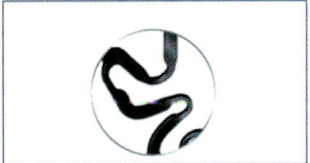

Fig. 12.12 NEXT study. The aim was to demonstrate non-inferiority in late lumen loss of the CRE8 vs. the Taxus and Liberté stents

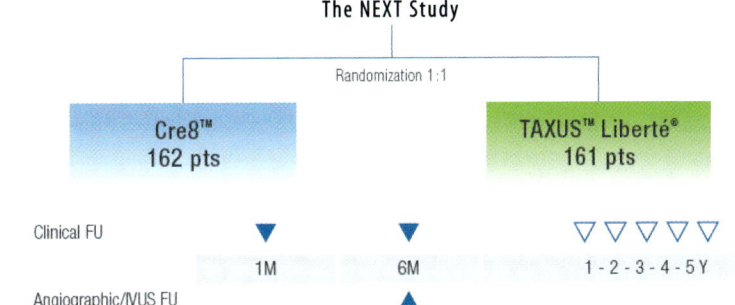
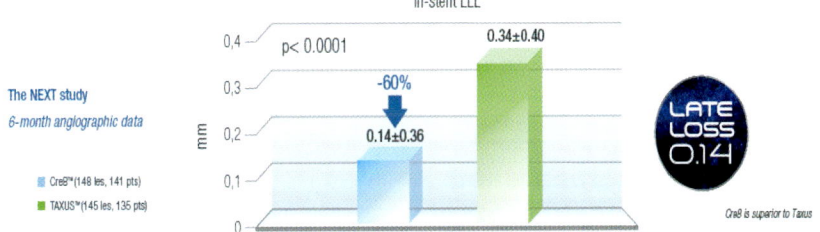

elution, with an amphilimus formulation (formulated sirolimus with an organic acid), which results in improved homogeneous drug distribution, and a bioinducer surface that helps to accelerate endothelialization and strut coverage (Fig. 12.11). Six-month angiographic data from the NEXT study showed that for the CRE8, the in-stent late lumen loss was 0.14 ± 0.36 whereas it was 0.34 ± 0.40 for the Taxus stent ($p < 0.0001$) (Fig. 12.12). With Avantgarde, the bioinducer surface I carbofilm showed optimal results in terms of endothelialization and strut coverage, based on optical coherence tomographic results at 4–7 days follow-up. The exclusive polymer-free ART (abluminal reservoir technology) allows consistent drug loading onto the stent platform, providing directed elution to the vessel wall and eliminating any interaction with the blood.

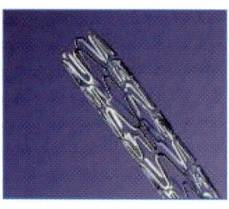
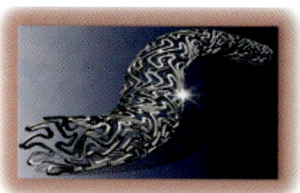
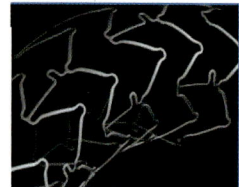

Fig. 12.13 Boston Scientific: stents available between 2003 and 2009

Stent Taxus Express 2   Stent Taxus Libertè   Stent Promus

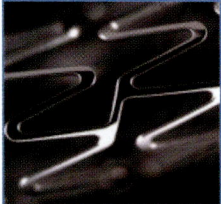
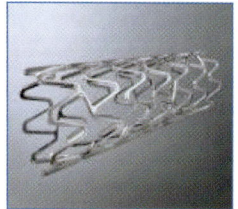

Stent Taxus Element   Stent Promus Element

12.4.3 Stent Coating

Stents with an active coating of gold, a highly radiovisible and biocompatible material, were shown to be inferior to plain stainless steel stents in four randomized trials. Coating stents with silicon carbide, a potentially less thrombogenic and more compatible material than stainless steel, also did not improve angiographic and clinical outcomes compared with BMS in two recent randomized trials. Other randomized trials reported similar results with phosphorylcholine-and heparin-coating. Indeed, in all these studies there was no angiographic or clinical benefit compared to BMS.

12.5 Bioabsorbable and Biocompatible Stents

Promising results have been obtained with DESs designed with biodegradable polymer technologies. An attractive alternative to these stents is certainly represented by the bioabsorbable stents; however, it remains to be determined whether this technology will address the issues of delayed endothelialization and late thrombosis, re-stenosis at the edges, unavoidable inflammatory reaction, and impaired vessel healing, all of which are normally encountered after stent implantation. Novel materials used as stent coatings include biocompatible though not biodegradable phosphorylcholine, a natural component of the cell membrane, and biodegradable PLLA and polylactic-co-glycolic acid (PLGA). As noted above, the latter two are fully metabolized to water and carbon dioxide, leaving in situ a BMS after the active compound is released. Promising results have been reported in the CREATE and CU-RAMI trials on three different stainless steel stents covered with PLLA and sirolimus (Table 12.2). Biolimus A9, a potent rapamycin derivative, has been evaluated in two PLLA-coated stainless steel stents: the Biomatrix (Biosensors International, Singapore) and the Nobori (Terumo, Japan).

12.5.1 Polymer-Free Solutions

Data on the possible pro-thrombotic effects, by delayed endothelial healing, of the permanent polymers integrated into first-generation DESs has motivated research into new stent platforms along two directions: (1) the development of biocompatible polymers and (2) the search for modern stent platforms that do not include a polymer coating. In a randomized trial examining the titanium-nitric oxide-coated stent (TiNOX), quantitative coronary angiography at 6 months revealed lower late lumen loss (0.55 ± 0.63 vs. 0.90 ± 0.76 mm, $p = 0.03$) and percent diameter stenosis ($26 \pm 17\%$ vs. $36 \pm 24\%$,

Table 12.2 Novel biodegradable and biocompatible stents

	Stent name	DES/BMS	Active drug	Stent platform	Manufacturer	Study
Biodegradable/biocompatible polymer						
PLLA	Exel	DES	Sirolimus	SS	JW Medical Systems	CREATE
	Cura	DES	Sirolimus	SS	Orbus Neich	CURAMI
	Supralimus	DES	Supralimus	Matrix SS	Sahajanand	PAINT
	Infinnium	DES	Paclitaxel	Matrix SS	Sahajanand	PAINT
	Biomatrix	DES	Biolimus A9	SS	Biosensors Int.	UI
	Nobori	DES	Biolimus A9	SS	Terumo	NOBORI
	S-stent	DES	Biolimus A9	SS	Biosensors	
PLGA	CoStar	DES	Paclitaxel	SS	Conor Medsystems	
	Mahoroba	DES	Tacrolimus	CoCr	Keneka	UI
	SymBio	DES	Pimecrolimus+Paclitaxel	SS	Conor Medsystems	UI
	Synchronnium	DES	Sirolimus+heparin	SS	Sahajanand	UI
No polymer	Tinox	BMS		SS+Ti/NO alloy		TiNOX
	Nanoporous AlO	DES	Tacrolimus	SS+AlO		UI
	Nanoporous hydroxyapetite	BMS		SS		UI
Biodegradable platform						
No PDLLA	Igaki-Tamai	BMS	Self-expandible	PLLA	Igaki Medical Planning	
	Absorb	DES	Everolimus	PLLA	Abbott	ABSORB
	Dreams	DES	Pimecrolimus	Mg	Biotronik	UI
PDTECI	REVA	DES	Paclitaxel	Tyrosine poly-carbonate	REVA	RESORB

PLLA polylactic acid, *DES* drug-eluting stent, *PLGA* polylactic-co-glycolic acid, *CoCr* cobalt chromium, *BMS* bare metal stent, *SS* stainless steel, *PDLLA* DL polylactic acid

$p = 0.04$) in lesions treated with the TiNOX-coated rather than with the control stents. To avoid polymer application, micro- and nanoporous stent platforms have been designed with the aim of allowing impregnation with active drug, thus customizing drug doses and/or combinations of different drugs. A nanoporous hydroxyapatite (a biocompatible crystalline derivative of calcium phosphate) coating is currently under investigation.

12.5.2 Biodegradable Platforms

Fully degradable stents are an attractive alternative to stents with a novel polymer coating. However, important characteristics need to be fulfilled in order to meet the expectations of modern interventional cardiology, such as the ability of controlled, sustained drug release and sufficient mechanical strength to prevent negative vessel re-modeling and to avoid stent deformity/strut fractures. The major theoretical advantage of this type of stent should, hopefully, be a lower risk of stent thrombosis and, subsequently, the possibility to eliminate prolonged dual anti-platelet therapy. In addition, vasomotion is restored after stent degradation, which may be an advantage in case of the necessity for repeat percutaneous or surgical revascularization.

12.5.3 Magnesium Alloy

An absorbable metal stent (AMS, Biotronik, Bülach, Switzerland) composed of a magnesium alloy is a promising alternative to polymer platforms. Unlike traditional metallic stents, the AMS is completely radiolucent, with two radio-opaque markers at its ends, and erodes completely in 30–60 days. However, the results of the first-in-humans study with the non-drug-eluting AMS were disappointing. In the "Biotronik Absorbable Metal Stent Below the Knee" (BEST-BTK) trial, the rate of re-stenosis in peripheral arteries was approximately 50%.

12.6 Impact of Stent Design on Clinical Outcome

12.6.1 Acute Outcome

Lesion-related (vessel diameter and length, ostial or bifurcational position, implantation technique, IVUS-guidance), and patient-related (diabetes, clinical presentation) variables are major determinants of acute, sub-acute, and long-term clinical outcomes. Although the immediate performance of the stent may be improved by increasing strut thickness (which increases radio-opacity, radial strength, and arterial-wall support), excessive strut thickness may impart greater vascular injury, trigger more extensive intimal hyperplasia, and engender a higher risk for re-stenosis than thinner struts. In recent years, active drug coating (e.g., with sirolimus or paclitaxel) has emerged as a major determinant in the reduction of angiographic re-stenosis and repeated revascularization of the target lesion. The choice of a particular type of stent design is mainly influenced by the specific familiarity of the surgeon with one device or another and by the potential performance of that device in a specific lesion. Indeed, the observation that different lesions behave in different ways after stent deployment supports the use of a different stent type with each type of lesion. For example, tortuous lesions necessitate the use of particularly conformable and flexible stents, while in ostial lesions stents with strong radial support and good radiological visibility are often preferable. For bifurcation lesions, the possibility to rewire the side branch through the stent struts after stent deployment in the main branch is a major factor determining a good result, while chronic total occlusions constitute a subset of lesions in which good lesion coverage and favorable radial support are important. Furthermore, small vessels require stents with good flexibility, very thin strut structure, and good trackability in the case of very distal lesions.

The most threatening acute complication of a stenting procedure, stent thrombosis, has been reduced to < 1–2% (compared to 5–7% in the initial trials) due to the introduction of high-pressure deployment of the device and double anti-platelet therapy. However, there are substantial differences in the hemodynamic and wall rheological characteristics of implanted stents of different designs; accordingly, the "hydrodynamic compatibility" of a stent is now recognized as an important feature of ideal stent design.

12.6.2 Long-Term Outcome

The wire-mesh stent, e.g., the self-expanding Wallstent (Boston Scientific), and the coil stent, e.g., the older Gianturco-Roubin Flex/GR-II (Cook) and Wiktor (Medtronic) stents, have a high propensity for thrombosis and re-stenosis, because of the high metal to surface area ratio of the former and the high degree of elastic recoil (associated with poor radial strength) and tissue prolapse of the latter. Better results have been obtained with other stent designs, such as the tubular Palmaz-Schatz (Johnson & Johnson, NIR, Boston Scientific) and Crown (Cordis, Johnson & Johnson) stents and the multicellular model (Multi-Link, Guidant, Boston Scientific), than with wire-mesh and coil stents. However, none of these stents are still used in clinical practice. Clinical studies have confirmed the direct relationship between strut thickness and arterial-wall reaction. In the ISAR-STEREO-2 trial, the ACS RX Multi-Link stent (Guidant, Advanced Cardiovascular Systems), with 0.05-mm struts, elicited less angiographic and clinical re-stenosis than the BX Velocity stent (Cordis, Johnson & Johnson), with a strut thickness of 0.14 mm.

The ideal DES should have a large surface area of contact with the vascular wall, minimal interfilament gaps, robust radial support, and symmetrical expansion to ensure uniform drug elution. At the same time, the stent needs to be slim, flexible, and conformable to enable successful deployment in complex lesions. The potential for long-term adverse effects of the synthetic polymers often used as carriers for anti-mitotic drugs is a major concern. Synthetic polymers may induce an enhanced inflammatory reaction and, possibly, a pro-thrombotic response. Late stent thrombosis, late stent apposition, and coronary aneurysm formation are thus real possibilities.

12.7 Conclusions

Although stents are currently considered the "gold standard" for the treatment of narrowed coronary arteries, there is experimental and clinical evidence to indicate that "a stent is not just a stent". Different stent models have different structural properties, with their own inherent advantages. Tubular or corrugated stents are better than coil or wire-mesh stents in terms of better acute and mid-term outcomes. Stents with thinner struts and lower metal density are associated with a lower risk of re-stenosis than stents with thicker struts and should be used for high-risk lesions such as those located in small vessels, where the risk of re-stenosis is often magnified. The availability of new, highly biocompatible, and more radiovisible alloys with the same if not superior tensile strength as stainless steel will enable the production of low metal density stents that may further improve the anatomical and clinical outcomes obtained with current stainless steel stents. Furthermore, stents coated with anti-proliferative agents, in particular sirolimus and paclitaxel, have opened a new era in interventional cardiology. The re-stenosis rates of these stents are unrivaled by other BMS models. However, several important questions regarding their cost-effectiveness, long-term safety, and durability need to be addressed in order to clearly understand their potential impact on daily practice. Moreover, as even these devices may be unsuccessful, the progressive understanding of the causes of their failures and of their different performances in various anatomical and biochemical settings becomes of pivotal importance. As scientists and companies continue to develop new types of stents containing different anti-proliferative drugs, it is entirely foreseeable that most interventional procedures will eventually involve DESs – containing sirolimus, paclitaxel, or even more effective drugs, with both anti-mitotic and anti-thrombotic actions – impregnated onto highly biocompatible carrier vehicles and mounted onto a stent design with uniform expansion and programmable, controllable drug-eluting capability. It is also possible that a co-action of different drugs, i.e., a paclitaxel-eluting stent and oral rapamycin given systemically, will further improve the clinical outcome in terms of re-stenosis. Finally, new stent platforms, such as biodegradable stents or endothelial progenitor cell capturing stents, may soon provide a more "physiological" answer to stent implantation, thus reducing vascular injury and accelerating vessel healing with consequent improvements in clinical outcome. Given the wide variety of devices currently under investigation and the prompt response of the industry to the requests of interventional cardiologists looking for their "Holy Grail", the road to finding the "ideal stent" is gradually becoming shorter.

Suggested Reading

Achenbach S (2006) Top 10 indications for coronary CTA. Applied Radiology 35:22-31

Cademartiri F, Mollet N, Lemos PA et al (2005) Usefulness of multislice computed tomographic coronary angiography to assess in-stent restenosis. Am J Cardiol 96:799-802

Maintz D, Juergens KU, Wichter T et al (2003) Imaging of coronary artery stents using multislice computed tomography: in vitro evaluation. Eur Radiol 13:830-835

Maintz D, Seifarth H, Flohr T et al (2003) Improved coronary artery stent visualization and in-stent stenosis detection using 16-slice computed-tomography and dedicated image reconstruction technique. Invest Radiol 38:790-795

Maseri A (2000) Ischemic heart disease. Churchill Livingstone and Saunders, New York

Schuijf JD, Bax JJ, Jukema JW et al (2004) Feasibility of assessment of coronary stent patency using 16-slice computed tomography. Am J Cardiol 94:427-430

Seifarth H, Raupach R, Schaller S et al (2005) Assessment of coronary artery stents using 16-slice MDCT angiography: evaluation of a dedicated reconstruction kernel and a noise reduction filter. Eur Radiol 15:721-726

CT Angiography of Coronary Stents

13

Gorka Bastarrika, Carlo Nicola De Cecco and U. Joseph Schoepf

13.1 Introduction

Coronary heart disease is a challenging socio-epidemiological problem in developed countries. In the United States, for example, the total prevalence of coronary heart disease in adults is 7.0%, with an annual incidence of myocardial infarction of 610,000 new attacks and 325,000 recurrent attacks. In 2007, mortality due to coronary heart disease was 406,351, with an estimated direct and indirect cost of $177.5 billion to the American healthcare system [1].

Percutaneous coronary intervention (PCI) was first performed in 1977 [2]. Since then its use has continuously grown such that it has become the coronary artery revascularization procedure of choice for an increasing number of clinical conditions [3]. Indeed, PCI has replaced traditional coronary artery bypass surgery for specific indications [4, 5], especially after the development of coronary artery stent implantation [6]. Compared with balloon angioplasty, coronary artery stenting has been shown to reduce the incidence of coronary re-stenosis, improve the rate of procedural success, and reduce the need for revascularization of the original coronary lesion [7]. Advances in stent technology have led to the development of drug-eluting stents [8, 9] and biodegradable drug-eluting stents [10]. Both types of devices are coated with pharmacological agents to diminish the occurrence of re-stenosis, which remains the primary problem of percutaneous revascularization [11]. The long-term results of an implanted coronary artery stent depend on several factors, including the clinical setting, coronary anatomy, morphology of the coronary lesion, associated medical therapy, and stent manufacturing material and design. Stents are made of various materials: stainless surgical steel, cobalt-chromium alloy, elgiloy (cobalt alloy), nitinol, tantalum, etc. The majority are balloon-expandable but some are self-expandable. Stent strut thickness may vary from 0.064 to 1 mm while the diameters and lengths range from 2.5 to 5 mm and from 4 to 35 mm, respectively [12]. In 2007, an estimated 622,000 patients underwent PCI procedures in the United States, with coronary stent placement accounting for 560,000 of these [1]. Approximately 76% of stents implanted during those PCIs were drug-eluting stents, with the remaining 24% being bare-metal stents [13].

Not infrequently, patients with previous coronary stent implantation develop recurrent symptoms, which may reflect intra-stent re-stenosis or coronary atherosclerosis progression. Due to its high spatial and temporal resolution, conventional coronary angiography remains the standard of reference to establish coronary stent patency. Among non-invasive imaging techniques, computed tomography (CT), first with electron-beam CT systems [14] and more recently in the form of multi-detector computed tomography (MDCT) [15], has proven to be a valuable tool in the assessment of stent patency and in establishing the presence of in-stent re-stenosis. Magnetic resonance imaging

G. Bastarrika (✉)
Cardiothoracic Imaging Division
Department of Medical Imaging
Sunnybrook Health Sciences Centre, Toronto, Canada
e-mail: bastarrika@unav.es

(MRI) has also shown promise in coronary status determination after PCI, although its use is still under vigorous research [16, 17].

13.2 Indications for Percutaneous Coronary Intervention

Large controlled randomized trials previously demonstrated the superiority of stent implantation over percutaneous transluminal angioplasty in native coronary arteries [7, 18] and by-pass grafts [19] with respect to long-term vessel patency. Since those initial steps, the use of PCI for the treatment of coronary artery disease has increased significantly and the number of indications has expanded dramatically. Two guidelines summarize the most recent indications for coronary revascularization, one published under the auspices of the European Society of Cardiology and the European Association for Cardio-Thoracic Surgery (EACTS) [5] and the other by the American Heart Association together with key specialty and subspecialty societies [4]. The clinical indications for PCI include the entire range of coronary heart disease, from stable coronary artery disease to acute coronary syndromes with or without ST segment elevation. The latest recommendations and appropriateness criteria for PCI are reviewed in [4, 5].

13.3 Technical Advances in the CT Assessment of Coronary Stents

From the initial electron-beam CT systems, non-invasive cardiac CT has rapidly evolved. The development of mechanical MDCT systems was accompanied by retrospective ECG synchronization and high acquisition speeds, advantages that have allowed high-resolution coronary artery imaging. The 4-detector-row systems have now been surpassed such that 64-detector-row MDCT technology is the current benchmark for cardiac CT imaging. With these newest-generation machines, volumetric acquisition of data is achieved in < 10 s, with isotropic voxels of 0.4 mm spatial resolution, a 165-ms temporal resolution, and a gantry rotation time of 330 ms [20].

More recently, technical development in MDCT equipment has progressed along two different lines. Complete volume coverage of the heart within a single heartbeat is now possible as the number of detector rows has continued to increase. The latest 320-detector-row scanner enables complete coverage of the heart in a single heartbeat and eliminates stair-step artifacts, reducing patient radiation dose and the amount of contrast agent required for cardiac studies [21, 22]. At the same time, with the addition of a second X-ray tube into 64-row MDCT scanners, so-called dual-source computed tomography (DSCT), the temporal resolution of CT has significantly improved [23]. This device provides a constant temporal resolution of 83 ms with a gantry rotation time of 330 ms, obviating the need for pharmacological heart rate control prior to cardiac CT examinations [24] and expanding the ability of CT to study individuals with high resting heart rates [25]. The combination of wide detector coverage and a two-tube configuration has opened up new pathways in the assessment of cardiac function, myocardial perfusion [26], and the simultaneous acquisition of high and low X-ray energy spectra within a single examination that also allows tissue characterization [27, 28]. The recent development of a second-generation DSCT system with two 128-slice acquisition detectors, a 280-ms gantry rotation time, and a temporal resolution of 75 ms has introduced the single heartbeat, prospectively ECG-triggered, high-pitch (3.4) spiral acquisition mode for cardiac CT imaging [29, 30]. Examinations performed with this technique in stent phantom models have shown that the high-pitch mode allows visualization of the coronary in-stent lumen with a quality comparable to that obtained with standard-pitch mode [31]. However, even with this system in-stent lumen narrowing is still too high for routine stent evaluation in clinical practice [32].

Nonetheless, in terms of image acquisition, new strategies have been developed to reduce the radiation dose necessary for cardiac CT imaging. In this setting, sequential CT acquisition with prospective ECG-synchronization yields coronary CT angiograms of high diagnostic accuracy but

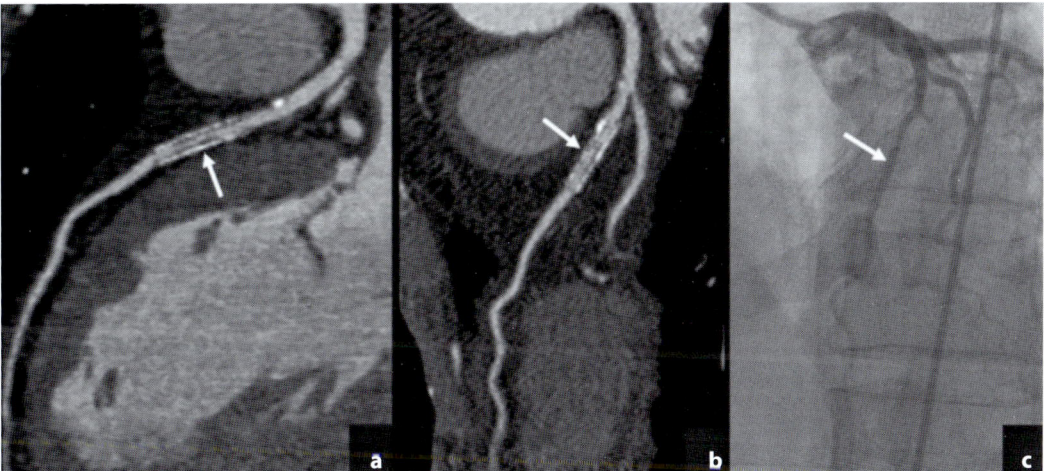

Fig. 13.1 Contrast-enhanced prospectively ECG-triggered coronary CT angiography in a 74-year-old man with previous stent implantation in the left anterior descending coronary artery (LAD) and atypical chest pain. **a**, **b** Curved multiplanar reformats and **c** conventional coronary angiography. The CT examination revealed in-stent re-stenosis, confirmed by conventional coronary angiography (*arrow*)

with a low radiation dose [33-35]. During this acquisition mode, the table remains stationary while the X-ray tube rotates around the patient and the tube current is restricted to predefined time points of the cardiac cycle: ordinarily diastole in patients with low heart rates and systole in those with fast heart rates [36]. The table is advanced for the following acquisition only when data acquisition is completed, thus preventing slice overlap. The major drawbacks of ECG-synchronization include the inability to evaluate cardiac function and the restricted use in patients with severe arrhythmia. Moreover, the ability to retrospectively change the reconstruction interval to more suitable phases of the cardiac cycle is limited. Minor heart rhythm irregularities that may occur during the study acquisition may be solved partially with the use of recently developed adaptive online monitoring of the ECG [37]. In the field of coronary stent imaging, phantom experiments [38, 39] as well as human studies demonstrated that, compared with the traditional retrospectively ECG-gated technique, prospective coronary CT angiography offers improved image quality and reduces the effective radiation dose in evaluations of in-stent re-stenosis [40, 41] (Fig. 13.1). In a study by Andreini et al. [40], both the occurrence of blooming artifacts and the radiation dose were significantly lower in the prospectively ECG-triggered coronary CT angiography group than in the retrospectively ECG-gated group. Reduction of the blooming effect is due to the sequential nature of the prospectively ECG-triggered acquisition mode. Moreover, with 140-kVp prospectively ECG-triggered coronary CT angiography protocols, coronary in-stent re-stenosis is visible at a lower radiation dose than is possible with conventional 120-kVp retrospectively ECG-gated examinations [42].

Finally, in the field of image reconstruction, development of iterative reconstruction algorithms may provide better detection of the intra-stent luminal area than is the case with conventional filtered back-projection reconstruction techniques, thus improving the assessment of coronary stents [43].

13.4 Cardiac CT Acquisition Protocols for Stent Imaging

Coronary CT examinations for stent evaluation are acquired with the patient in the supine position and at end inspiration. Although the more recently developed scanners allow patients with high and irregular heart rates to undergo scanning, the regular use of premedication to control the heart rate before the examination significantly improves diagnostic quality and minimizes radiation exposure during 64-row MDCT scanning. For coronary CT angiography using conventional MDCT systems a heart rate of < 65 beats per minute is usually recommended [44]. In the clinical setting this is achieved by oral and/or intravenous administration of selective 1-adrenoreceptor antagonists, such as metoprolol tartrate; alternatively, calcium-channel blockers may be used. Sublingual administration of a tablet of 0.4 mg nitroglycerin is recommended to obtain significant dilation of the coronary arteries, allowing more distal and smaller-caliber vessels to be visualized [45], thus further improving the diagnostic accuracy of coronary CT angiography [46].

Coronary CT examinations are usually performed with 120 kVp. The tube current is specifically adjusted to the patient size but is typically 750–850 mAs for conventional 64-row MDCT scanners. For DSCT, a current of 330 mAs for each tube is used. Tube-current modulation techniques allow significant lowering of the radiation dose and should be employed whenever possible. The thinnest possible collimation (0.6 mm) and the fastest gantry rotation time are required for adequate imaging of coronary stents. The use of ECG-gated tube-current dose modulation is mandatory to maintain the radiation dose at a reasonable level [47].

High and homogeneous enhancement of the coronary arteries requires appropriate contrast dynamics [48]. Contrast material should be administered continuously through a right antecubital vein at a high injection flow rate (4–6 ml/s). Regardless of the technique used for contrast timing (automated bolus tracking or test bolus technique), the contrast should reach its peak attenuation during the acquisition and the contrast plateau should last for the duration of the entire study. Intravenous contrast should be followed by a saline flush chaser to compact the contrast bolus, extend the plateau phase of contrast enhancement, and avoid streaks artifacts that may hamper coronary artery evaluation [49]. A bolus consisting of a mixture of saline and contrast material may be used if opacification of the right heart chamber is advantageous [50]. As a general rule, the contrast volume for a coronary CT angiography examination is calculated as follows: Volume of contrast (ml) = scan time (s) × flow (ml/s) [51].

Image reconstruction is performed with a field of view confined to the heart, using 0.75-mm section thickness and a 0.4- to 0.5-mm increment within the optimal reconstruction window [52]. The reconstruction window is usually set in a diastolic phase in individuals with low heart rates and in a systolic phase in patients with high heart rates [53]. For the evaluation of coronary artery stents, a high convolution kernel (B46f) is recommended. This provides stronger edge-enhancement with better delineation of metallic stent struts. Consequently, beam-hardening artifacts are minimized and in-stent intimal hyperplasia and re-stenosis may be identified more accurately [54]. Examples of coronary CT acquisition protocols for 64-row MDCT and DSCT are shown in Table 13.1.

13.5 Coronary Stent Imaging with CT

Accurate depiction of the in-stent lumen is necessary to establish stent patency and to diagnose in-stent re-stenosis secondary to intimal hyperplasia. Reliable assessment of re-stenosis requires, however, appropriate knowledge of the inherent limitations of CT technology, which may hamper coronary stent evaluation [55].

The most common types of artifacts that may impede accurate coronary stent evaluation are those due to motion, partial-volume averaging, and beam hardening. Motion artifacts are the most frequent reason for non-assessable stented segments. As a general rule, CT systems with high temporal resolution are mandatory for coronary stent imaging. Fast gantry rotation speed allows image reconstruction at optimal time points of the cardiac cycle, thereby avoiding cardiac motion and image blurring. Equally important is the appropriate selection of candidates with regular sinus rhythm, which is necessary to obtain high-quality coronary CT angiograms. If the available CT equipment is of relatively low temporal resolution, then premedication of the patient with a β-blocker may be necessary to control the heart rate prior to exami-

Table 13.1 Coronary 64-row MDCT and dual-source CT acquisition protocols for coronary stent evaluation

			64-row MDCT	Dual-source CT
Preparation	Venous access	Injection site	Right antecubital vein	Right antecubital vein
		Needle size	18 G	18 G
	Medication	Beta-blockers	If heart rate >65 bpm	Not necessary
		Nitroglycerine	0.4 mg sublingual (spray or tablet)	0.4 mg sublingual (spray or tablet)
CT parameters	Exam	Range	Carina to diaphragm	Carina to diaphragm
		Direction	Craniocaudal	Craniocaudal
		Duration	~ 9-12 s	~ 8-10 s
	Tube settings	Tube voltage	120 kVp	120 kVp
		Tube current	850 mAs	330 mAs for each tube
		Dose modulation	ECG-pulsing	ECG-pulsing
	Acquisition	Slice collimation	0.6 mm	0.6 mm
		Acquisition	64 x 0.6 mm	64 x 0.6 mm
		Rotation time	330 ms	330 ms
		Pitch	0.2	0.2-0.5, depending on heart rate
	Reconstruction	Slice thickness	0.75 mm	0.75 mm
		Reconstruction increment	0.4 mm	0.4 mm
		Reconstruction kernel	B46f	B46f
Contrast	Contrast administration	Iodine concentration	400 mg I/ml	400 mg I/ml
		Volume	80 ml	80 ml
		Flow rate	4-5 ml/s	5-6 ml/s
		Triphasic	50 ml mixture (30% CM / 70% S) + 50 ml S at 4-5 ml/s	50 ml mixture (30% CM / 70% S) + 50 ml S at 5-6 ml/s

bpm Beats per min, *CM* contrast medium, *FR* flow rate, *S* saline.

nation. Partial-volume averaging may adversely affect in-stent luminal evaluation by providing incorrect CT attenuation values, which may result in a loss of the sharp border delineating the stent and the lumen. This artifact is more pronounced in small-caliber (< 3 mm) coronary stents. The beam-hardening artifact is produced by the X-ray beam as it penetrates the metal of the stent and results in blooming artifacts. Consequently, as demonstrated by in vitro studies, the stent struts appear thicker than they actually are, the diameters of the visible stent lumen decrease, and attenuation values inside the stent lumen increase, thus interfering with the ability to assess the presence and severity of disease [12, 56-58]. These limitations may be partially overcome by reducing the voxel size, selecting a field of view confined to the heart, using the thinnest collimation available for image acquisition, and employing sharp, edge-enhancing convolution filters (kernels) for image reconstruction (Fig. 13.2). A sharp coronary reconstruction filter improves lumen visibility [54, 59] and stenosis delineation but at the expense of a higher noise level [57]. High intraluminal contrast enhancement may compensate for the increased image noise [60]. From a technical point of view, dedicated specific noise-reduction filters [54] or the newly developed advanced iterative reconstruction algorithms [43] can be used to resolve this problem.

13.6 Coronary Stent Imaging Interpretation

The interpretation of cardiac CT examinations performed for coronary stent assessment does not significantly differ from the interpretation of

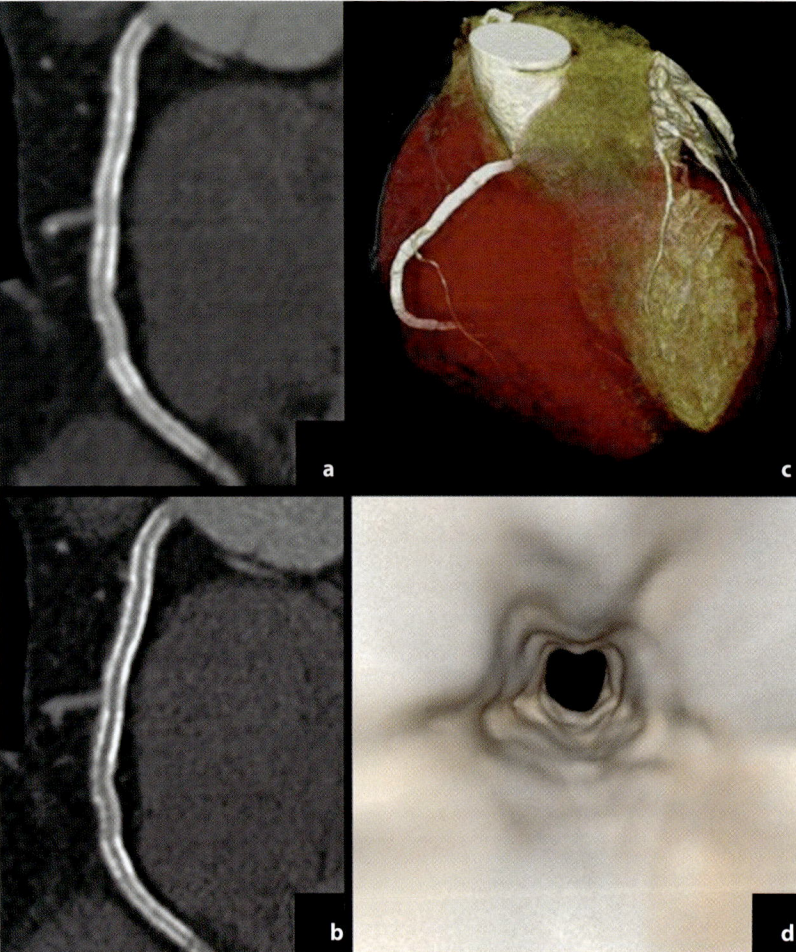

Fig. 13.2 Contrast-enhanced coronary CT angiography in a 51-year-old asymptomatic man with prior implantation of four coronary stents in the right coronary artery. **a** Curved multiplanar reformat of a reconstruction performed with a regular soft-tissue convolution filter (B26f). **b** Curved multiplanar reformat of a reconstruction performed using a sharp edge-enhancing convolution filter (B46f). **c** Three-dimensional volume-rendered image and **d** virtual endoscopic view of the inner vessel surface. Note the superiority of the edge-enhancing reconstruction filter in the assessment of the in-stent lumen. This examination ruled out significant in-stent re-stenosis

conventional coronary CT angiograms. The stented coronary segments are initially assessed using axial source images with wide window settings. Narrow window settings will preclude accurate evaluation of the in-stent lumen [60]. Various post-processing techniques are then applied for comprehensive evaluation of the stent as well as the non-stented coronary segments. These techniques include multiplanar reformats (MPR), curved MPR, and 3D-volume rendered (VR) images (Fig. 13.3). Virtual endoscopy may be useful in particular cases. In particular, curved MPR and sectional images acquired perpendicular to these curved reformats become very helpful in determining stent patency and establishing the degree of intimal hyperplasia and re-stenosis. Three dimensional VR images well-demonstrate the location of the stent and are especially useful for further therapeutic planning. Unlike conventional CT angiograms, maximum intensity projection images are not suitable for in-stent lumen assessments as the stent material has a higher attenuation than the contrast in the vessel.

As noted above, due to imaging artifacts associated with coronary MDCT angiography, the stent struts tend to appear significantly thicker than their actual size, such that there is a density increment all along the lumen, with lower attenuation in the center of the stented coronary segment and higher attenuation at the vessel wall [58]. Sharp coronary reconstruction filters should be used routinely to improve visualization of the in-stent lumen, as they minimize beam-hardening artifacts and maintain an optimal degree of edge enhancement for visu-

Fig. 13.3 Contrast-enhanced coronary CT angiography in a 65-year-old asymptomatic man with prior stent implantation in the LAD 6 years earlier due to acute coronary syndrome. **a** Curved multiplanar reformat and **b** detail. **c-f** Three-dimensional volume-rendered images. The study revealed the patency of the coronary stent

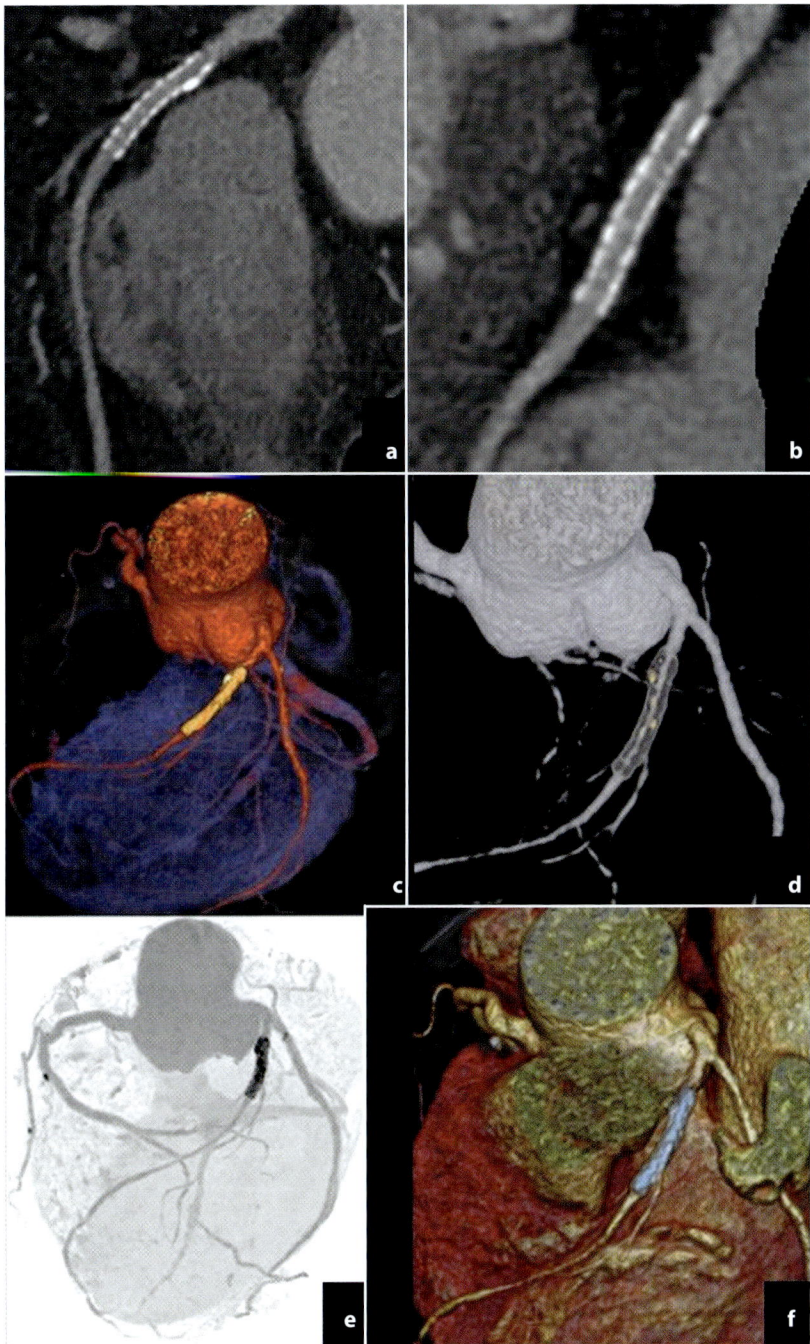

alization of the vessel lumen and wall, with adequate contrast resolution [54].

In coronary CT imaging, the stent occlusion usually appears as an area of low-density inside the lumen, compared with the high attenuation values of the contrast-enhanced proximal coronary segment. In initial studies performed with electron-beam CT, the coronary stent was defined as patent if the distal segments of the same vessel were opacified and their attenuation values were similar to those of other segments of comparable size [14]. Similarly, initial observations with MDCT

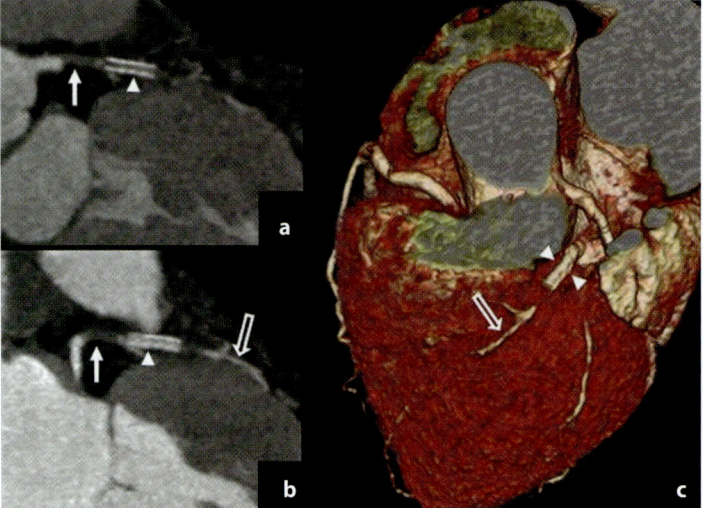

Fig. 13.4 Contrast-enhanced coronary CT angiography in a 71-year-old asymptomatic heart transplant recipient. The patient underwent stent implantation in the proximal segment of the LAD due to cardiac allograft vasculopathy. **a** Curved multiplanar reformat, **b** with maximum intensity projection. **c** Three-dimensional volume rendered image. The CT examination revealed complete occlusion of the LAD proximal to the stent (*arrow*), which also appeared occluded (*arrowhead*). Note the presence of contrast in the distal run-off of the LAD secondary to retrograde filling by collateral vessels (*open arrow*)

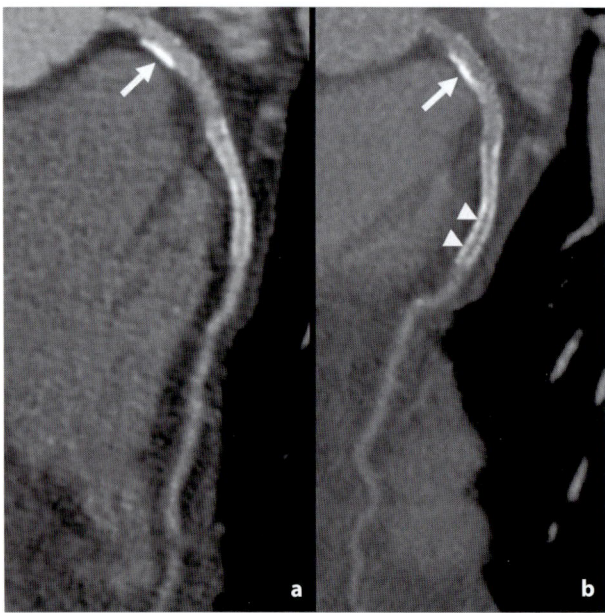

Fig. 13.5 Contrast-enhanced coronary CT angiography in a 39-year-old woman with hypertension and diabetes who was admitted for atypical chest pain. She had a past history of PCI consisting of the placement of two stents in the proximal and mid segments of the LAD. **a** Curved multiplanar reformat of the coronary CT angiography performed one year earlier. **b** Curved multiplanar reformat of the follow-up examination. The most recent study revealed patency of the coronary stent implanted in the proximal segment of the vessel (*arrow*). The stent located in the mid segment of the LAD developed significant in-stent intimal hyperplasia (*arrowheads*). Conventional coronary angiography confirmed the CT findings

suggested that the absence of contrast material in the distal portions of the stented vessel reflected severe in-stent re-stenosis or occlusion; conversely, the presence of intravenous contrast in the coronary segments distal to the implanted stent was interpreted as stent patency. However, this definition does not consider that the presence of contrast in the distal run-off does not necessarily mean stent patency and could instead be secondary to retrograde filling by collateral vessels (Fig. 13.4).

Nowadays, with newer-generation CT scanners, providing sub-millimeter spatial resolution, a coronary stent evaluation should include an assessment of in-stent luminal narrowing. In-stent intimal hyperplasia is seen as a low-attenuation rim located between the stent wall and the contrast-enhanced vessel lumen (Fig. 13.5). In-stent re-stenosis presents as a localized lesion, commonly associated with vessel size, lesion length [61], discontinuity in stent coverage [62], and

Table 13.2 Accuracy of 16-row MDCT vs. conventional coronary angiography for the assessment of stent patency (in-stent re-stenosis)

Author	Total number of stents	Number of assessable stents	Sensitivity (%)	Specificity (%)
Schuijf [77]	65	50	78	100
Cademartiri [70]	76	2	83	99
Kitagawa [75]	61	42	100	100
Gilard [73]	29	27	100	92
Kefer [74]	73	73	67	98
Chabbert [71]	134	121	92	67
Watanabe [78]	42	35	83	90
Ohnuki [76]	20	19	75	88
Gilard [72]	232	126	54	100

stent type [63]. Edge re-stenosis may occur more frequently in the proximal stent border [62], is frequently associated with local trauma outside the stent, and may be influenced by incomplete lesion coverage by the stent. As a general rule in coronary CT examinations, a reduction in luminal diameter > 50% is defined as significant in-stent re-stenosis.

13.7 Accuracy of CT in Assessing Coronary Stent Patency

The successful implementation into clinical practice of coronary artery stent placement in the treatment of coronary artery disease requiring revascularization has markedly increased the number of patients considered for PCI. However, a substantial number of patients with coronary stents will develop in-stent intimal hyperplasia and therefore in-stent re-stenosis or complete obstruction [64]. While conventional coronary angiography is the standard of reference for the evaluation of stent patency and the exclusion of in-stent re-stenosis, CT has emerged as a potentially valid alternative for this purpose.

Preliminary studies performed with electron-beam CT showed modest sensitivity and specificity values for the evaluation of stent patency compared with conventional coronary angiography [14, 65, 66]. MDCT revolutionized non-invasive cardiac imaging by allowing submillimeter section-thicknesses and dedicated ECG-gated reconstruction algorithms capable of accurately assessing the coronary tree. Preliminary studies performed with 4-row MDCT systems, however, failed to demonstrate the reliability of this approach in the detection of in-stent re-stenosis in percutaneously treated coronary vessels [58, 67-69]. The advent of 16-row MDCT scanners with 420-ms rotation times increased the potential for the detection of in-stent re-stenosis, with reported sensitivity and specificity values in the ranges of 54–100% and 67–100%, respectively [70, 78] (Table 13.2). Nonetheless, the number of assessable segments remained relatively low, with up to 51.2% of the lumens being non-interpretable in detectable stents [72].

The higher spatial and temporal resolutions of 64-row MDCT scanners increased the sensitivity and specificity for the detection of in-stent re-stenosis [79-94] (Table 13.3). A recent meta-analysis designed to define the role of 16-row and 64-row MDCT scanners for the diagnosis of coronary in-stent re-stenosis demonstrated a pooled sensitivity of 82% and 85% and a specificity of 92% and 91% for studies performed using 16-row and 64-row MDCT, respectively [15]. Similarly, other meta-analyses analyzing the diagnostic performance of 64-row MDCT angiography for the detection of in-stent re-stenosis in the coronary arteries showed sensitivity and specificity values of 86–90% and 84–93%, respectively [95, 97]. Consequently, since a large proportion of stents remains non-interpretable with 64-MDCT, the use of this technology may not be generalized to rule-out in-stent luminal narrowing; rather, it may serve as a potentially non-invasive alternative to exclude in-stent re-stenosis only in selected patients.

Table 13.3 Accuracy of 64-row MDCT vs. conventional coronary angiography for the assessment of stent patency (in-stent re-stenosis). Modified from [104]

Author	Total number of stents	Number of assessable stents	Sensitivity (%)	Specificity (%)
Van Mieghem [90]	70	70	100	91
Cademartiri [79]	192	14	95	93
Carrabba [81]	87	87	84	100
Rist [87]	46	45	75	92
Oncel [86]	39	39	89	95
Manghat [84]	114	103	85	86
Ehara [83]	125	110	92	81
Rixe [88]	102	59	86	98
Das [82]	110	107	97	88
Schuijf [89]	76	65	100	100
Carbone [80]	74	21	75	86
Hecht [91]	132	132	94	74
Nakamura [85]	75	64	67	92
Andreini [92]	179	170	87	98
Wykrzykowska [93]	75	48	33	92
Abdelkarim [94]	122	106	91	95

Better visualization of coronary artery stents was achieved with DSCT. Oncel et al. [98] evaluated 35 consecutive patients with 48 stents, all of which were found to be assessable. The authors reported 100% sensitivity, 94% specificity, 89% positive predictive value, 100% negative predictive value, and 96% accuracy for the detection of in-stent re-stenosis and occlusion. In a similar study, Pugliese et al. [99] analyzed 100 patients with chest pain subsequent to coronary artery stent implantation. For stents ≥ 3.5 mm in diameter, 100% sensitivity and specificity were determined whereas for stents ≤ 2.75 mm in diameter the corresponding values declined to 84% and 64%, respectively. Pflederer et al. [100] examined a total of 112 patients with 150 previously implanted coronary stents (≥ 3 mm diameter). All stents > 3 mm were found to be assessable by DSCT whereas 19% of the stents 3 mm in diameter were not. Among the assessable stents, a sensitivity of 84%, specificity of 95%, positive predictive value of 73%, and negative predictive value of 97% were determined for the detection of in-stent re-stenosis compared with quantitative coronary angiography. Finally, in a recent study. a volumetric 320-row MDCT system was used to evaluate 53 patients with 89 stents [101]. Seven of the stents were of non-diagnostic image quality; overall, the sensitivity, specificity, and positive and negative predictive values on a stent basis were 92%, 83%, 46%, and 98%, respectively.

Thus, given these results it currently seems reasonable to confine the use of coronary CT angiography to patients in whom the patency of proximal and large-diameter coronary stents must be established.

13.8 Summary and Current Indications for Stent Imaging with MDCT

Coronary stents continue to pose a technical challenge for non-invasive coronary CT imaging. The current literature suggests that in individuals with large-diameter stents and good image quality examinations, 64-row MDCT systems or newer-generation CT scanners can be used to assess stent patency and to exclude with confidence significant in-stent re-stenosis [102].

The most recent appropriateness criteria for the use of non-invasive cardiac imaging with CT are those of the American College of Cardiology Foundation [103]. In their report, a technical panel scored each indication on a numerical scale of 1 to 9, considering a score of 7–9 as appropriate (test is generally acceptable and is a reasonable approach

Table 13.4 Summary of the criteria for the appropriate use of cardiac multidetector computed tomography (MD-CT) imaging in patients with prior coronary stent implantation. Modified from [103]

	Clinical scenario	Appropriate use score (1–9)	
Symptomatic (ischemic equivalent)	Stent diameter < 3 mm or not known Stent diameter ≥ 3 mm	I (3) U (6)	
Asymptomatic	Left main coronary stent with stent diameter Time since percutaneous coronary intervention Stent diameter < 3 mm or not known Stent diameter ≥ 3 mm	≥3 mm < 2 years I (2) I (3)	A (7) ≥2 years I (2) U (4)

I inappropriate, *U* uncertain.

for the indication), a score of 4–6 as uncertain (test may be generally acceptable and may be a reasonable approach for the indication, more research and/or patient information are needed to classify the indication definitively), and a score of 1–3 as inappropriate (test is not generally acceptable and is not a reasonable approach for the indication). According to this document, MDCT evaluation of coronary stent status is considered a function of several conditions, including the patient's clinical symptoms, the time from revascularization, and stent size. Non-invasive stent imaging with MDCT is considered appropriate only in asymptomatic patients with a prior left main coronary stent of diameter ≥ 3 mm. In non-symptomatic individuals at least 2 years from the PCI and with large-caliber stents (≥ 3 mm), and in symptomatic patients with a prior coronary stent of diameter ≥ 3 mm, coronary MDCT imaging is considered uncertain. In asymptomatic patients with coronary stent implantation less than 2 years earlier or with coronary stents <3 mm diameter and in symptomatic patients with stent caliber < 3 mm or unknown diameter, non-invasive coronary MDCT imaging is considered inappropriate [103]. Table 13.4 summarizes the criteria for the appropriate use of cardiac MDCT imaging in patients with prior coronary stent implantation.

References

1. Roger VL, Go AS, Lloyd-Jones DM et al (2011) Heart disease and stroke statistics-2011 update: a report from the American Heart Association. Circulation 123(4):e18-e209
2. Gruntzig AR, Senning A, Siegenthaler WE (1979) Nonoperative dilatation of coronary-artery stenosis: percutaneous transluminal coronary angioplasty. N Engl J Med 301(2):61-68
3. Chan PS, Patel MR, Klein LW et al (2011) Appropriateness of percutaneous coronary intervention. JAMA 306(1):53-61
4. Patel MR, Dehmer GJ, Hirshfeld JW et al (2009) ACCF/SCAI/STS/AATS/AHA/ASNC 2009 Appropriateness Criteria for Coronary Revascularization: a report by the American College of Cardiology Foundation Appropriateness Criteria Task Force, Society for Cardiovascular Angiography and Interventions, Society of Thoracic Surgeons, American Association for Thoracic Surgery, American Heart Association, and the American Society of Nuclear Cardiology Endorsed by the American Society of Echocardiography, the Heart Failure Society of America, and the Society of Cardiovascular Computed Tomography. J Am Coll Cardiol 53(6):530-553
5. Wijns W, Kolh P, Danchin N et al (2010) Guidelines on myocardial revascularization: The Task Force on Myocardial Revascularization of the European Society of Cardiology (ESC) and the European Association for Cardio-Thoracic Surgery (EACTS). Eur Heart J 20:2501-2555
6. Sigwart U, Puel J, Mirkovitch V et al (1987) Intravascular stents to prevent occlusion and restenosis after transluminal angioplasty. N Engl J Med 316(12):701-706
7. Fischman DL, Leon MB, Baim DS et al (1994) A randomized comparison of coronary-stent placement and balloon angioplasty in the treatment of coronary artery disease. Stent Restenosis Study Investigators. N Engl J Med 331(8):496-501
8. Moses JW, Leon MB, Popma JJ et al (2003) Sirolimus-eluting stents versus standard stents in patients with stenosis in a native coronary artery. N Engl J Med 349(14):1315-1323

9. Stone GW, Ellis SG, Cox DA et al (2004) A polymer-based, paclitaxel-eluting stent in patients with coronary artery disease. N Engl J Med 350(3):221-231
10. Windecker S, Serruys PW, Wandel S et al (2008) Biolimus-eluting stent with biodegradable polymer versus sirolimus-eluting stent with durable polymer for coronary revascularisation (LEADERS): a randomised non-inferiority trial. Lancet 372(9644):1163-1173
11. Lemos PA, Serruys PW, van Domburg RT et al (2004) Unrestricted utilization of sirolimus-eluting stents compared with conventional bare stent implantation in the "real world": the Rapamycin-Eluting Stent Evaluated At Rotterdam Cardiology Hospital (RESEARCH) registry. Circulation 109(2):190-195
12. Maintz D, Seifarth H, Raupach R et al (2006) 64-slice multidetector coronary CT angiography: in vitro evaluation of 68 different stents. Eur Radiol 16(4):818-826
13. US Food and Drug Administration CSDPMm, December 8, 2006, Washington, DC. Available at: http://www.fda.gov/ohrms/dockets/ac/06/transcripts/2006-4253t2.rtf
14. Pump H, Mohlenkamp S, Sehnert CA et al (2000) Coronary arterial stent patency: assessment with electron-beam CT. Radiology 214(2):447-452
15. Hamon M, Champ-Rigot L, Morello R, Riddell JW. Diagnostic accuracy of in-stent coronary restenosis detection with multislice spiral computed tomography: a meta-analysis. Eur Radiol 2008 Feb;18(2):217-225
16. Spuentrup E, Ruebben A, Mahnken A et al (2005) Artifact-free coronary magnetic resonance angiography and coronary vessel wall imaging in the presence of a new, metallic, coronary magnetic resonance imaging stent. Circulation 111(8):1019-1026
17. Gilbert G, Soulez G, Beaudoin G (2009) Improved in-stent lumen visualization using intravascular MRI and a balanced steady-state free-precession sequence. Acad Radiol 16(12):1466-1474
18. Erbel R, Haude M, Hopp HW et al (1998) Coronary-artery stenting compared with balloon angioplasty for restenosis after initial balloon angioplasty. Restenosis Stent Study Group. N Engl J Med 339(23):1672-1678
19. Savage MP, Douglas JS Jr., Fischman DL et al (1997) Stent placement compared with balloon angioplasty for obstructed coronary bypass grafts. Saphenous Vein De Novo Trial Investigators. N Engl J Med 337(11):740-747
20. Flohr T, Stierstorfer K, Raupach R et al (2004) Performance evaluation of a 64-slice CT system with z-flying focal spot. Rofo 176(12):1803-1810
21. Rybicki FJ, Otero HJ, Steigner ML et al (2008) Initial evaluation of coronary images from 320-detector row computed tomography. Int J Cardiovasc Imaging 24(5):535-546
22. Dewey M, Zimmermann E, Deissenrieder F et al (2009) Noninvasive coronary angiography by 320-row computed tomography with lower radiation exposure and maintained diagnostic accuracy: comparison of results with cardiac catheterization in a head-to-head pilot investigation. Circulation 120(10):867-875
23. Flohr TG, McCollough CH, Bruder H et al (2006) First performance evaluation of a dual-source CT (DSCT) system. Eur Radiol 16(2):256-268
24. Johnson TR, Nikolaou K, Wintersperger BJ et al (2006) Dual-source CT cardiac imaging: initial experience. Eur Radiol 16(7):1409-1415
25. Weustink AC, Neefjes LA, Kyrzopoulos S et al (2009) Impact of heart rate frequency and variability on radiation exposure, image quality, and diagnostic performance in dual-source spiral CT coronary angiography. Radiology 253(3):672-680
26. Bastarrika G, Ramos-Duran L, Rosenblum MA et al (2010) Adenosine-stress dynamic myocardial CT perfusion imaging: initial clinical experience. Invest Radiol 45(6):306-313
27 Weininger M, Schoepf UJ, Ramachandra A et al (2010) Adenosine-stress dynamic real-time myocardial perfusion CT and adenosine-stress first-pass dual-energy myocardial perfusion CT for the assessment of acute chest pain: Initial results. Eur J Radiol Dec 30 2010
28. Ruzsics B, Schwarz F, Schoepf UJ et al (2009) Comparison of dual-energy computed tomography of the heart with single photon emission computed tomography for assessment of coronary artery stenosis and of the myocardial blood supply. Am J Cardiol 1 104(3):318-326
29. Lell M, Marwan M, Schepis T et al (2009) Prospectively ECG-triggered high-pitch spiral acquisition for coronary CT angiography using dual source CT: technique and initial experience. Eur Radiol 19(11):2576-2583
30. Leschka S, Stolzmann P, Desbiolles L et al (2009) Diagnostic accuracy of high-pitch dual-source CT for the assessment of coronary stenoses: first experience. Eur Radiol 19:2896-2903
31. Donati OF, Burg MC, Desbiolles L et al (2010) High-pitch 128-slice dual-source CT for the assessment of coronary stents in a phantom model. Acad Radiol 17(11):1366-1374

32. Wolf F, Leschka S, Loewe C et al (2010) Coronary artery stent imaging with 128-slice dual-source CT using high-pitch spiral acquisition in a cardiac phantom: comparison with the sequential and low-pitch spiral mode. Eur Radiol 20(9):2084-2091
33. Scheffel H, Alkadhi H, Leschka S, et al (2008) Low-dose CT coronary angiography in the step-and-shoot mode: diagnostic performance. Heart 94(9):1132-1137
34. Stolzmann P, Scheffel H, Schertler T et al (2008) Radiation dose estimates in dual-source computed tomography coronary angiography. Eur Radiol 18(3):592-599
35. Husmann L, Valenta I, Gaemperli O et al (2008) Feasibility of low-dose coronary CT angiography: first experience with prospective ECG-gating. Eur Heart J 29(2):191-197
36. Bastarrika G, Broncano J, Arraiza M et al (2011) Systolic prospectively ECG-triggered dual-source CT angiography for evaluation of the coronary arteries in heart transplant recipients. Eur Radiol 21:1887-1894,
37. Earls JP, Berman EL, Urban BA et al (2008) Prospectively gated transverse coronary CT angiography versus retrospectively gated helical technique: improved image quality and reduced radiation dose. Radiology 246(3):742-753
38. Yang WJ, Pan ZL, Zhang H et al (2011) Evaluation of coronary artery in-stent restenosis with prospectively ECG-triggered axial CT angiography versus retrospective technique: a phantom study. Radiol Med 116(2):189-196
39. Suzuki S, Furui S, Kuwahara S et al (2009) Coronary artery stent evaluation using a vascular model at 64-detector row CT: comparison between prospective and retrospective ECG-gated axial scans. Korean J Radiol 10(3):217-226
40. Andreini D, Pontone G, Bartorelli AL et al (2011) High diagnostic accuracy of prospective ECG-gating 64-slice computed tomography coronary angiography for the detection of in-stent restenosis: in-stent restenosis assessment by low-dose MDCT. Eur Radiol 21(7):1430-1438
41. Zhao L, Zhang Z, Fan Z et al (2011) Prospective versus retrospective ECG gating for dual source CT of the coronary stent: comparison of image quality, accuracy, and radiation dose. Eur J Radiol 77(3):436-442
42. Horiguchi J, Fujioka C, Kiguchi M et al (2009) Prospective ECG-triggered axial CT at 140-kV tube voltage improves coronary in-stent restenosis visibility at a lower radiation dose compared with conventional retrospective ECG-gated helical CT. Eur Radiol 19(10):2363-2372
43. Min JK, Swaminathan RV, Vass M et al (2009) High-definition multidetector computed tomography for evaluation of coronary artery stents: comparison to standard-definition 64-detector row computed tomography. J Cardiovasc Comput Tomogr 3(4):246-251
44. Giesler T, Baum U, Ropers D et al (2002) Noninvasive visualization of coronary arteries using contrast-enhanced multidetector CT: influence of heart rate on image quality and stenosis detection. AJR Am J Roentgenol 179(4):911-916
45. Decramer I, Vanhoenacker PK, Sarno G et al (2008) Effects of sublingual nitroglycerin on coronary lumen diameter and number of visualized septal branches on 64-MDCT angiography. AJR Am J Roentgenol 190(1):219-225
46. Chun EJ, Lee W, Choi YH et al (2008) Effects of nitroglycerin on the diagnostic accuracy of electrocardiogram-gated coronary computed tomography angiography. J Comput Assist Tomogr 32(1):86-92
47. Jakobs TF, Becker CR, Ohnesorge B et al (2002) Multislice helical CT of the heart with retrospective ECG gating: reduction of radiation exposure by ECG-controlled tube current modulation. Eur Radiol 12(5):1081-1086
48. Bae KT (2010) Intravenous contrast medium administration and scan timing at CT: considerations and approaches. Radiology 256(1):32-61
49. Kim DJ, Kim TH, Kim SJ et al (2008) Saline flush effect for enhancement of aorta and coronary arteries at multidetector CT coronary angiography. Radiology 246(1):110-115
50. Kerl JM, Ravenel JG, Nguyen SA et al (2008) Right heart: split-bolus injection of diluted contrast medium for visualization at coronary CT angiography. Radiology 247(2):356-364
51. Schoepf UJ, Zwerner PL, Savino G et al (2007) Coronary CT angiography. Radiology 244(1):48-63
52. Flohr TG, Schaller S, Stierstorfer K et al (2005) Multi-detector row CT systems and image-reconstruction techniques. Radiology 235(3):756-773
53. Leschka S, Husmann L, Desbiolles LM et al (2006) Optimal image reconstruction intervals for non-invasive coronary angiography with 64-slice CT. Eur Radiol 16(9):1964-1972
54. Seifarth H, Raupach R, Schaller S et al (????) Assessment of coronary artery stents using 16-slice MDCT angiography: evaluation of a dedicated reconstruction kernel and a noise reduction filter. Eur Radiol 15(4):721-726

55. Sheth T, Dodd JD, Hoffmann U et al (2007) Coronary stent assessability by 64 slice multidetector computed tomography. Catheter Cardiovasc Interv 69(7):933-938
56. Maintz D, Burg MC, Seifarth H et al (2009) Update on multidetector coronary CT angiography of coronary stents: in vitro evaluation of 29 different stent types with dual-source CT. Eur Radiol 19(1):42-49
57. Maintz D, Seifarth H, Flohr T et al (????) Improved coronary artery stent visualization and in-stent stenosis detection using 16-slice computed-tomography and dedicated image reconstruction technique. Invest Radiol 38(12):790-795
58. Maintz D, Juergens KU, Wichter T et al (2003) Imaging of coronary artery stents using multi-slice computed tomography: in vitro evaluation. Eur Radiol 13(4):830-835
59. Hong C, Chrysant GS, Woodard PK, Bae KT (2004) Coronary artery stent patency assessed with in-stent contrast enhancement measured at multi-detector row CT angiography: initial experience. Radiology 233(1):286-291
60. Pugliese F, Cademartiri F, van Mieghem C et al (2006) Multidetector CT for visualization of coronary stents. Radiographics 26(3):887-904
61. Lee CW, Suh J, Lee SW et al (2007) Factors predictive of cardiac events and restenosis after sirolimus-eluting stent implantation in small coronary arteries. Catheter Cardiovasc Interv 69(6):821-825
62. Lemos PA, Saia F, Ligthart JM et al (2003) Coronary restenosis after sirolimus-eluting stent implantation: morphological description and mechanistic analysis from a consecutive series of cases. Circulation 108(3):257-260
63. Kastrati A, Dibra A, Mehilli J et al (2006) Predictive factors of restenosis after coronary implantation of sirolimus- or paclitaxel-eluting stents. Circulation 16 113(19):2293-2300
64. Dangas GD, Claessen BE, Caixeta A et al (2010) In-stent restenosis in the drug-eluting stent era. J Am Coll Cardiol 30 56(23):1897-1907
65. Schmermund A, Haude M, Baumgart D et al (1996) Non-invasive assessment of coronary Palmaz-Schatz stents by contrast enhanced electron beam computed tomography. Eur Heart J 17(10):1546-1553
66. Knollmann FD, Moller J, Gebert A et al (2004) Assessment of coronary artery stent patency by electron-beam CT. Eur Radiol 14(8):1341-1347
67. Maintz D, Grude M, Fallenberg EM et al (2003) Assessment of coronary arterial stents by multislice-CT angiography. Acta Radiol 44(6):597-603
68. Ligabue G, Rossi R, Ratti C et al (2004) Noninvasive evaluation of coronary artery stents patency after PTCA: role of multislice computed tomography. Radiol Med 108(1-2):128-137
69. Kruger S, Mahnken AH, Sinha AM et al (2003) Multislice spiral computed tomography for the detection of coronary stent restenosis and patency. Int J Cardiol 89(2-3):167-172
70. Cademartiri F, Mollet N, Lemos PA et al (2005) Usefulness of multislice computed tomographic coronary angiography to assess in-stent restenosis. Am J Cardiol 96(6):799-802
71. Chabbert V, Carrie D, Bennaceur M et al (2007) Evaluation of in-stent restenosis in proximal coronary arteries with multidetector computed tomography (MDCT). Eur Radiol 17(6):1452-1463
72. Gilard M, Cornily JC, Pennec PY et al (2006) Assessment of coronary artery stents by 16 slice computed tomography. Heart 92(1):58-61
73. Gilard M, Cornily JC, Rioufol G et al (2005) Noninvasive assessment of left main coronary stent patency with 16-slice computed tomography. Am J Cardiol 95(1):110-112
74. Kefer JM, Coche E, Vanoverschelde JL, Gerber BL (2007) Diagnostic accuracy of 16-slice multidetector-row CT for detection of in-stent restenosis vs detection of stenosis in nonstented coronary arteries. Eur Radiol 17(1):87-96
75. Kitagawa T, Fujii T, Tomohiro Y et al (2006) Noninvasive assessment of coronary stents in patients by 16-slice computed tomography. Int J Cardiol 10 109(2):188-194
76. Ohnuki K, Yoshida S, Ohta M et al (2006) New diagnostic technique in multi-slice computed tomography for in-stent restenosis: pixel count method. Int J Cardiol 4 108(2):251-258
77. Schuijf JD, Bax JJ, Jukema JW et al (2004) Feasibility of assessment of coronary stent patency using 16-slice computed tomography. Am J Cardiol 94(4):427-430
78. Watanabe M, Uemura S, Iwama H et al (2006) Usefulness of 16-slice multislice spiral computed tomography for follow-up study of coronary stent implantation. Circ J 70(6):691-697
79. Cademartiri F, Schuijf JD, Pugliese F et al (2007) Usefulness of 64-slice multislice computed tomography coronary angiography to assess in-stent restenosis. J Am Coll Cardiol 5 49(22):2204-2210
80. Carbone I, Francone M, Algeri E et al (2008) Non-invasive evaluation of coronary artery

stent patency with retrospectively ECG-gated 64-slice CT angiography. Eur Radiol Feb 18(2): 234-243

81. Carrabba N, Bamoshmoosh M, Carusi LM et al (2007) Usefulness of 64-slice multidetector computed tomography for detecting drug eluting in-stent restenosis. Am J Cardiol 100(12):1754-1758

82. Das KM, El-Menyar AA, Salam AM et al (2007) Contrast-enhanced 64-section coronary multidetector CT angiography versus conventional coronary angiography for stent assessment. Radiology 245(2):424-432

83. Ehara M, Kawai M, Surmely JF et al (2007) Diagnostic accuracy of coronary in-stent restenosis using 64-slice computed tomography: comparison with invasive coronary angiography. J Am Coll Cardiol 49(9):951-959

84. Manghat N, Van Lingen R, Hewson P et al (2008) Usefulness of 64-detector row computed tomography for evaluation of intracoronary stents in symptomatic patients with suspected in-stent restenosis. Am J Cardiol 101(11):1567-1573

85. Nakamura K, Funabashi N, Uehara M et al (2008) Impairment factors for evaluating the patency of drug-eluting stents and bare metal stents in coronary arteries by 64-slice computed tomography versus conventional coronary angiography. Int J Cardiol 28 130(3):349-356

86. Oncel D, Oncel G, Karaca M (2007) Coronary stent patency and in-stent restenosis: determination with 64-section multidetector CT coronary angiography--initial experience. Radiology 42(2):403-409

87. Rist C, von Ziegler F, Nikolaou K et al (2006) Assessment of coronary artery stent patency and restenosis using 64-slice computed tomography. Acad Radiol 13(12):1465-1473

88. Rixe J, Achenbach S, Ropers D et al (2006) Assessment of coronary artery stent restenosis by 64-slice multi-detector computed tomography. Eur Heart J 27(21):2567-2572

89. Schuijf JD, Pundziute G, Jukema JW et al (2007) Evaluation of patients with previous coronary stent implantation with 64-section CT. Radiology 245(2):416-423

90. Van Mieghem CA, Cademartiri F, Mollet NR et al (2006) Multislice spiral computed tomography for the evaluation of stent patency after left main coronary artery stenting: a comparison with conventional coronary angiography and intravascular ultrasound. Circulation 15 114(7):645-653

91. Hecht HS, Zaric M, Jelnin V et al (2008) Usefulness of 64-detector computed tomographic angiography for diagnosing in-stent restenosis in native coronary arteries. Am J Cardiol 101(6):820-824

92. Andreini D, Pontone G, Bartorelli AL et al (2009) Comparison of feasibility and diagnostic accuracy of 64-slice multidetector computed tomographic coronary angiography versus invasive coronary angiography versus intravascular ultrasound for evaluation of in-stent restenosis. Am J Cardiol 15 103(10):1349-1358

93. Wykrzykowska JJ, Arbab-Zadeh A, Godoy G et al (2010) Assessment of in-stent restenosis using 64-MDCT: analysis of the CORE-64 Multicenter International Trial. AJR Am J Roentgenol 194(1):85-92

94. Abdelkarim MJ, Ahmadi N, Gopal A et al (2010) Noninvasive quantitative evaluation of coronary artery stent patency using 64-row multidetector computed tomography. J Cardiovasc Comput Tomogr 4(1):29-37

95. Carrabba N, Schuijf JD, de Graaf FR et al (2010) Diagnostic accuracy of 64-slice computed tomography coronary angiography for the detection of in-stent restenosis: a meta-analysis. J Nucl Cardiol 17(3):470-478

96. Kumbhani DJ, Ingelmo CP, Schoenhagen P et al (2009) Meta-analysis of diagnostic efficacy of 64-slice computed tomography in the evaluation of coronary in-stent restenosis. Am J Cardiol 15 103(12):1675-1681

97. Sun Z, Almutairi AM. Diagnostic accuracy of 64 multislice CT angiography in the assessment of coronary in-stent restenosis: a meta-analysis. Eur J Radiol 2010 Feb 73(2):266-273

98. Oncel D, Oncel G, Tastan A, Tamci B (2008) Evaluation of coronary stent patency and in-stent restenosis with dual-source CT coronary angiography without heart rate control. AJR Am J Roentgenol 191(1):56-63

99. Pugliese F, Weustink AC, Van Mieghem C et al (2008) Dual source coronary computed tomography angiography for detecting in-stent restenosis. Heart 94(7):848-854

100. Pflederer T, Marwan M, Renz A et al (2009) Noninvasive assessment of coronary in-stent restenosis by dual-source computed tomography. Am J Cardiol 15 103(6):812-817

101. de Graaf FR, Schuijf JD, van Velzen JE et al (2010) Diagnostic accuracy of 320-row multidetector computed tomography coronary angiography to noninvasively assess in-stent restenosis. Invest Radiol 45(6):331-340

102. Mark DB, Berman DS, Budoff MJ et al (2010) ACCF/ACR/AHA/NASCI/SAIP/SCAI/SCCT 2010 expert consensus document on coronary computed tomographic angiography: a report of the American College of Cardiology Foundation Task Force on Expert Consensus Documents. J Am Coll Cardiol 55(23):2663-2699
103. Taylor AJ, Cerqueira M, Hodgson JM et al (2010) ACCF/SCCT/ACR/AHA/ASE/ASNC/NASCI/SCAI/SCMR 2010 appropriate use criteria for cardiac computed tomography. A report of the American College of Cardiology Foundation Appropriate Use Criteria Task Force, the Society of Cardiovascular Computed Tomography, the American College of Radiology, the American Heart Association, the American Society of Echocardiography, the American Society of Nuclear Cardiology, the North American Society for Cardiovascular Imaging, the Society for Cardiovascular Angiography and Interventions, and the Society for Cardiovascular Magnetic Resonance. J Am Coll Cardiol 56(22):1864-1894
104. Bastarrika G, Lee YS, Ruzsics B, Schoepf UJ (2009) Coronary CT angiography: applications. Radiol Clin North Am 47(1):91-107

X-Ray Exposure in Coronary CT Angiography

Paolo Pavone and Roberto Leo

In coronary CT angiography (CTA), X-ray radiation is delivered through an X-ray tube from which the amount of radiation emitted can be carefully controlled. Recently, the use of X-rays for diagnostic purposes has been the subject of important and renewed attention, with the aim of limiting radiation exposure and thus its negative consequences on human health. The potential oncological impact of X-rays is well-known. Earlier generations of radiologists used diagnostic equipment often without the protection that has since become routine. Consequently, they often suffered dermatological problems on their hands as well as an increased frequency of tumors, mostly of the hematopoietic series. In the following, we focus on the unintentional exposure that occurs during a diagnostic evaluations, i.e., for coronary artery disease.

14.1 Damage from Ionizing Radiation

The damage induced by ionizing radiation can lead to tumor development. While this is a well-known fact, neither a definitive and consistent cause-andeffect relationship nor the incidence of tumors induced by exposure to diagnostic examinations can be measured or defined properly. In fact, the low amount of X-rays used in diagnostic examinations cannot have an immediate effect on human tissues (unless there has been continuous exposure, as in repeated and prolonged exposure during cardiac catheterizations). Direct damage by ionizing radiation can, however, be exactly forecasted and documented for therapeutic irradiation in radiotherapy, in the use of nuclear weapons (Hiroshima and Nagasaki), and in the course of unforeseen events at nuclear power stations (Chernobyl). In these cases, the immediate or delayed effect of ionizing radiation can be defined with precision, with the more radiosensitive organs, i.e., those with more active metabolism and high cellular turnover, being the most vulnerable.

In the diagnostic use of ionizing radiation, the damage is hypothetical and cannot be evaluated immediately. Brenner and Hall, in a study published in 2007, concluded that, following the atomic bombing of Hiroshima, approximately 25,000 people who were far from the central area of atomic fall-out were exposed to an amount of radiation similar to that used during diagnostic CT. However, the comparison is not entirely valid, since radiation exposure due to atomic fall-out is continuous in time and involves the entire body uniformly; the exposure during diagnostic CT, by contrast, is controlled, with X-ray exposure of only a limited part of the body (collimated exposure) and for a very short time (in the range of seconds). Thus, such claims have to be evaluated with extreme care, and scientific proof of the damage caused by diagnostic exposure to X-rays remains to be definitively determined.

P. Pavone (✉)
Radiology Department
Casa di Cura Mater Dei
Rome, Italy
e-mail: paolo.pavone@materdei.it

Table 14.1 Typical organ radiation dose from various cardiological diagnostic examinations (from Dowe D (2006) Radiological Society of North America)

Procedure	Dose (mSv)
Coronary catheter angiography	6-9
Coronary CTA	7-13
Interventional coronary procedure	20
SPECT Thallium, Persinakis et al (2002)	25.3
SPECT sesta-MIBI, Persinakis et al (2002)	12.2

14.2 X-Ray Dose During CT

Table 14.1 provides a direct comparison of the X-ray dose used in frequently performed cardiac diagnostic procedures, including coronary CTA, as measured in mSievert (m Sv). Overall, coronary CTA exposes patients to a high dose of X-rays, in the range of 7–13 mSv. In fact, with current procedures, X-rays are emitted throughout cardiac image acquisition, despite the fact that the computer, during image reconstruction, utilizes only a small portion of the data acquired, i.e., those obtained in the telediastolic part of the ECG. Therefore, for clinical purposes, a consistent part of cardiac irradiation is unnecessary and corresponds to an excess X-ray dose of over 80%.

14.3 Techniques for Limiting X-Ray Exposure in Coronary CT Angiography

New techniques aimed at drastically reducing the amount of X-ray exposure during coronary CTA have recently been proposed. Here, we consider three that have been used successfully.

The first technique is available as part of every type of CT equipment and allows a proportional reduction of X-ray exposure according to the patient's size and weight. The procedure is fully automated and evaluates body thickness and tissue consistency (in terms of X-ray penetration) in order to reduce, slice by slice and moment by moment, the amount of X-rays emitted, measured in milliamperes. For example, higher doses are required for the abdomen than for the chest, which contains air. This technique reduces unnecessary X-ray exposure by 30–40%. Furthermore, for thinner patients, the radiologist can manually reduce X-ray exposure by reducing the kV values.

In the second, recently proposed technique, X-ray exposure is controlled and it is limited to the telediastolic phase through the use of a prospective gating procedure. In this so-called snap and shoot approach, each data packet, corresponding to an anatomic area containing a thick slice of the heart (4 cm for 64-slice CT), is acquired during an axial rotation of the X-ray tube, with emission only in the telediastolic phase. Immediately afterwards, the table is moved to the next anatomic area and the data are again acquired (the spiral procedure is therefore not used during data acquisition). These steps are repeated four to five times until the entire anatomical area containing the heart has been scanned (Fig. 14.1). This technique reduces the X-ray dose from 15–20 mSv to 2–3 mSv, according to patient configuration. Its one major limitation is that it excludes the use of spiral acquisition and instead requires single axial acquisitions, possibly leading to overlap artifacts in the single thick slices acquired during each telediastolic phase.

An alternative to this technique uses a prospective gating procedure, but rather than obtaining axial slices with stepwise movement of the patient table, it allows spiral acquisition of the data. The X-ray tube continuously emits radiation during the acquisition procedure, but emission is very low during the cardiac cycle (only 4% of the standard emission) and increases to the amount needed for diagnostic imaging only in the telediastolic phase (Fig. 14.2). There are no artifacts arising from the overlap of each thick volume (as in the previous technique), since the acquisition is fully spiral. A dose reduction of 50–60% has been estimated.

Figure 14.3 illustrates a case in which, with the patient's consent, a snap and shoot acquisition was followed by a second acquisition using spiral technique with dose reduction. In the three-dimensional and bi-dimensional images, there are no major differences in the image quality and diagnostic evaluation of the coronary arteries. The dose exposure was 2 mSv with snap and shoot and 12 mSv using the spiral procedure.

Fig. 14.1 Snap and shoot axial acquisition: X-rays are emitted by the tube only during telediastole (blue stripe in the ECG gating scheme of the console)

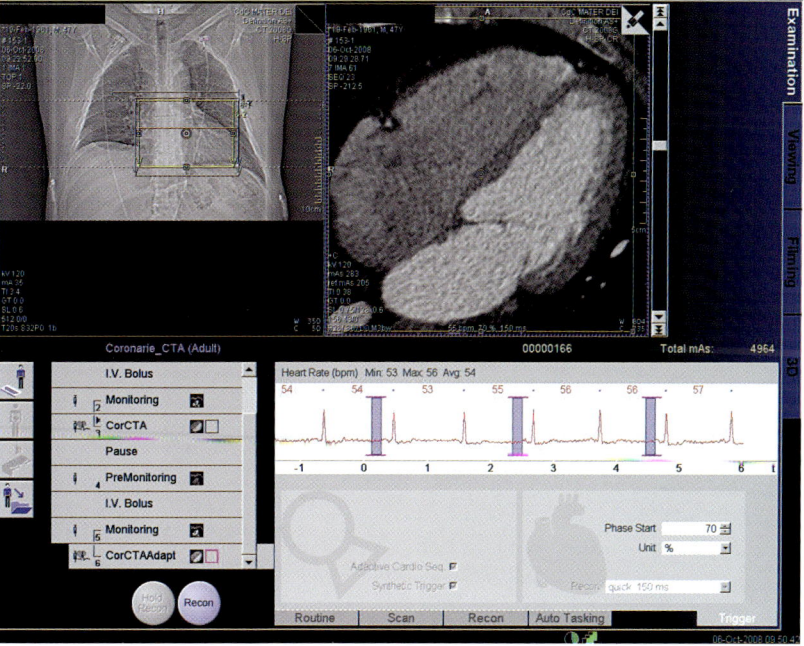

Fig. 14.2 Spiral acquisition with reduced X-ray exposure. During systole, 4% of the radiation dose is emitted, whereas during the time frame when telediastole is expected (light blue area in the scheme) the full dose is emitted. Thus, it is possible to define the width of the area of maximal exposure

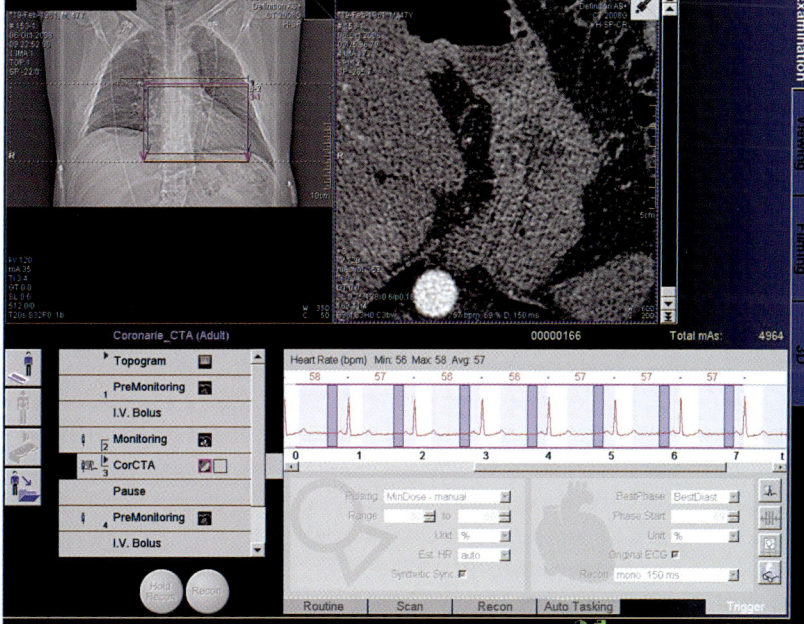

Large-array detectors, with single-slice acquisition of the entire anatomical area containing the heart, modulate X-ray emission, limiting patient exposure to the telediastolic phase and avoiding overlap-type artifacts in the acquisition of thick volumes.

Lately a new raw-data reconstruction technique, referred to as "iterative reconstruction", has been developed to reduce the radiation dose and to increase image quality. In CT, iterative reconstruction achieves both an improvement in

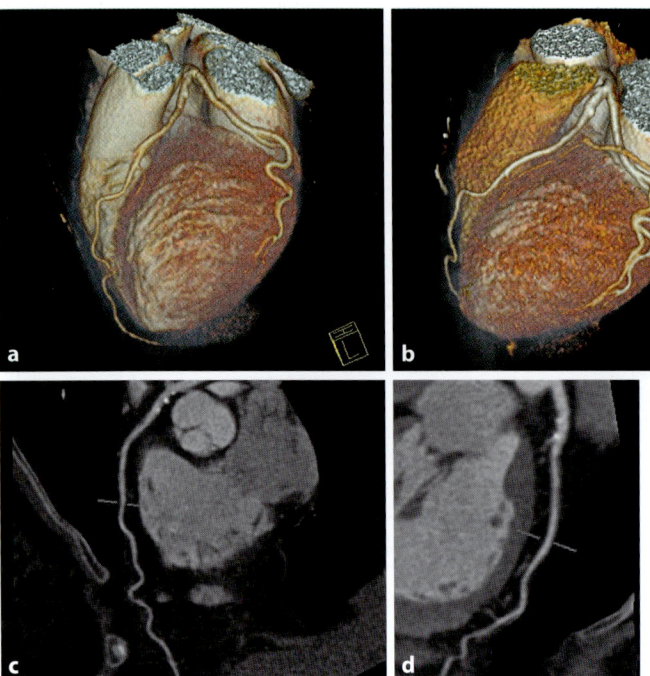

Fig. 14.3 a-d A 74-year-old female patient. Data acquisition using (**a**, **c**) snap and shoot technique (2 mSv exposure) and (**b**, **d**) spiral acquisition (12 mSv exposure). Image quality is basically the same. **a**, **b** Three-dimensional volume-rendering image. **c**, **d** Bi-dimensional images of the same data sets

image quality and a reduction in the radiation dose relative to the currently used filtered back projection techniques. The most noticeable benefit of iterative reconstruction is that it is able to incorporate into the reconstruction process a physical model of the CT system that can accurately characterize the data acquisition process, including noise, beam hardening, and scatter. This ability allows for dramatic improvements in image quality, especially in the case of low-dose CT scans, in which the propagation of non-ideal data during image reconstruction becomes more significant than in routine CT scanning. Iterative reconstruction is also superior to filtered back projection in handling insufficient data. Recent advances in iterative reconstruction allow a significant reduction in the number of required projection views, while still producing acceptable image quality. The use of iterative reconstruction techniques thus has the potential to substantially reduce the radiation dose in CT. With computational power growing quickly, the clinical implementation of iterative reconstruction algorithms is within delivery.

14.4 X-Ray Exposure and Patient Age

The damage caused by X-rays is directly related to the age of the patient. In children, the radiosensitivity of growing organs and the fact that exposure has occurred before the patient reaches his or her adult years, together with the fact that he or she will almost inevitably undergo further X ray diagnostic procedures in the future, allow a more definitive cause-and-effect relationship to be established. Pediatric radiologists are fully aware of this problem and thus of the need to use alternative diagnostic procedure, e.g., magnetic resonance imaging and ultrasound.

In elderly patients, damage due to ionizing radiations is statistically less relevant and the statistical incidence of oncological problems is correspondingly lower. In the evaluation of the heart by coronary CTA, only a limited area of the body is exposed and X-ray emission is controlled and collimated, with protection of contiguous anatomic areas through the use of more effective diaphragms that exclude the irradiation of nearby tissues. Thus, in coronary CTA, irradiation is limited to the portion of the lungs surrounding the heart, and, for female patients, the breast tissues. To further reduce unwanted irradiation, bismuth-based mildly radio-opaque breast shields are available.

14.5 Conclusion

In considering the relationship between coronary CTA and the tissue damage ensuing from the radiation exposure that is an integral part of this examination, several points must be mentioned.

Firstly, there is the option of using less radiation. Initial techniques employed a high dose of X-ray radiation, with exposures similar to those incurred with cardiac catheterization and nuclear medicine procedures. Nowadays, prospective gating procedures allow a dose reduction of 60–80%, resulting in the controlled and limited exposure of a defined anatomic area and to exposure amounts that are similar to those of other current and widely used CT diagnostic procedures.

Secondly, there is the matter of exam repetition. In the USA, patients are frequently and repeatedly exposed to X-rays due to repetitions of diagnostic examinations (this is particularly true in traumatology and oncology). It has been calculated that, during a patient's recovery in the hospital, the total X-ray radiation exposure is 20–40 mSv. CTA, however, is an examination that is performed only once, to evaluate the anatomic status of the coronary arteries. If repetition of the exam is deemed necessary, it will not be until many years later.

Thirdly, the patient's age must be considered. Coronary CTA is indicated for the evaluation of atherosclerotic disease; thus, the patients are older, usually 55–65 years. In this population, the radiosensitivity of the organs is reduced and the potential oncological risk due to ionizing-radiation exposure is limited if not irrelevant, when careful exposure is performed.

Finally, there are risk-benefit considerations. When proposing CTA to a patient, the cardiologist and the radiologist have to evaluate the benefit that may come from a proper evaluation of the atherosclerotic burden on the coronary arteries, the advantage gained by properly characterizing a plaque in terms of the correct pharmaceutical approach, and the possibility to identify vascular stenosis, which may be amenable to stenting or re-vascularization procedures. Therefore, the proper, limited use of ionizing radiation is to be proposed in the presence of well-defined clinical indications for this procedure.

Suggested Reading

Park EA, Lee W, Kim KW et al (2011) Iterative reconstruction of dual-source coronary CT angiography: assessment of image quality and radiation dose. Int J Cardiovasc Imaging. 2011 Dec 21. [Epub ahead of print] PubMed PMID: 22187198

Renker M, Ramachandra A, Schoepf UJ et al (2011) Iterative image reconstruction techniques: Applications for cardiac CT. J Cardiovasc Comput Tomogr 5(4):225-230. Epub 2011 May 25. PubMed PMID: 21723513

Renker M, Nance JW Jr, Schoepf UJ et al (2011) Evaluation of heavily calcified vessels with coronary CT angiography: comparison of iterative and filtered back projection image reconstruction. Radiology 260(2):390-399. Epub 2011 Jun 21. PubMed PMID: 21693660

Optical Coherence Tomography in the Cathlab

15

Francesco Prati and Luca Di Vito

15.1 Physical Principles of OCT and Technical Issues

Optical coherence tomography (OCT) is an imaging modality that uses light instead of sound and offers significantly better resolution than obtained with intravascular ultrasound (IVUS) [1, 2]. In fact, as a result of the very short wavelength of the imaging light, OCT resolution is 10–15 µm and thus about 10 times higher than that of IVUS. There are two main technologies that can be used to obtain OCT images: time domain (TD) and frequency domain (FD) [2-4].

TD is the older technology; it consists of long and complicated procedures to clear the vessel of blood and has a lower resolution than FD-OCT (Table 15.1). Images are obtained with the M3 LightLab OCT wire (Imagewire), which has an outer diameter of 0.048 cm and contains a 0.015-cm fiber-optic imaging core (< 0.4 mm in diameter). The distal radio-opaque spring tip of the TD-OCT image-wire is similar to conventional guide-wires.

The FD-OCT catheter is designed for rapid-exchange delivery and is compatible with a conventional 0.036-cm angioplasty guide-wire, inserted in a short monorail lumen at the tip. The main advantage of FD-OCT is that the technology enables rapid imaging of the coronary artery, with long coronary segments scanned in a few seconds at a maximum pull-back speed of 25 mm/s.

F. Prati (✉)
Interventional Cardiology
San Giovanni Hospital, Rome, Italy
e-mail: fprati@hsangiovanni.roma.it

Table 15.1 The main differences between TD-OCT and FD-OCT

	TD-OCT	FD-OCT
Pull-back speed, mm/s	3	20
Frame rate, fps	20	100
Lines per frame	240	500
Axial resolution, µm	10–20	10–20
Lateral resolution, µm	25–30	25–30
Penetration depth, mm	1.5–2	1.5–2
Scan diameter, mm	7	10

The penetration depth of OCT is between 0.5 and 2.0 mm in most tissue types and remains the chief limitation of the technique, because optical scattering losses and tissue attenuation limit light penetration and focusing in vascular tissues. Nevertheless, many OCT experts agree that a slight improvement in the penetration depth of FD-OCT compared to TD-OCT can be appreciated in most tissues.

15.1.1 Image Acquisition

As TD-OCT will soon be universally replaced by FD-OCT, the focus here is restricted to aspects of OCT acquisition obtained with the latter system.

The main obstacle to the adoption of OCT imaging in clinical practice is that OCT cannot image through a blood field, as infrared light cannot penetrate red blood cells. Therefore, unlike IVUS, OCT requires the clearing or flushing of blood from the lumen.

The acquisition technique of FD-OCT has been optimized following the concept specifically de-

Table 15.2 Differences in plaque assessment between IVUS and OCT

	Resolution (μ)	Fibrous cap	Lipid	Calcium	Thrombus
IVUS	150-200	+	++	+++	+
OCT	15-20	+++	+++	++	++

veloped for the non-occlusive modality of acquisitions carried out with TD-OCT [2]. Contrast solution, due to its viscosity, can displace blood cells for a sufficient period of time such that OCT images can be recorded from the coronary segment of interest. Obviously, the fact that FD-OCT images can be obtained at speeds up to 25 mm/s implies the acquisition of long coronary segments in a very short time. The size of the OCT image is first calibrated by adjusting the z-offset, i.e., the zero-point setting of the system. In FD-OCT systems, the calibration procedure can be done in a fully automated modality. To maintain accurate measurements, the z-offset must be readjusted prior to off-line analysis and monitored throughout the longitudinal segment.

The OCT probe is first positioned over a regular guide-wire, distal to the region of interest. Identification of the pull-back starting point is a simple task, as a dedicated marker identifies the exact position of the OCT lens, located 10 mm proximal to the marker itself. The acquisition of a rapid OCT image sequence with fast pull-back can be automatically started by the injection of a bolus of contrast medium through the guiding catheter, with the acquisition speed set between 5 and 25 mm/s. The infusion rate of contrast is usually set to 3–4 ml/s for the left coronary artery and 2–3 ml/s for the right coronary, but it can be modified based on vessel run-off and size.

Pull-back can begin automatically when blood clearance is distally recognized, but manual activation is also possible. At an acquisition speed of 20 mm/s, 200 cross-sectional image frames can be obtained over a 4- to 5-cm length of artery in 3.5 s, with a total infused volume of 14 ml of contrast. In percutaneous interventions (PCIs), this is a definite advantage of FD-OCT since both the stent and the landing zones can be evaluated quickly. Since the FD-OCT pull-back speed is too fast to interpret the run during the acquisition, the recorded images are stored digitally for later review in a slow playback loop.

15.1.2 Comparison with IVUS

The assessment of target lesions by IVUS is frequently demanding. IVUS probes tend to occlude the lumen in tight lesions during the time required to acquire pull-back images at low pull-back speed (0.5–1.0 mm/s); consequently, symptoms and signs of myocardial ischemia may develop, while blood stagnation can complicate subsequent image interpretation. In OCT, however, the high acquisition speed and the miniaturization of the OCT probes, which have a slightly thinner profile than IVUS probes, make vessel imaging more user-friendly (Table 15.2).

Although recent papers have shown the ability of FD-OCT to image the left main coronary artery, this tract of the coronary tree still represents a limitation of the technique, due to the relatively wide dimension of this artery, which complicates the clearing of blood from the vessel during image acquisition.

15.2 Safety and Effectiveness

Previous experiences with TD-OCT technology, either occlusive or non-occlusive, showed OCT acquisition to be safe and effective [2]. OCT provides excellent differentiation between the lumen and the arterial wall, facilitating the determination of lumen areas and volumes as well as the depiction of stent struts with high accuracy [2]. Furthermore, early studies in which lumen, stent, and neointimal areas were quantitatively measured revealed a high reproducibility, primarily driven by the high resolution of the technology [2].

Preliminary data on the safety of FD-OCT technology are even more promising. In an early study based on 14 patients [4] and a more recent one on 90 patients with coronary artery disease no complications were reported. In fact, no ischemic ECG changes or arrhythmias developed during the short injection period. This was attributed to the marked simplification of the acquisition procedures and the consequent reduction in the required contrast volume [4, 5]. Thus, FD-OCT was judged to be highly effective, as it allows the study of longer segments with clearer images than obtained with TD-OCT [4, 5]. However, as with TD-OCT, FD-OCT image quality depends on an accurate acquisition technique and proper guiding-catheter engagement in order to optimize directional contrast flushing.

In general, OCT can negotiate tortuous calcific arteries better than IVUS. In our experience, comprising over 400 vessels imaged with OCT, only very diffuse calcific arteries are not suitable for OCT imaging. Also, after stenting, the OCT probe may become stuck at the proximal edge due to a non-complete apposition. In such cases, gentle maneuvers are often successful in pushing the probe downward, unless there is a very tortuous and calcific anatomy.

15.3 Assessment of the Vessel Wall and Atherosclerosis

15.3.1 Normal Coronary Morphology

Unlike IVUS, OCT can both clearly distinguish the intimal from the medial layer of the coronary arterial wall and measure its thickness, which is 125–350 μm (mean 200 μm) [2]. The media appears as a dark band, delimited by the internal elastic lamina and external elastic lamina. However the assessment of a normal intima is beyond the resolution of OCT because the intimal layer is only approximately 4 μm thick, which corresponds to a small sub-endothelial collagen layer and a single layer of endothelial cells that in the normal vessels of children and young people is flattened. This limitation is of utmost importance in the study of stent follow-up, as OCT can identify the presence of strut coverage but not the presence of a physiologic stent surface covered with endothelial cells.

The limited penetration of OCT does not consistently enable the study of vessel remodeling, which is well addressed by IVUS. Remodeling is defined as medial thinning in the areas of plaque accumulation as a result of asymmetric expansion of the vessel wall.

Nearly all coronary arteries of adults show some grade of intimal thickness, as it increases with age.

15.3.2 Assessment of Atherosclerosis

As noted above, OCT allows the study of plaque components at a very high resolution, however, this comes at the cost of limited penetration such that the assessment of deeper structures is difficult. Jang et al., in one of the first comparisons between OCT and IVUS, found that the former led to a more precise measurement of the thickness of the fibrous cap and improved the study of structures located behind superficial macro-calcification [2]. Furthermore, OCT was able to identify with high accuracy tissue components such as intimal hyperplasia and lipid-rich plaques.

It is well known that angiography is of poor sensitivity in the detection of calcific deposits, especially when their radial extension is < 180°. IVUS is able to identify calcium with a high degree of accuracy, although the shadowing effect caused by these deposits prevents measurement of their thickness. Infrared light better penetrates calcium, but calcific components with a thickness > 1–1.3 mm can prove impossible to penetrate. Thus, calcium deposits with a deep intra-plaque location may be missed with OCT. However this event is rather uncommon as calcium deposits are often sub-endothelial.

Unlike angiography or IVUS, however, OCT is able to identify thrombi, measuring their dimensions and guiding their removal (Fig. 15.1) [6].

15.3.3 Qualitative Descriptions

The distinction at OCT between calcium and a lipid pool is not easy as these tissue components have a similar appearance. Calcifications are seen

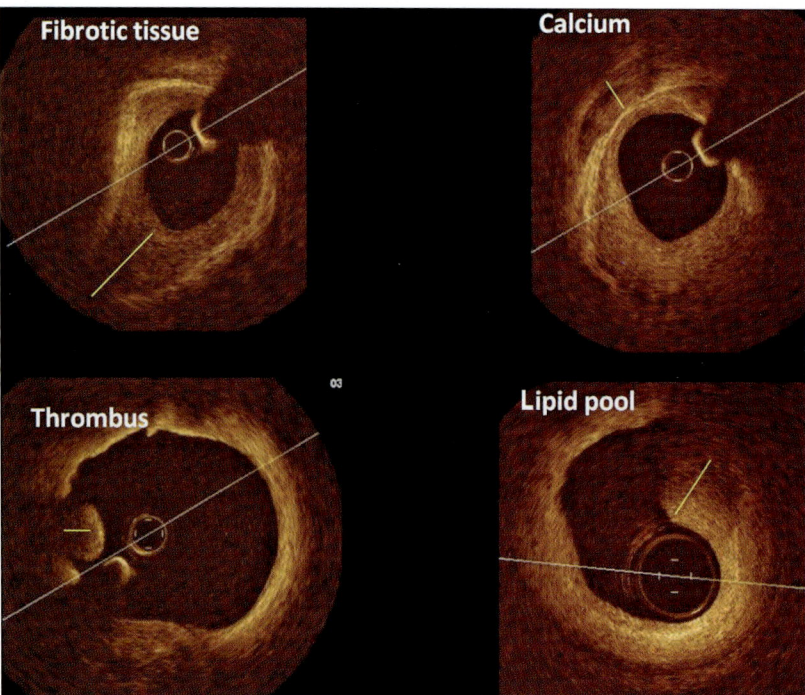

Fig. 15.1 Examples of plaque components at OCT. OCT penetration (lines in all quadrants) is affected by plaque composition

as well-delineated, low back-scattering heterogeneous regions [2] whilst necrotic lipid pools most often appear as diffusely-bordered, signal-poor regions (lipid pools) with overlying signal-rich bands, corresponding to fibrous caps [2]. Fibrous plaques consist of homogeneous high back-scattering areas [2]. OCT can also identify superficial micro-calcifications, as small calcific deposits that subtend an angle < 90° and are separated from the lumen by a rim of tissue < 100-μm thick [2].

In contrast to IVUS, OCT identifies thrombi with high accuracy. The appearance of thrombi on IVUS is similar to that of lipid components but thrombi may be recognized as relatively echolucent formations. However, a stagnant blood flow can simulate a thrombus such that the diagnosis of thrombus by IVUS should always be considered presumptive [7]. The ability of OCT to identify thrombi is extremely important as they are the ultimate events leading to acute coronary syndrome, and OCT is the ideal technique to identify culprit lesions in uncertain cases.

Thrombi are identified by OCT as masses protruding into the vessel lumen that are discontinuous from the surface of the vessel wall. Red thrombi consist mainly of red blood cells; the relevant OCT images show high-backscattering protrusions with signal-free shadowing. White thrombi consist mainly of platelets and white blood cells and are characterized by signal-rich, low-backscattering billowing projections protruding into the lumen [2].

15.3.4 Quantitative Descriptions

It must be emphasized that the identification and quantification of atherosclerotic plaque components by OCT both depend on the penetration depth of the incident light beam into the vessel wall. The depth of penetration is greatest for fibrous tissue and least for thrombi, with calcium and lipid tissue having intermediate values.

OCT is able to penetrate superficial calcium deposits and measure their thicknesses if they do not exceed 1.0–0.5 mm. As OCT does not penetrate superficial necrotic lipid pools as well as it does calcified and fibrous tissues, the thickness of lipid pools cannot be measured in the majority of lesions

[2]. However, OCT does allow measurement of the thickness of the fibrous cap that delimits superficial lipid pools. Fibrous-cap thickness can be obtained either as a single measurement at the cross-section where its thickness is considered minimal or as the average of multiple (three or more) samples [2].

The arc (in degrees) and the longitudinal extent of calcific deposits or superficial necrotic lipid pools can be measured (in degrees) with a protractor positioned in the center of the lumen [2]. A semi-quantitative grading system is used to classify these plaque components according to the number of quadrants they subtend [1-4].

OCT can also be applied to identify inflammatory cells, such as clusters of macrophages. Streaks of macrophages or foam cells are seen as bands of high reflectivity in OCT images. When they are located in a plaque with a lipid pool, macrophage streaks become visible within the fibrous cap covering the lipid pool. To identify inflammatory cells with sufficient specificity and sensitivity, dedicated algorithms should be applied [8].

15.5 Localization of Plaques with High-Risk Morphology

Pathological studies carried out in patients who died due to acute coronary syndromes identified the morphology of vulnerable plaques. In line with previous data, OCT studies confirmed that culprit plaques of patients with acute coronary syndrome (ACS) have a higher lipid content, a thinner fibrous cap, and greater macrophage concentration than non-culprit sites [9]. In addition, patients with acute myocardial infarction were more likely to have thrombus and thin cap fibrous atheromas in the non-culprit lesion. OCT confirmed the histological finding that ruptured plaques are mainly located in the proximal segments (proximal 30 mm) of the vessel [2].

Moreover, morphological differences are not restricted to patients with or without ACS, but are also present between different presentations of ACS. According to Tanaka et al., plaque rupture in exertion-onset ACS is associated with greater fibrous cap thickness and is more often located at the shoulder of the plaque [10].

15.4 Pathophysiology of Acute Coronary Syndromes

Acute plaque ulceration or rupture can be detected by OCT as a ruptured fibrous cap that connects the lumen with the lipid pool. These ulcerated or ruptured plaques may occur with or without a superimposed thrombus. When signs of ulceration are present without evidence of thrombosis, the lesion cannot be defined as a "culprit" with certainty, unless clinical criteria provide evidence that the lesion is responsible for the acute events. The use of thrombolysis, IIb-IIIa GP inhibitors, or other antithrombotic drugs facilitates clot degradation and in some circumstances will lead to the complete disappearance of the clot.

The identification of erosion as a mechanism of plaque instability is a challenge even for a technique with a resolution below 20 μm. A thrombosis with an apparently normal endothelial lining underneath may be indicative of erosion.

15.6 Plaque Morphology, Vulnerability and Progression

Changes in plaque volume in response to specific treatments aimed at regression or the cessation of progression are mainly identified by IVUS. In this setting, OCT may prove to be an important addition because it can discriminate among the different plaque components, whose changes may be important in serial studies.

Preliminary data indicate that statin therapy is associated with certain plaque characteristics. In fact, patients under statin therapy have a lower incidence of plaque rupture than control patients. Furthermore, in a prospective study with 3-month follow-up OCT examination, statin therapy was shown to increase the thickness of the fibrous cap in the culprit lesions of patients with stable angina. This occurred only in the presence of a thin fibrous cap at baseline assessment [11].

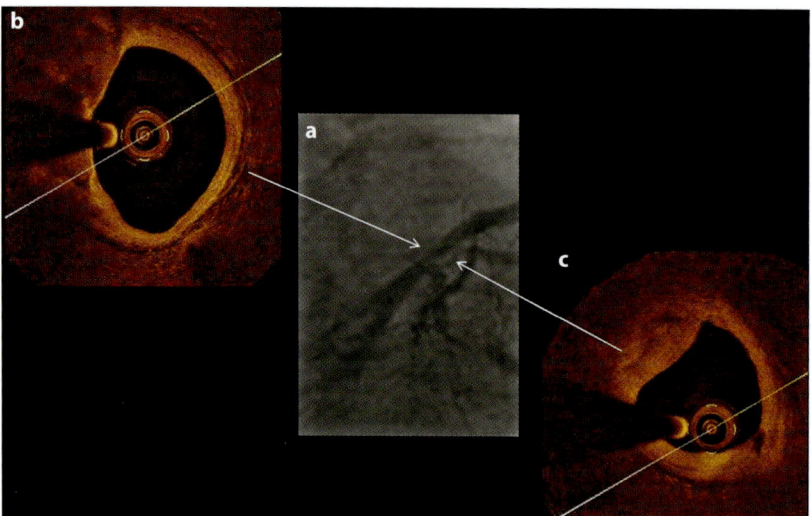

Fig. 15.2 OCT details vessel anatomy of a moderate distal left main disease at angiography (**a**). OCT shows a significant lesion of the distal left main, with a minimal lumen area of 5.4 mm^2 (**b**), and reveals a non-significant lesion (3.7 mm^2) at the left circumflex ostium

However, robust validation studies are needed to verify whether OCT is capable of measuring serial changes in plaque components indicative of vulnerability, such as fibrous cap thickness or lipid pool extension. It is possible that OCT will one day play a role in assessing the risk of myocardial infarction. Also, due to its ability to address plaque components, OCT can be used to relate plaque morphology to clinical characteristics. Surprisingly, plaque composition is similar among diabetics and non-diabetics.

15.7 Current Clinical Applications. Advantages and Disadvantages of OCT vs. IVUS

15.7.1 Evaluation of Intermediate Stenoses and Ambiguous Lesions

Normal angiograms or angiograms with minimal irregularities are found in around 10–15% of patients undergoing coronary angiography for suspected coronary artery disease. Like IVUS, OCT can confirm the absence of significant atherosclerosis or indicate the degree of subclinical atherosclerotic lesion formation. This is of importance to defer coronary intervention.

Suboptimal angiographic visualization impairs the accurate assessment of stenosis severity. This may happen in the presence of intermediate lesions of uncertain severity, very short lesions, pre- or post-aneurysmal lesions, ostial or left main stem stenoses, disease at branching sites, sites with focal spasm, or angiographically hazy lesions. OCT has the potential to become a routine clinical tool to guide interventional procedures as it provides accurate luminal measurements of lesion severity due to a better delineation of the lumen-wall interface than achieved with IVUS.

Like IVUS, OCT is able to quantify lesion severity more accurately than quantitative coronary angiography by measuring a minimal lumen area < 2.4–3.0 mm^2. This should be considered the significant cut-off threshold for flow-limiting stenosis in appropriately sized (> 3 mm) vessels, excluding the left main coronary artery [12]. In the presence of left main disease, the most commonly used threshold is 6.0 mm^2. Further validation studies may be needed to corroborate these values (Fig. 15.2).

In particular, OCT is indicated for the assessment of angiographically hazy lesions and focal vessel spasm. In the former, OCT often detects ruptured plaques with thrombus attached to the site of rupture of the fibrous cap over a partially emptied lipid pool. Under these circumstances the decision to proceed with treatment is

Fig. 15.3 Deployment of a drug-eluting stent in the right coronary artery. OCT shows a well expanded stent (**b**) and a dissection distal to the stent edge (**c**), that was missed by angiography (**a**)

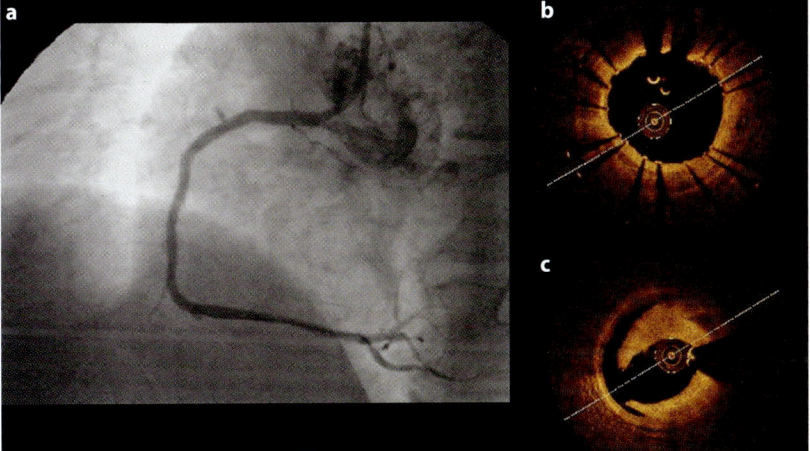

more often based on these morphologic observations than on the absolute measurement of lumen area.

15.7.2 Post-intervention Assessment: The Rationale for Using Imaging Modalities

Optimization of stent expansion is of critical importance in the prevention of late in-stent re-stenosis, based on the concept that measurement of minimum stent area is the most powerful predictor of long-term patency and clinical outcomes. For bare metal stents, multiple studies have addressed the use of IVUS-guided expansion to reduce re-stenosis and thrombosis. While the results have been conflicting, meta-analyses identified a potential advantage, particularly in complex lesions [13]. The same considerations apply to drug-eluting stents (DESs); in fact, a threshold of absolute minimal lumen cross-sectional area within the stent of at least 5.0–5.5 mm^2 has been advocated as the target minimum stent area to prevent failure. A significant difference in mortality was also observed between IVUS and angiographic guidance after left main stenting [13].

A further motivation to rely on intravascular imaging modalities to improve clinical results and safety is the fact that stents, including DES, rarely achieve the nominal area, with the average being 66 ± 17% of the predicted minimal lumen area [13].

15.7.3 The Potential of OCT in Stent Guidance

Using OCT, the minimal stent area can be easily compared with the reference area, which is the most-often used IVUS criterion for optimal stent expansion. Unlike IVUS, OCT has sufficient resolution to detect mild levels of malapposition, to visualize small intra-stent thrombotic formations, and to perform a per-strut analysis of the thickness of intimal coverage. In the presence of stent under-expansion or haziness within the stent or at the stent edges, which may be due to plaque prolapse or edge dissection, OCT can precisely identify and quantify these phenomena (Figs. 15.3, 15.4).

Malapposition can contribute to stent thrombosis by disturbing the normal laminar blood flow along the vessel wall and promoting the deposition of platelets and fibrin. Also, the persistence of acute and late-acquired malapposition is associated with reduced re-endothelialization and neointima formation, which may lead to platelet adhesion and subsequent thrombotic stent occlusion. However, to date, the role of malapposition as a cause of stent thrombosis is unclear. Based on IVUS data, stent malapposition does not increase the risk of major adverse cardiac events . This may be due to the fact that IVUS identifies only gross malapposition.

OCT is capable of detecting very small thrombotic depositions on stent struts, a common finding in patients with ACS after stenting of the

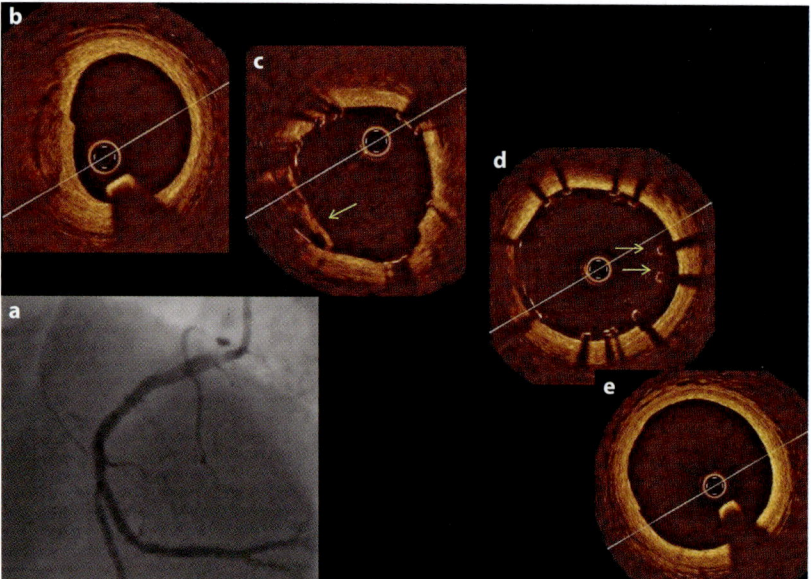

Fig. 15.4 Optimal angiographic result after deployment of a drug-eluting stent in the right coronary artery (**a**). OCT shows an under-expanded stent. At the site of minimal stent area (**c**), the stent is smaller than the distal reference (**b**) and the proximal reference (**e**) and exhibits some tissue prolapse (*arrows*). In the proximal portion, the stent appears non-apposed (*arrows* in **d**)

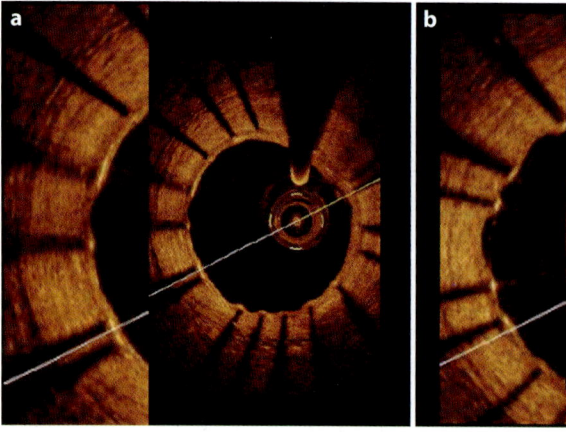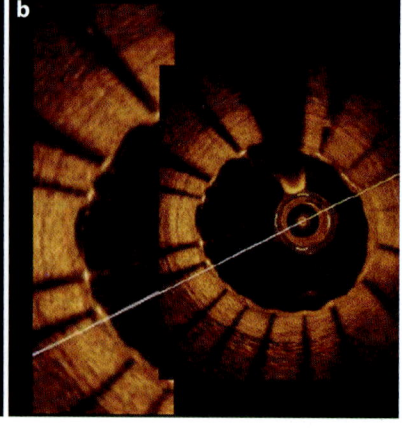

Fig. 15.5 OCT detection of covered stent struts (**a**), and uncovered stent struts (**b**)

culprit lesion [1]. Although the clinical significance of this finding is still unknown, it is reasonable to hypothesize that the presence of thrombus after stenting elevates the risk for acute and sub-acute stent thrombosis. This may also influence the decision to use adjuvant pharmacological therapies, including glycoprotein IIb/IIIa receptor antagonists, at the time of stenting.

15.7.4 Stent Follow-Up

Conventional stents develop circumferential coverage with an average thickness of 500 mm or more and are thus well visualized with IVUS and angiography. By contrast, in DESs the hyperplastic response is delayed or even prevented, so that the average late lumen loss for these stents can be < 100 mm, which means that this amount of intimal thickening will not be detectable by IVUS. Further, although coronary angioscopy is able to visualize strut tissue coverage, this highly specialized technique is not quantitative and is therefore not used in practice, except in a few research centers in Japan. Hence, OCT is an attractive alternative as it is able to circumvent many of these limitations and to assess the in-vivo tissue response following stent implantation (Fig. 15.5).

DES technology has been associated with a small but statistically significant increase in late and very late stent thrombosis. Delayed healing and poor endothelialization are common findings in pathologic specimens of vessels treated with DES. In addition, recent post-mortem studies demonstrated that late stent thrombosis is highly associated with the ratio of uncovered/total stent struts [14]. OCT anecdotal studies in patients with stent thrombosis revealed a high incidence of strut non-coverage. OCT is now an established method to verify the presence of stent coverage despite the fact that it is unable to identify the endothelium [1]. Follow-up OCT data revealed that most of the DESs were covered with a thin neointima, but complete coverage was rare [15]. The DETECTIVE study [16] reported a high percentage of stent coverage in the early phase (4–7 days after implantation). OCT follow-up studies showed that the frequency of uncovered stent struts was 15% at 3 months but only 5% two years after stenting with sirolimus-eluting stents. Zotarolimus-eluting stents showed a very high incidence of strut coverage at 6 months on a per patient analysis [15].

Recent data revealed that incomplete stent apposition and the absence of tissue coverage are more frequently detected by OCT in patients presenting with ACS. This finding likely reflects the presence of thrombus, a milieu that facilitates the malapposition of stent struts and hampers the process of vessel healing. Furthermore, in patients with ST elevation myocardial infarction, DES deployment was shown to increase the risk of incomplete strut apposition and lack of coverage.

It is difficult to offer any recommendation at this stage for the use of OCT in the late follow-up of individual patients. Instead, these are anecdotal cases of OCT applications to rule out the prolongation of dual antiplatelet treatment in patients requiring non-deferrable surgery. Currently, the main application is the comparison of different stent platforms, assuming that a more uniform strut coverage is expected to improve late outcome.

Acknowledgement We are thankful to the CLI Foundation for supporting this manuscript.

References

1. Jang IK, Tearney GJ, MacNeill B et al (2005) In vivo characterization of coronary atherosclerotic plaque by use of Optical Coherence Tomography. Circulation 111:1551-1555
2. Prati F, Regar E, Mintz GS et al for the Expert's OCT Review Document (2010) Expert review document on methodology and clinical applications of OCT. Physical principles, methodology of image acquisition and clinical application for assessment of coronary arteries and atherosclerosis. Eur Heart J 31:401-415
3. Tearney GJ, Waxman S, Shishkov M et al (2008) Three-dimensional coronary artery microscopy by intracoronary Optical Frequency Domain Imaging. J Am Coll Cardiol Img 1:752-761
4. Takarada S, Imanishi T, Liu Y et al (2010) Advantage of next-generation frequency-domain optical coherence tomography compared with conventional time-domain system in the assessment of coronary lesion. Catheter & Cardiovasc Interv 75:202-206
5. Imola F, Mallus MT, Ramazzotti V et al (2010) Safety and feasibility of frequency domain Optical Coherence Tomography to guide decision making in percutaneous coronary intervention. EuroInterv 6:575-581
6. Mintz GS, Nissen SE, Anderson WD et al (2001) ACC Clinical Expert Consensus Document on Standards for the acquisition, measurement and reporting of intravascular ultrasound studies: a report of the American College of Cardiology Task Force on Clinical Expert Consensus Documents (Committee to Develop a Clinical Expert Consensus Document on Standards for Acquisition, Measurement and Reporting of Intravascular Ultrasound Studies [IVUS]. J Am Coll Cardiol 37:1478-1492
7. Prati F, Capodanno D, Pawlowski T et al (2010) Local versus standard intracoronary infusion of abciximab in patients with acute coronary syndromes. J Am Coll Cardiol Intv 3:928-934
8. Tearney GJ, Yabushita H, Houser SL et al (2003) Quantification of macrophage content in atherosclerotic plaques by optical coherence tomography. Circulation 107:113-119
9. Fujii K, Masutani M, Okumura T et al (2008) Frequency and predictor of coronary thin-cap fibroatheroma in patients with acute myocardial infarction and stable angina pectoris a 3-vessel optical coherence tomography study. J Am Coll Cardiol 52:787-788

10. Tanaka A, Imanishi T, Kitabata H et al (2008) Morphology of exertion-triggered plaque rupture in patients with acute coronary syndrome: an optical coherence tomography study. Circulation 118:2368-2373
11. Takarada S, Imanishi T, Kubo T et al (2009) Effect of statin therapy on coronary fibrous-cap thickness in patients with acute coronary syndrome: assessment by optical coherence tomography study. Atheroscler 202:491-497
12. Kang Y, Mintz GS. IVUS vs. FFR for the assessment of intermediate lesions. Circ Card Interv, in press
13. Mintz GS, Weissman NJ (2006) Intravascular ultrasound in the drug-eluting stent era. J Am Coll Cardiol 48:421-429
14. Finn AV, Joner M, Nakazawa G et al (2007) Pathological correlates of late drug-eluting stent thrombosis: strut coverage as a marker of endothelialization. Circulation 115:2435-2441
15. Bezerra HG, Costa MA, Guagliumi G et al (2009) Intracoronary optical coherence tomography: a comprehensive review clinical and research applications. J Am Coll Cardiol Intv 2:1035-1046
16. Prati F, Stazi F, Dutary J et al (2011) Detection of very early stent healing after primary angioplasty: an optical coherence tomographic observational study of chromium cobaltum and first generation drug eluting stents. The DETECTIVE study. Heart 97:1841-1846

Triple Rule Out: the Use of Cardiac CT in the Emergency Room

16

Giulio Speciale and Vincenzo Pasceri

16.1 Introduction

Acute chest pain is one of the most frequent symptoms reported by patients evaluated in emergency departments (EDs). In the USA, approximately 8 million people with acute chest pain are seen annually in an emergency setting [1, 2]. The diagnosis of an acute coronary syndrome (ACS) is often difficult, and studies have suggested that 2–6% of ACS patients are inappropriately sent home from the ED, leading to increased morbidity and mortality. This is also an increasing motive for malpractice claims. The protocol for the evaluation of this group of patients includes ECG and the assessment of myocardial damage markers (including CK/MB and troponin) [1]. Unfortunately, there is also a minority of patients with normal ECG and cardiac enzymes at admission who still have an ACS. These patients require a time-consuming and expensive protocol, with serial ECG and cardiac enzyme assessments [1-3]. In case of persistently negative results, patients often undergo a stress test. Sometimes additional tests are also performed to rule out other, possibly fatal causes of chest pain, including aortic dissection and lung embolism. Nonetheless, mistakes are still possible even after this complex protocol, which has an estimated annual cost of $10–13 billion in the USA alone [3]. Finally, a large number of patients with no serious disease are kept for many hours in the ED, leading to overwork, the need for more staff, and a longer waiting time for other patients.

Recently, integration of the diagnostic triage of chest pain with coronary CT scan has been proposed [4] in order to obtain an anatomic assessment of the coronary arteries that may allow a quick diagnosis and thus an early discharge [5]. A coronary CT scan may also help in identifying patients with other serious conditions, including aortic dissection and lung embolism [6]. This chapter provides a review of the current evidence regarding the use of multislice CT in this setting and its pro and cons compared with other widely used diagnostic techniques.

16.2 Causes of Acute Chest Pain

In clinical practice, only 15–20% of patients coming to the ED for acute chest pain have a final diagnosis of heart disease, whereas the large majority do not (Table 16.1). On the other hand, the ECG may be non-diagnostic in many patients

Table 16.1 Final diagnosis of patients with acute chest pain who were seen by a general practitioner or at an emergency department. Modified from [6]

	General Practitioner	Emergency Department
Cardiac	20%	45%
Musculoskeletal	43%	14%
Gastrointestinal	5%	6%
Psychiatric	11%	8%
Pulmonary	4%	5%
Other	16%	26%

G. Speciale (✉)
Chief Interventional Cardiology, San Filippo Neri Hospital, Rome, Italy
e-mail: giuliospeciale@yahoo.it

Table 16.2 Diagnostic accuracy of non-invasive tests for identifying coronary disease (results adjusted for referral bias) [7-9]

	Sensitivity	Specificity
CECG-stress test	45%	85%
Echo-stress test	78%	85%
Myocardial perfusion imaging	82%	59%

with acute myocardial infarction and in most patients with unstable angina. According to the ACC/AHA guidelines, all patients presenting to the ED with acute chest pain should be assessed with both ECG and a cardiac biomarker (preferably a cardiac-specific troponin, i.e., troponin-I or troponin-T). Patients with a negative ECG should undergo a serial ECG assessment to evaluate dynamic ECG changes (initially at 15- to 30-min intervals). Similarly, patients with normal cardiac biomarkers should undergo a repeat blood test 8–12 h after symptom onset [7]. Negative ECG and normal troponin identify a low-risk population; however, even patients with persistently normal troponin may have significant coronary disease. In this group, the diagnosis of coronary disease may require functional tests, such as ECG stress test, a stress-echocardiogram, or nuclear imaging. However, none of these tests has optimal sensitivity or specificity (Table 16.2) [8-10]. Accordingly, 10–15% of patients with a diagnosis of ACS who are submitted to coronary angiography have normal coronary arteries, which underlines the limits of the current diagnostic methods.

16.3 Multislice CT Scan in Acute Chest Pain

Over 30 studies assessing the diagnostic accuracy of CT scan in identifying coronary disease have been published, with over 2,000 patients enrolled. Studies using a per-patient analysis (1,329 patients, examined by 16- or 64-slice CT scan) reported a mean sensitivity and specificity of 97% and 84%, respectively [11], with a sensitivity and specificity of 98% and 93%, respectively, for 64-slice CT studies (Table 16.3). However, the most interesting result was the negative predictive value (NPV) of over 97%, which is much better than that reported for any other non-invasive diagnostic test. This excellent NPV makes CT a very attractive modality for ruling out coronary disease in patients seen in the ED. Nonetheless, it should be kept in mind that CT may have a lower diagnostic accuracy in patients with pre-existing coronary disease, who often have extensive coronary calcifications and coronary stents (which may produce artifacts on CT scan). These patients are already considered to be at high-risk when they come to the ED. Thus, instead, CT may be an invaluable asset for the evaluation of low-intermediate risk patients with acute chest pain (which are the large majority of ED patients).

These observations have formed the basis of several studies aimed at assessing the specific role of CT in patients with acute chest pain. Thus far, seven studies on the use of 64-slice CT, enrolling a total of 376 ED patients, have been published [12]. All of them included low- to intermediate-risk patients with acute chest pain, normal cardiac

Table 16.3 Diagnostic accuracy of 64-row CT scan for identifying >50% coronary stenoses

	Patients (n)	Sensitivity	Specificity	Negative predictive value
Leshka	67	97%	94%	99%
Raff	70	95%	86%	98%
Leber	59	97%	88%	99%
Mollet	52	95%	99%	99%
Ropers	82	93%	95%	99%
Fine	66	96%	95%	95%
Budoff	230	95%	83%	99%
Meijboom	360	99%	64%	97%

Table 16.4 Comparison of 64-row CT scan and a standard diagnostic protocol in the emergency department (data from [13])

	CT scan	Standard protocol	P
Time to diagnosis (h)	3.4	15	<0.001
Total cost (US$)	1586	1872	<0.001
Need for re-evaluation at 6 months	2%	7%	0.29

Table 16.5 Comparison of 64-row CT scan and nuclear imaging for identifying coronary disease in patients with acute chest pain in the emergency department (data from the CT-STAT Trial)

	CT scan	Nuclear imaging	P
Time to diagnosis (h)	2.9	6.2	<0.001
Total cost (US$)	2137	3458	<0.001
Cardiac events in patients with negative tests (%)	0.8	0.4	0.29

biomarkers, and no ischemic ECG changes (two studies excluded patients with a previous history of coronary disease). The results of the CT examination allowed significant coronary disease to be correctly excluded, with a mean NPV of 99%. These findings strongly support the use of CT to identify low-risk patients who can be safely discharged. In particular, a study from William Beaumont Hospital (Royal Oak, MI) reported a trial consisting of 197 patients randomized to early CT in the ED vs. a standard diagnostic protocol (serial cardiac biomarkers, etc.): patients with no stenosis as determined on CT (< 25%) were immediately discharged; patients with significant stenosis (> 75%) underwent early coronary angiography; and patients with intermediate stenosis (25–75%) received a stress test [13]. In the CT group, two-thirds of the patients were discharged immediately after the CT scan and none of them had any adverse event at 6 months follow-up (NPV: 100%). CT was non-diagnostic due to the presence of intermediate lesions or suboptimal imaging in 24% of patients, who then received a stress test; while in 8%. CT identified significant coronary lesions (with a positive predictive value of 85%). The CT-based approach was much quicker (time to diagnosis 3.4 h vs. 15.0 h in the standard diagnosis group) and significantly reduced costs (-15%) (Table 16.4) [13].

Recently, the CT-STAT trial compared CT with rest-stress myocardial perfusion imaging in the evaluation of acute low-risk chest pain in over 700 patients presenting to the ED [14]. The results showed that CT allows a more rapid and cost-efficient, safe diagnosis than obtained with rest-stress myocardial perfusion imaging. Interestingly, median costs were reduced from $3,548 to $2,137, while the incidence of cardiac events remained very low in both groups (0.8% with CT scan and 0.4% with myocardial perfusion imaging). These recent findings support the use of CT for ruling out coronary disease in lower risk patients presenting to the ED.

Conversely, a simple assessment of the calcium score by CT is insufficient to correctly identify patients who present in the ED with coronary disease, since patients with acute chest pain have mostly noncalcified coronary plaques, which can be identified only by multislice CT scan [15]. The possible limits of this latter technique (discussed in other chapters of this volume) include its contraindication in patients with a fast heart rate (> 65 bpm) and arrhythmias (in particular, atrial fibrillation). Although it is common to treat patients undergoing multislice CT with beta-blockers to reduce the heart rate to < 65 bpm, these drugs are contraindicated in up to 15% of patients seen in the ED. Finally, all patients should be screened for a history of iodine allergy and for renal failure.

16.4 The Triple Rule-Out Protocol

Multislice CT scan (64-slice and more) allows rapid scanning not only of the heart and coronary arteries, but also of the entire lung and thoracic aorta, as a complete scan of all these areas can be performed in less than 20 s. These technical improvements have led to the use of multislice CT to identify coronary disease, aortic dissection, and lung embolism as well [12]. Thus, a single scan

can rule out three potentially fatal causes of acute chest pain, referred to as the "triple rule-out." However, these scans can be technically challenging because they require optimal and simultaneous contrast intensity in both the left (coronary and aorta) and the right (pulmonary) circulation, while avoiding artifacts due to the presence of contrast in the right atrium and ventricle, which may reduce the accuracy of coronary imaging. The use of a dedicated protocol of contrast injection with two contrast boluses, one for the coronary arteries and the other for the pulmonary arteries, followed by a saline injection to clear contrast from the right heart chambers can yield good imaging of all three arteries in a single scan. While this protocol is very attractive and has been introduced in several hospitals, it has not yet been tested in clinical trials. In particular, since aortic dissection and lung embolism are much less frequent than coronary disease, it is unclear whether the large-scale use of this protocol, especially since it requires an increased radiation dose, has a positive risk/benefit ratio in unselected populations. Nonetheless, it may be a very important asset in patients in whom aortic dissection or lung embolism is clinically suspected.

From a technical point of view a triple rule-out protocol requires the use of a 64-slice CT scanner (or better). A 16-slice scanner would require a patient breath-hold > 30 s in order to acquire images of both the heart and the lungs (from the apices to the diaphragm), whereas with a 64-slice scan the breath-hold is reduced to < 15–20 s [12,16]. It is also technically challenging to obtain optimal contrast intensity in both the pulmonary and the coronary system. Several protocols of contrast injection have been developed to optimize visualization of the pulmonary and coronary arteries while reducing artifacts. Usually these entail a bolus of saline to quickly remove contrast from the right heart. The protocol of Vrachliotis et al. [17] consisted of a triphasic injection with a total of 100 ml of contrast at 5 ml/s, then an injection of 30 ml at 3 ml/s (for optimal visualization of the pulmonary arteries), followed by a saline injection. The authors performed a caudal-cranial scan rather than the usual cranial-caudal sequence in order to improve visualization of the distal pulmonary branches at the base of the lungs, which are the most difficult to visualize.

As noted above, the use of a triple rule-out protocol may increase radiation exposure. In fact, the radiation dose is about 50% higher than that associated with a standard coronary CT scan [12, 16]. This increase in exposure must be taken into account, especially in younger patients. Clearly, the risk/benefit of a triple rule-out scan must be weighed according to individual risk. The identification of patients who will benefit most from this technique should be addressed in further studies. However, an important consideration is that with the new high-yield scanners (128-slice or even 320-slice) the total radiation exposure can be significantly reduced; in some settings, exposure is even lower than that of a simple coronary scan with a 64-slice CT.

The clinical benefit of a triple rule-out scan compared with a simple coronary scan should be carefully considered for each patient. Among patients with acute chest pain, the incidence of coronary disease is overwhelming compared with the incidence of lung embolism, aortic dissection, or other conditions that can be assessed with a triple rule-out scan. Whether the routine use of this protocol vs. a simple coronary scan in an unselected population presenting with chest pain is of clinical benefit remains to be determined. In a recent study, Madder et al. [18], compared 272 patients assessed with triple rule-out scan vs. 1796 patients examined with a standard coronary CT scan. No significant differences were found between the two groups (diagnosis of lung embolism of 1.1% with triple rule-out vs. 0.2% with coronary CT, with no cases of aortic dissection in either group). Triple rule out scans resulted in increased radiation exposure (12±5.6 mSv vs. 8.2±4 mSv) and, somewhat surprisingly, an increased request for a standard pulmonary CT scan to rule out lung embolism [18]. There was no difference in clinical events. Thus, with current technologies, it seems appropriate to limit the triple rule-out scan to patients with a higher risk of non-coronary disease. However, with further technological advances and the routine use of high-speed scans (128 and 320-slice), the benefits of this protocol over a coronary CT scan may increase the appeal of this comprehensive approach.

16.5 Conclusions

Multislice CT scan is an ideal diagnostic test to rule-out coronary and possibly other vascular thoracic diseases in low-risk patients. Diagnostic assessment of acute chest pain in the ED may be an optimal setting to use this new diagnostic method. Randomized studies have confirmed that integrating multislice CT scan into the diagnostic protocols in the ED not only results in excellent diagnostic accuracy, but also in shorter hospital stay and reduced costs. Although the CC/AHA guidelines for the assessment of patients with acute chest pain do not yet include multislice CT, there is evidence supporting its use as a diagnostic tool in ED protocols. The potential of a triple rule-out scan to rule out aortic and pulmonary diseases awaits the development of well-defined diagnostic protocols regarding its application.

Patients coming to the ED with acute chest pain should first undergo a complete clinical assessment, with ECG and cardiac biomarkers. High-risk patients with an ECG suggestive of ischemia and/or positive biomarkers do not require multislice CT and should be immediately admitted and treated. Patients with a negative ECG and biomarkers at admission may benefit from a diagnostic CT scan, as it would avoid the waiting time associated with serial ECG and biomarkers, thus allowing the early identification of patients without coronary disease who could therefore be safely discharged. The traditional diagnostic protocol, consisting of serial ECG, biomarkers and possible stress test, should be reserved for patients with suboptimal imaging at multislice CT or with intermediate-grade stenosis.

References

1. Amsterdam EA, Kirk JD, Bluemke DA et al (2010) Testing of low-risk patients presenting to the emergency department with chest pain. A Scientific Statement from the American Heart Association. Circulation 122:1756-1776
2. Pitts SR, Niska RW, Xu J, Burt CW (2008) National Hospital Ambulatory Medical Care Survey: 2006 emergency department summary Natl Health Stat Report 7:1-38
3. Tatum JL, Jesse RL, Kontos MC et al (1997) Comprehensive strategy for the evaluation and triage of the chest pain patient Ann Emerg Med 29:116-125
4. Arbab-Zadeh A, Hoe J (2011) Quantification of coronary arterial stenoses by multidetector CT angiography in comparison with conventional angiography methods, caveats, and implications. JACC Cardiovasc Imaging 4(2):191-202
5. Goldstein JA, Chinnaiyan KM, Abidov A et al (2011) The CT-STAT (Coronary Computed Tomographic Angiography for Systematic Triage of Acute Chest Pain Patients to Treatment) trial J Am Coll Cardiol 58:1414-1422
6. Erhardt L, Herlitz J, Bossaert L et al (2002) Task Force on the management of chest pain. Eur Heart J 23:1153-1176
7. Wright RS, Anderson JL, Adams CD et al (2011) 2011 ACCF/AHA Focused Update Incorporated Into the ACC/AHA 2007 Guidelines for the Management of Patients With Unstable Angina/Non–ST-Elevation Myocardial Infarction. J Am Coll Cardiol 57:215-367
8. Froelicher VF, Lehmann KG, Thomas R et al (1998) The electrocardiographic exercise test in a population with reduced workup bias: diagnostic performance, computerized interpretation, and multi- variable prediction. Veterans Affairs Cooperative Study in Health Services #016 (QUEXTA) Study Group. Quantitative Exercise Testing and Angiography. Ann Intern Med 128:965-974
9. Roger VL, Pelikka PA, Bell MR et al (1997) Sex and test verification bias: impact on the diagnostic value of exercise echocardiography. Circulation 95:405-410
10. Cecil MP, Kosinski AS, Jones MT et al (1996) The importance of work-up (verification) bias correction in assessing the accuracy of SPECT thallium-201 testing for the diagnosis of coronary artery disease. J Clin Epidemiol 49:735-742
11. Raff GL, Goldstein JA (2007) Coronary angiography by computed to- mography: Coronary imaging evolves. J Am Coll Cardiol 49:1830-1833
12. Gallagher MJ, Raff GL (2008) Use of multislice CT for the evaluation of emergency room patients with chest pain: the so-called "triple rule-out". Cardiovasc Interv 71:92-99
13. Goldstein JA, Gallagher MJ, O'Neill WW et al (2007) A randomized controlled trial of multislice coronary computed tomography for evaluation of acute chest pain. J Am Coll Cardiol 49:863-871

14. Goldstein JA, Chinnaiyan KM, Abidov A et al (2011) The CT-STAT (Coronary Computed Tomographic Angiography for Systematic Triage of Acute Chest Pain Patients to Treatment) trial J Am Coll Cardiol 58:1414-1422
15. Henneman MM, Schuijf JD, Pundziute G et al (2008) Noninvasive evaluation with multislice computed tomography in suspected acute coronary syndrome: plaque morphology on multislice computed tomography versus coronary calcium score. J Am Coll Cardiol 52:216–222
16. Yoon YE, Wann S. Evaluation of acute chest pain in the emergency department: "triple rule-out" computed tomography angiography. Cardiol Rev 2011) 19:115-121
17. Vrachliotis TG, Bis KG, Haidary A et al (2007) Atypical chest pain: coronary, aortic, and pulmonary vasculature enhancement at biphasic single-injection 64-section CT angiography. Radiology 243:368-376
18. Madder RD, Raff GL, Hickman L et al (2011) Comparative diagnostic yield and 3-month outcomes of "triple rule-out" and standard protocol coronary CT angiography in the evaluation of acute chest pain. J Cardiovasc Comput Tomogr 5:165-171

Contraindications to Coronary CT Angiography

17

David A. Dowe

17.1 Introduction

Computed tomography (CT) technology has undergone major advances over the last decade, with no advance being more important than the development of 64-slice multidetector CT (MDCT) scanners. In parallel, the contraindications to coronary CT angiography (CCTA) have decreased, although there are still several absolute contraindications to this procedure. This chapter addresses the absolute contraindications to CCTA with respect to the medical/technical aspects of the exam, as well as the clinical absolute contraindications.

17.2 Medical/Technical Absolute Contraindications

The most important medical contraindication is a known hypersensitivity to current-generation, non-ionic contrast agent. In patients with a hypersensitivity to the older ionic versions of contrast, this history can be largely ignored. Instead, these patients should be interviewed regarding the nature of the hypersensitivity reaction. If it occurred prior to 1990, it can safely be assumed that it was secondary to an injection of ionic contrast; these patients

---

D.A. Dowe (✉)
Coronary CTA, Program Director
Atlantic Medical Imaging
Galloway, NJ, USA
e-mail: ddowe@atlanticmedicalimaging.com

should not be prepped with steroids. Patients with a history of a reaction to one of the current-generation non-ionic contrast agents should be prepped with oral steroids and an antihistamine. If there is a history of a reaction including symptoms of airway compromise, the patient should have his or her exam, with a steroid prep, in a hospital setting with respiratory therapy on site.

Renal insufficiency can be an absolute contraindication. The cutoff point varies with the institution [1]. Hoffman et al. use a serum creatinine cutoff of > 1.5 mg/dl. An alternative, less conservative approach is a cutoff of >2.0 mg/dl or a creatinine clearance <3 0 ml/min/1.73 m^2. This cutoff of creatinine clearance mirrors the guidelines used for magnetic resonance imaging (MRI) gadolinium contrast agents in order to avoid the complication of nephrogenic systemic sclerosis. In this author's experience, these MRI-based cutoffs of serum creatinine and/or creatinine clearance have proven to be extremely safe and are highly recommended.

Patients with a history of recent pulmonary emboli or strong suspicion of pulmonary emboli may decompensate if given beta-blockers, as tachycardia may occur in response to the decreased stroke volume caused by the obstruction emboli. This poses some risk when a triple rule-out CCTA is contemplated.

Acute congestive heart failure may be an absolute contraindication, depending on the severity. These patients may have difficulty handling the volumes of contrast agent and saline necessary for CCTA. Accordingly, great care should be taken to determine that the patient can tolerate the administration of beta-blockers or additional beta-blockers. The use of beta-blockers may need to be omitted and the exam instead performed with retrospective gating.

The patient's inability to perform a breath-hold for 6 s is also an absolute contraindication. However, this is mostly a theoretical limitation, as even patients with severe COPD can perform a breath-hold for this brief interval.

Severe arrhythmias may be an absolute contraindication, although the definition of severe in regards to performing CCTA has changed over time secondary to the development of sophisticated algorithms that allow post-exam editing of the ECG tracing. Thus, a rogue premature ventricular contraction can be easily deleted and the images reconstructed without it. However, in the presence of numerous aberrant beats, such as occurs with bigeminy or trigeminy, deletion of all of them will obviously hinder image reconstruction. In addition, these algorithms have removed atrial fibrillation from the absolute contraindication territory. Consequently, patients with atrial fibrillation can be scanned by applying retrospective gating, which provides a sufficient number of phases to reconstruct the entire coronary artery circulation.

17.3 Absolute Clinical Contraindications

The recently published 2010 Appropriateness Criteria for Performing Cardiac Computed Tomography provide excellent guidance regarding the appropriate conditions for CCTA [2]. It is important to note that these guidelines have been agreed upon by multiple societies from both disciplines, radiology and cardiology. The published guidelines consider the use of CCTA in different clinical scenarios as (1) appropriate, (2) inappropriate, and (3) uncertain. The following discussion critically considers only the inappropriate indication category.

The guidelines define an inappropriate indication as the detection of coronary artery disease (CAD) in symptomatic patients without known heart disease if the patient has an interpretable ECG, is able to exercise, and has a high probability of having CAD based on the Framingham Risk Evaluation. In this author's opinion, this definition is questionable as even in high-risk patients chest pain and shortness of breath are just as likely, or even more likely, to be caused by conditions other than CAD. Based on personal experience, many of these patients will have a CCTA consistent with negative or mild disease (stenosis < 50%), which is very helpful in streamlining their subsequent workup.

The most important absolute contraindication is the use of CCTA for the detection of CAD in a symptomatic patient with a proven myocardial infarction, by ECG and/or serum enzyme markers for myocardial necrosis, e.g. troponin. These patients do not need a diagnostic CCTA as their diagnosis has been reached with near certainty by clinical means. Instead, they should undergo catheter coronary angiography, which brings with it the option of a percutaneous coronary intervention.

Currently considered an absolute contraindication is the detection of CAD in low- and intermediate-risk asymptomatic patients. This is based on the low probability of their having significant CAD. Perhaps in the future, CCTA will be instituted as a screening test for CAD [3].

While CCTA may be used for pre-operative clearance, it is not recommended in patients in need of this procedure for non-cardiac surgery if they are at high risk. Once again, however, in this author's opinion a negative CCTA can greatly influence and streamline the workup for suspected CAD in these patients.

CCTA has a limited role in the evaluation of patients with new-onset atrial fibrillation as it has a very low yield in this category. Instead, cardiac CT plays a role mainly in pre-ablation mapping of the pulmonary veins.

If there are prior tests, their results can limit the utility of CCTA. If a patient has had an exercise ECG test with low-risk findings, it may be more appropriate to halt further testing if the clinical suspicion for CAD is low. Alternatively, if this test yields high-risk findings with a high clinical suspicion, then proceeding to catheter angiography rather than pursuing a diagnostic CCTA may be more prudent.

If the prior stress test is an imaging stress test it is considered inappropriate to pursue CCTA in patients with moderate or severe ischemia. However, in this author's opinion, if the test was a single photon emission CT (SPECT) myocardial perfusion study, there is considerable overlap between ischemia and well-known artifacts such as breast or diaphragm attenuation. Thus, if there is no urgent clinical fact supporting immediate catheter angiography, CCTA can have great value in preventing a negative, diagnostic catheterization.

CCTA is considered contraindicated in the repeat testing of patients who are asymptomatic or have stable symptoms and have undergone prior stress imaging or coronary angiography, regardless of risk category as well as the date of the prior exam.

CCTA, even with the latest generation of high-definition CT scanners, has difficulty imaging the lumen of small stents. For this reason, it is contraindicated in symptomatic patients with a prior coronary stent with a diameter < 3 mm. This recommendation also applies to asymptomatic patients regardless of when the stent was placed.

CCTA with retrospective gating can yield functional information. However, since retrospective gating cannot be done with lowest radiation techniques, CCTA is not indicated as the initial test, as functional information can be obtained without any radiation exposure with echocardiography. Likewise, CCTA is not indicated as the initial test for the workup of intra- or extra-cardiac masses, as these can also be evaluated without radiation by echocardiography and/or MRI.

References

1. Hoffman U, Ferenik M, Cury R, Pena A (2006) Coronary CT angiography. J Nuc Med 47:797-806
2. Taylor A, Cerqueira M, Hodgson J et al (2010) ACCF/SCCT/ACR/AHA/ASE/ASNC/NASCI/SCAI/SCMR 2010 Appropriate use criteria for cardiac computed tomography. J Am Coll Card 56(27):1863-1894
3. Dowe D (2007) The case in favor of screening for coronary artery disease with coronary CT angiography. JACR 4(5):289-294

Prognostic Value of Coronary CT

18

Bruno Pironi, Antonio Lucifero and Massimo Fioranelli

18.1 Introduction

Multidetector computed tomography (MDCT) with the latest-generation scanners (64- and 128-slice) allows evaluation of the entire coronary tree (main vessels and their collateral and marginal branches). Validation studies performed to date have focused on patient populations with a high pretest likelihood of coronary disease (range: 50–80%). However, several concepts that conflict with those results are emerging in clinical practice, influencing the indications and recommendations for the clinical use of MDCT. Both the recent guidelines of the European Society of Cardiology and a recent consensus statement on the appropriateness criteria for cardiac CT and cardiac magnetic resonance imaging (MRI) suggest that the appropriate use of MDCT includes patients at low to intermediate risk and with a doubtful, unfeasible, or inconclusive stress test.

In the last few years, several studies have examined the role of MDCT in diagnosing coronary stenosis and in the prognosis of patients with ischemic cardiomyopathy, to prevent the development of acute coronary syndrome. Specifically, CT may have a role in evaluating the prognosis and in guiding therapy, both of which are influenced, in turn, by its diagnostic capability.

B. Pironi (✉)
Cardiology and Hemodynamics
Madre Giuseppina Vannini Hospital, Rome, Italy
e-mail: pironib@hotmail.com

18.2 Diagnosis

Invasive coronary angiography is the current reference standard diagnostic test for defining the presence and severity of obstructive coronary artery disease (CAD) based on luminal stenosis. However, this refers more to the demonstrated value of coronary angiography in defining prognosis and guiding treatment than to its documented ability to provide an accurate and reproducible assessment of the extent and severity of coronary atherosclerosis. Other technologies that can image the diseased vessel wall, such as intravascular ultrasound (IVUS), cardiac magnetic resonance imaging (CMRI), and optical coherence tomography (OCT), may actually be more appropriate reference standards in the assessment of some aspects of the diagnostic performance of CT angiography (CTA), given the latter's ability to image the vessel wall in addition to the lumen.

Noninvasive multidetector CT coronary angiography (MDCT-CA) is a technique with high diagnostic accuracy in the detection of significant coronary stenosis in patients with atypical pain or stable angina and low to intermediate risk. Given the low disease prevalence in this population, MDCT-CA may become an ideal screening tool to exclude the presence of critical coronary disease, thereby obviating the need for coronary angiography in a subset of patients.

The use of CTA raises two important safety issues: (1) the amount of radiation absorbed by the body tissues, and (2) the exposure to iodinated contrast agents, with the risk of allergic reaction

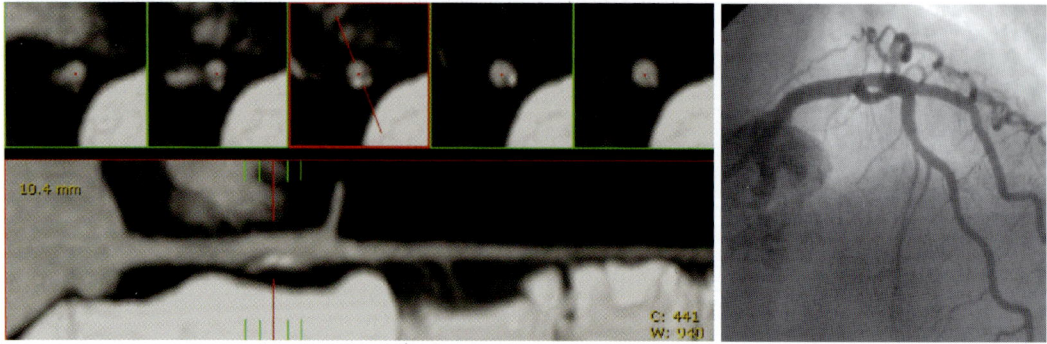

Fig. 18.1 Female patient with atypical chest pain and a non-diagnostic stress test; only coronary CT showed a plaque in the proximal left anterior descending artery

and acute renal injury. MDCT-CA may provide a means to "fill in the detection gap", defined as the difference between coronary heart disease cases or events currently detected and the total burden of disease or events among the population [1].

18.2.1 Asymptomatic and Low-Risk Patients

An intriguing possibility of coronary CT is its use in the determination of occult atherosclerosis and as a tool in the early detection of atherosclerosis in asymptomatic individuals. Since CT coronary imaging comprehensively evaluates the (calcific and non-calcific) composition of coronary plaques, it may be able to provide prognostic evidence independent of and incremental to simple CT calcium scoring. So far, MDCT has not been explored extensively in asymptomatic individuals, and only a few reports have been published indicating the feasibility of the technique [2, 3]. Since approximately 50% of all acute coronary syndromes occur in previously asymptomatic patients, there obviously is a need to identify these individuals before coronary atherosclerosis becomes clinically manifest and irreversible damage occurs by progression to myocardial infarction or cardiac death [4]. It is customary to initially estimate a risk of cardiovascular death or myocardial infarction with traditional risk factors, including age and gender, to derive a risk score, for instance, the Framingham Risk Score or the European Risk Score (Systemic Coronary Risk Evaluation). However, asymptomatic individuals generally have a low risk score while those with more than one risk factor may nonetheless be only at intermediate risk. In low-risk populations, the prognostic accuracy of screening is far from perfect and the incorporation of CT atherosclerotic imaging data into a CAD risk score might improve existing algorithms for risk stratification (Fig. 18.1).

18.3 Prognosis

Coronary CTA (CCTA) is a novel imaging modality with high sensitivity for the detection of atherosclerosis. Studies have suggested the superior prognostic value of CCTA in patients with traditional risk factors [5, 6]. While CCTA carries the risks inherent to contrast and radiation exposures [7], it may have a role in the noninvasive assessment of patients with symptoms [8] as well as in the screening of certain higher-risk asymptomatic subgroups. Nonetheless, the consequences of CCTA testing need to be considered [9].

Given the potential for the greater widespread use of CCTA in cardiac risk evaluation, River et al. evaluated the downstream implications of CCTA testing in a cohort of asymptomatic patients who had already undergone CCTA as part of a prior study [10, 11]. They prospectively followed this

CCTA group along with a matched control group drawn from the same screening program. This was the first study to examine the implications of CCTA screening in a large matched cohort study, including its effect on physicians' prescribing practices and patients' use of medications, as well as the impact on downstream secondary testing and cardiac events.

A screening CCTA suggesting coronary atherosclerosis was associated with a sustained increase in aspirin and statin use. However, an abnormal result was also associated with more intensive secondary tests and invasive revascularizations outside of evidence-based guidelines. The clinical implications of these results may add to the debate regarding the utility of statins and aspirin in primary prevention. Randomized trials of CCTA use with longer follow-up are needed to assess whether these effects can alter outcomes [12].

At present, data on the prognostic value of CCTA using 64-channel or greater systems are quite limited. Furthermore, there have been no large-scale studies directly comparing long-term outcomes following conventional diagnostic imaging strategies versus strategies involving CCTA. As with invasive coronary angiography, the results of CCTA are often not concordant with stress single-photon emission computed tomography (SPECT) myocardial perfusion imaging (MPI). The differences in the parameters measured by MPI (function or physiology) and CTA (anatomy) must be considered in patient-management decisions. Of note, a normal MPI does not exclude the presence of coronary atherosclerosis although it does signify a very low risk of future major adverse events over the short to intermediate term. Conversely, CCTA allows the detection of some coronary atherosclerotic plaques that are not hemodynamically significant. The optimal management of this disease aspect has not been established. At present, neither test can identify with any reasonable clinical probability the risk of future rupture of non-obstructive coronary plaques and therefore the subsequent likelihood of an acute myocardial infarction. Invasive coronary angiography has similar limitations [13].

18.3.1 Vulnerable Plaque and Thin-Capped Fibroatheroma

The role of CCTA may be important in the study and prevention of acute coronary syndrome (ACS). It is known that in the majority of cases ACS is the result of a complication in an atherosclerotic plaque that had not caused a reduction in the bloodstream prior to the episode. The presence of a stenosis, even if appreciable, does not necessarily lead to ischemia in the area supplied by the stenotic vessel. Even the presence of a complete obstruction does not automatically imply that the area downstream will become necrotic. In two-thirds of ACS patients, there is fragmentation of what is referred to as a "vulnerable plaque." About three-quarters of plaques complicated by rupture involve 50% of the vessel diameter and in approximately half of the cases > 75%. In two-thirds of the patients, the lipid core occupies > 25% of the volume of the lesion, while in 80% it expands to occupy > 50% of the thickness of the vessel wall. The situation is further complicated by the fact that enlargement of the necrotic core is associated with a high probability of rupture. Disruption of a vulnerable plaque characterized by a thin fibrous cap, large lipid pool, and macrophage infiltration, the so-called thin-capped fibroatheroma (TCFA), is a primary culprit in ACS. Detection of a TCFA before plaque rupture remains a challenge for cardiologists. The increased detection of vulnerable plaque rupture may allow better risk stratification in patients with known or suspected CAD.

Several imaging techniques have been applied for the detection of vulnerable plaques, including IVUS, OCT, and MDCT. Among these, OCT has recently emerged as a highly informative imaging method for plaque characterization in vivo. A histology-controlled study (Circulation 2002) has shown that OCT is well able to detect TCFAs and may therefore serve as a useful technique to assess vulnerable plaques. However, OCT as a diagnostic procedure is both invasive and costly, precluding its use in the routine clinical settings. MDCT has been proposed as a noninvasive imaging technique that not only can evaluate coronary artery stenosis but can also detect and classify coronary plaques in vivo. Several studies have suggested that MDCT findings can be related to plaque instability. These findings include a low CT density value, positive vessel remodeling, spotty calcification, and the signet-ring-like appearance of the suspected lesion. Such observations underline the diagnostic importance of a noninvasive method to identify the characteristics that make a plaque vulnerable.

In 1996, Agatston proposed the use of a CT electron beam to quantify coronary calcium. Many studies have since demonstrated that a high Agatston score, i.e., a high calcium content, is associated with a high incidence of coronary episodes. The annual incidence of adverse episodes in individuals without significant calcium content in the coronary tree is approximately 2 out of every 1000 such patients. With a coronary artery calcium (CAC) score > 400, however, the incidence of coronary episodes rises ten-fold, which translates into 20–50 episodes for every 1000 such patients. In a primary prevention study, Budoff et al. [14] analyzed the impact of the CAC score on the prognosis of 25,000 asymptomatic patients, with an average follow-up period of about 7 years. Six score classes, 0, 1–10, 11–100, 101–400, 401–1000, and > 1000 were defined. CAC proved to be an independent predictor of mortality. The relative risk of cardiovascular mortality was 2.2, 4.5, 6.4, 9.2, 10.4, and 12.5 times per score of 11, 100, 101, 299, 300–399, 400–699, 700–999, and > 1000, respectively ($p < 0.0001$), compared with a CAC score of 0. The 10-year survival rate was 99.4% for a score of 0 and 87.8% for a score > 1000 ($p < 0.0001$).

Autopsy and IVUS have indicated that positive vessel remodeling is associated with plaque vulnerability and ACS. Increased oxidative stress is closely associated with positive vessel remodeling and plaque vulnerability, as determined using simultaneous examination with IVUS and immunohistochemistry analyses. Recent studies reported that low CT attenuation and positive vessel remodeling, detected using MDCT, may be related to plaque vulnerability. Motoyama et al. [15] reported that a low-attenuation (30 HU) plaque and positive vessel remodeling were frequently observed in ACS culprit lesions and both were characteristics of plaques subsequently resulting in ACS. In a comparative study with IVUS, Tanaka et al. [16] reported that ruptured plaques had a low mean CT density of 46.8 HU and a large remodeling index of 1.11. In studies using OCT and IVUS, Raffel et al. [17] and Kashiwagi et al. [18] found that plaques exhibiting positive remodeling had a thinner fibrous cap and there was a significant association between positive remodeling and the presence of TCFA. In a serial IVUS and OCT study, Yamada et al. [19] reported that positive arterial remodeling was related to thinning of the fibrous cap. Tsuyoshi et al. [20] concluded that a higher lipid content was associated with a lower CT density and a larger remodeling index. Furthermore, fibrous cap thickness was negatively correlated with CT density value and positively correlated with the remodeling index, which confirmed published data suggesting that low CT attenuation and a large remodeling index are the CT characteristics of a vulnerable plaque. Tanaka et al. [16] reported that a semicircular thin enhancement around the plaque (ring-like) as seen on CT may be an indicator of a rupture-prone plaque. There are three possible explanations for this specific image: First, it may reflect the occupation of most of the plaque by lipid. Given that the CT density values of the vascular wall and fibrous plaque contents are higher, a vessel wall or fibrous component around a large lipid core may confer a signet-ring-like appearance to the plaque. Second, it may indicate intraplaque vaso vasorum, as previous studies have shown that new vessel formation is related to plaque vulnerability. Finally, it may be due to microcalcification within the plaque, which is thought to be associated with a vulnerable plaque.

In a recent study [20], a signet-ring-like appearance was more frequently observed in patients with TCFAs and was a potential predictor of TCFA formation, but there was no relation between spotty calcification and plaque vulnerability. In that study it was unclear whether the plaque observed in an ACS lesion was identical to a TCFA. Since some clinically stable patients have TCFAs, it is difficult to characterize these plaques precisely when based only on clinical status (Table 18.1).

Table 18.1 Diagnostic evaluation of thin-capped fiberoatheroma by MDCT (from [20])

Variable	Sensitivity	Specificity	Positive predictive value	Negative predictive value
Mean computed tomographic density ≤62.4	30/37 (81%)	61/85 (72%)	30/54 (55%)	61/68 (90%)
Remodeling index ≥1.08	28/37 (76%)	71/85 (84%)	28/42 (67%)	71/80 (89%)
Signet-ring-like appearance	24/37 (65%)	71/85 (84%)	24/38 (63%)	71/84 (85%)
Mean computed tomographic density ≤62.4 and remodeling index ≥1.08	24/37 (65%)	77/85 (91%)	24/32 (75%)	77/90 (86%)
Remodeling index ≥1.08 and signet-ring-like appearance	20/37 (54%)	81/85 (95%)	20/24 (83%)	81/98 (82%)
Mean computed tomographic density ≤62.4 and signet-ring-like appearance	19/37 (51%)	80/85 (94%)	19/24 (79%)	80/98 (82%)
Mean computed tomographic density ≤62.4, remodeling index ≥1.08, and signet-ring-like appearance	24/37 (65%)	77/85 (91%)	24/32 (75%)	77/90 (86%)

18.4 Conclusion

The potential of MDCT to identify TCFA is controversial. Density-based software is able to define the features of the plaque and identify the necrotic core. The best currently available low-contrast, high resolution, and minimum slice thickness (64 × 0.5) hardware should allow better differentiation of fibrous from soft plaques.

Coronary MDCT has an adequate sensitivity (83–99%), a high specificity (93–98%), a low positive predictive power (81%), and a high negative predictive power (95–100%) in its ability to diagnose coronary stenosis and is therefore adequate to diagnose coronary atherosclerosis as well; however, it is not efficient enough to evaluate the grade of coronary stenosis. In the quantification of stenosis, MDCT (64-slice scanner) has limitations due to its spatial resolution of 0.4 mm and temporal resolution of 164 ms. A high spatial and temporal resolution is a prerequisite for visualization of the coronary arteries. A more invasive technique, catheter coronary angiography has a spatial resolution of 0.2 mm, twice that of CTA, and a temporal resolution 8 ms, corresponding to the acquisition of 12–30 images/s. The implication is that the quantification of a stenosis by means of CCTA cannot be as precise as obtained through catheter angiography. However, with the new 128-slice machines, the entire heart can be imaged in 4–5 s, with a spatial resolution of 0.24 mm, sufficient to reveal small anatomic structures.

Cardiovascular risk is currently determined by the Framingham Risk Score, according to which around half the population is at low risk. This means that the chance of a coronary episode is < 5% over 10 years (< 0.5% per year); 40% of the population is considered at intermediate risk (5–20% in 10 years, 0.5–2% per year); and 10% is at high risk (> 20%, > 2% per year).

The gold standard of diagnostic tests is the combination of various exams. In the study of van Werkhoven et al. [21], the combined use of MDCT and MPI resulted in significantly improved prediction of the composite hard endpoint of all-cause mortality and nonfatal myocardial infarction (log-rank test, $p < 0.005$). In 256 patients with none or mild CAD (MDCT < 50% stenosis) and a normal MPI (summed stress score, SSS, < 4), the annualized event rate was 1.0%, with an annualized hard event rate of 0.6%. In 72 patients with none or mild CAD (MDCT < 50% stenosis) but an abnormal MPI (SSS ≥4), the corresponding values were 3.7% and 2.2%, whereas in the 57 patients with significant CAD (MDCT ≥ 50% stenosis) and a normal MPI (SSS < 4) they were 3.8% and 3.8%. Interestingly, the event rates between patients with none or mild CAD (< 50%) stenosis and an abnormal MPI and patients with significant CAD (MSCT ≥ 50% stenosis) did not differ significantly. In the 54 patients with both significant CAD (MDCT ≥ 50% stenosis) and an abnormal MPI (SSS < 4), the annualized event rate was 9.0% and the annualized hard event rate 6.0%) [21].

In conclusion MDCT may be able to detect vulnerable plaques and therefore to guide the choice of appropriate therapy. It should be kept in mind that the concept of the "vulnerable plaque" has been accompanied by the recognition of the "vulnerable patient." This is a person at high risk, with multiple pathologies, including coronary, peripheral, and cerebral vasculopathies and diabetes mellitus. In this setting, MDCT has the potential to diagnose vulnerable plaque and to determine an adjustment in therapy.

References

1. Taylor AJ, Merz CN, Udelson JE (2003) 34th Bethesda Conference: executive summary – can atherosclerosis imaging techniques improve the detection of patients at risk for ischemic heart disease? J Am Coll Cardiol 41:1860-1862
2. Bachar GN, Atar E, Fuchs S et al (2007) Prevalence and clinical predictors of atherosclerotic coronary artery disease in asymptomatic patients undergoing coronary multidetector computed tomography. Coron Artery Dis 18:353-360
3. Romeo F, Leo R, Clementi F et al (2007) Multislice computed tomography in an asymptomatic high-risk population. Am J Cardiol 99:325-328
4. Murabito JM, Evans JC, Larson MG, Levy D (1993) Prognosis after the onset of coronary heart disease. An investigation of differences in outcome between the sexes according to initial coronary disease presentation. Circulation 88:2548-2555)
5. Russo V, Zavalloni A, Bacchi Reggiani ML et al (2010) Incremental prognostic value of coronary CT angiography in patients with suspected coronary artery disease. Circ Cardiovasc Imaging 3(4):351-359
6. Min JK, Shaw LJ, Devereux RB et al (2007) Prognostic value of multidetector coronary computed tomographic angiography for prediction of all-cause mortality. J Am Coll Cardiol 50(12):1161-1170
7. Einstein AJ, Henzlova MJ, Rajagopalan S (2007) Estimating risk of cancer associated with radiation exposure from 64-slice computed tomography coronary angiography. JAMA. 298(3):317-323
8. Hecht HS (2009) A paradigm shift: coronary computed tomographic angiography before stress testing. Am J Cardiol 104(4):613-618
9. Becker MC, Galla JM, Nissen SE (2011) Left main trunk coronary artery dissection as a consequence of inaccurate coronary computed tomographic angiography [published online December 13, 2010]. Arch Intern Med 171(7): 698-701
10. Rivera JJ, Nasir K, Cox PR et al (2009) Association of traditional cardiovascular risk factors with coronary plaque sub-types assessed by 64-slice computed tomography angiography in a large cohort of asymptomatic subjects. Atherosclerosis 206(2):451-457
11. Choi EK, Choi SI, RiveraJ J et al (2008) Coronary computed tomography angiography as a screening tool for the detection of occult coronary artery disease in asymptomatic individuals. J Am Coll Cardiol 52(5):357-365
12. McEvoy JW, Blaha, MJ (2011) Impact of coronary computed tomographic angiography results on patient and physician behavior in a low-risk population. Arch Intern Med. Published online May 23, 2011. doi:10.1001/archinternmed. 2011.204
13. Mark DB, Berman DS, Budoff MJ et al (2010) ACCF/ACR/AHA/NASCI/SAIP/SCAI/SCCT 2010 expert consensus document on coronary computed tomographic angiography. JACC 55:2663-2699
14. Budoff MJ, Shaw LJ, Liu ST et al (2007) Long-term prognosis associated with coronary calcification. J Am Coll Cardiol 49:1860-1870
15. Motoyama S, Sarai M, Harigaya H et al (2009) Computed tomographic angiography characteristics of atherosclerotic plaques subsequently resulting in acute coronary syndrome. J Am Coll Cardiol 54:49-57
16. Tanaka A, Shimada K, Yoshida K et al (2008) Non-invasive assessment of plaque rupture by 64-slice multidetector computed tomography – comparison with intravascular ultrasound. Circ J 72:1276-1281
17. Raffel OC, Merchant FM, Tearney GJ et al (2008) In vivo association between positive coronary artery remodelling and coronary plaque characteristics assessed by intravascular optical coherence tomography. Eur Heart J 29:1721-1728

18. Kashiwagi M, Tanaka A, Kitabata H et al (2009) Relationship between coronary arterial remodeling, fibrous capthickness and high-sensitivity C-reactive protein levels in patients with acute coronary syndrome. Circ J 73:1291-1295
19. Yamada R, Okura H, Kume T et al (2010) Relationship between arterial and fibrous cap remodeling: a serial three-vessel intravascular ultrasound and optical coherence tomography study. Circ Cardiovasc Interv 3:484-490
20. Tsuyoshi I, Terashima M (2011) Comparison of in vivo assessment of vulnerable plaque by 64-slice multislice computed tomography versus optical coherence tomography. Am J Cardiol 107:1270-1277
21. van Werkhoven JM, Schuijf JD, Gaemperli O et al (2009) Prognostic value of multislice computed tomography and gated single-photon emission computed tomography in patients with suspected coronary artery disease. J Am Coll Cardiol 53:623-632

Clinical Cases 19

David A. Dowe, Paolo Pavone and Massimo Fioranelli

19.1 Asymptomatic or Mild Symptomatic CAD

Case 1
Severe Coronary Artery Disease in an Asymptomatic Football Referee with One Risk Factor

Patient: 52-year-old asymptomatic white male with hypercholesterolemia.

Case Description

Left main equivalent disease is depicted in Figure 1a-c. Asymptomatic, severe CAD is present in this athletic male patient. "Left main equivalent" refers to simultaneous disease of the proximal LAD and LCX.
Again, left main equivalent disease is seen in Figure 2a,b.

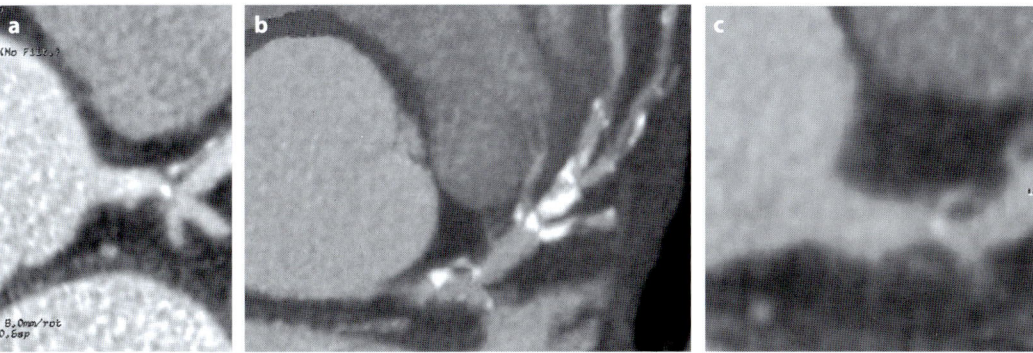

Fig. 1 a-c Left main equivalent disease

David A. Dowe
Atlantic Medical Imaging, Galloway, NJ, USA
e-mail: ddowe@atlanticmedicalimaging.com

Paolo Pavone
Radiology Department, Casa di Cura Mater Dei
Rome, Italy
paolo.pavone@materdei.it

Massimo Fioranelli
Heart Center
Casa di Cura Mater Dei
Rome, Italy
massimo.fioranelli@gmail.com

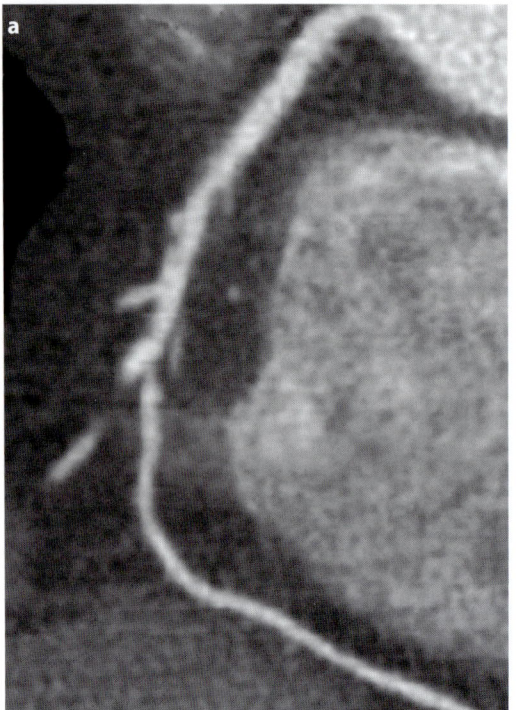
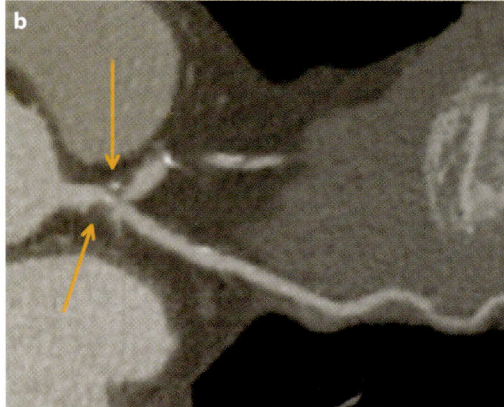

Fig. 2 a, b Left main equivalent disease

19 Clinical Cases

Case 2
Two-Vessel Severe Stenoses in a Completely Asymptomatic Patient

Patient: 63-year-old male, heavy smoker with a cholesterol of 280, hypertension and other generic risk factors. Coronary CTA was performed in the context of a screening protocol. He subsequently had an EKG and a treadmill test (up to 150 Watts).

Case Description

Figure 1a, b shows a focal segmental stenosis of the right coronary artery (a angiography, b coronary CTA). Diffuse LAD disease is seen in Fig. 1c, d. Multiple calcific plaques are evident but the focal severe (90%) stenosis is due to a fibrolipidic plaque (arrow). The two stenotic segments were stented soon after coronary CTA.

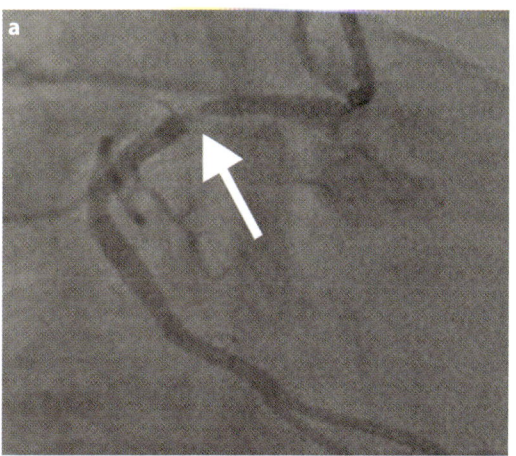
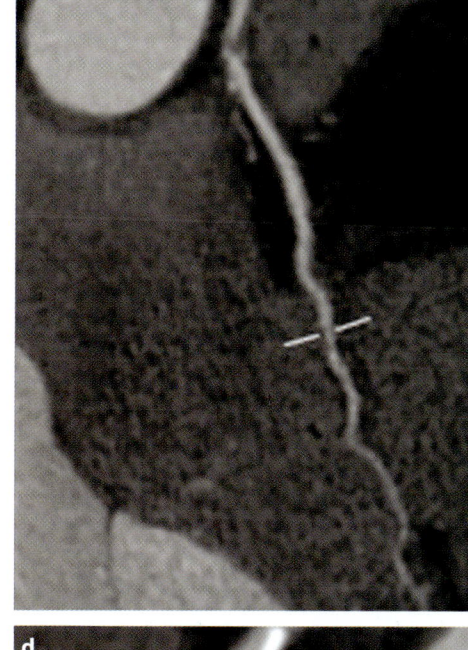
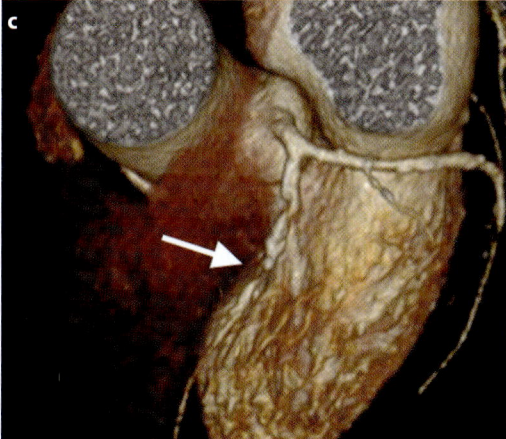
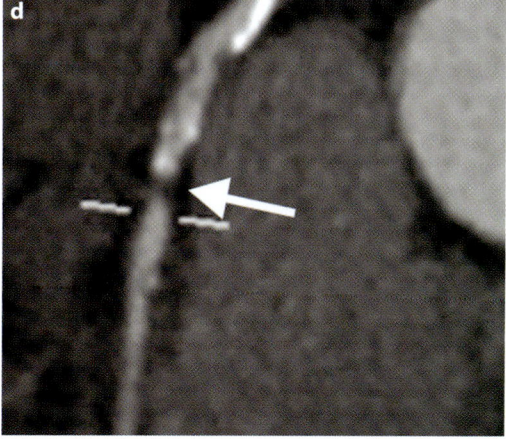

Fig. 1 a, b Soft plaque: severe stenosis of the right coronary artery. **c, d** Diffuse atheromas of the left anterior descending artery (LAD). Severe stenosis is caused by the soft plaque (hypodense at CT angiography)

Case 3
Three Asymptomatic Patients with Significant Stenosis Diagnosed in a Routine Screening Program

Patients: These three patients underwent coronary CTA in a standard screening procedure offered by a large electrical company. Every employee over 45 years of age was offered coronary CTA. None of these three patients had symptoms or important risk factors.

Case Description

As seen in Fig. 1a–f, the imaging findings in these three completely asymptomatic patients, none of whom had important risk factors, are very similar. There is focal atheromatous involvement of the LAD, with significant stenosis. Consistent with the very similar imaging findings, all three underwent stenting of the LAD, with positive clinical outcomes.

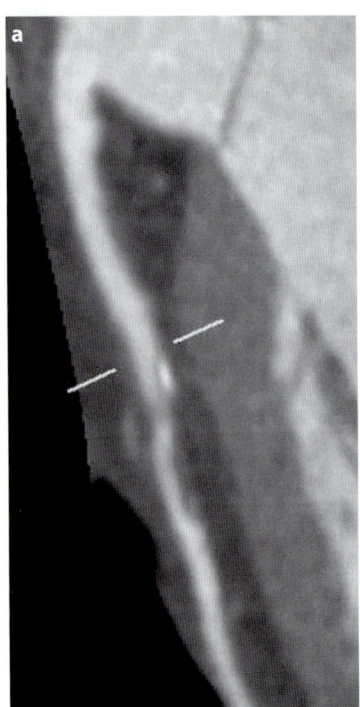
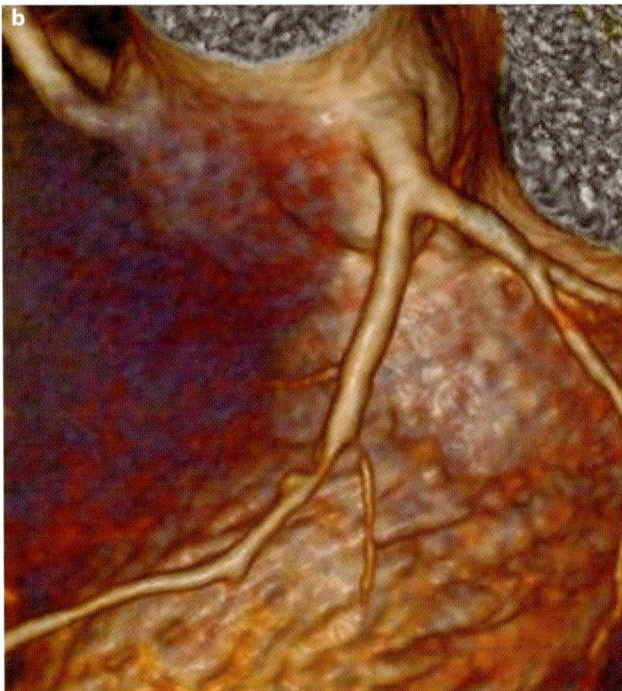
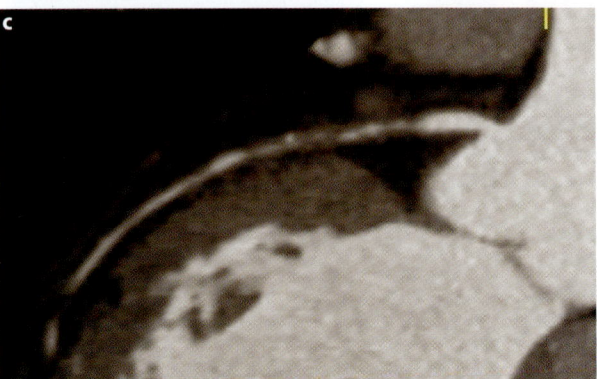

Fig. 1 a-f (*cont.* →)

19 Clinical Cases

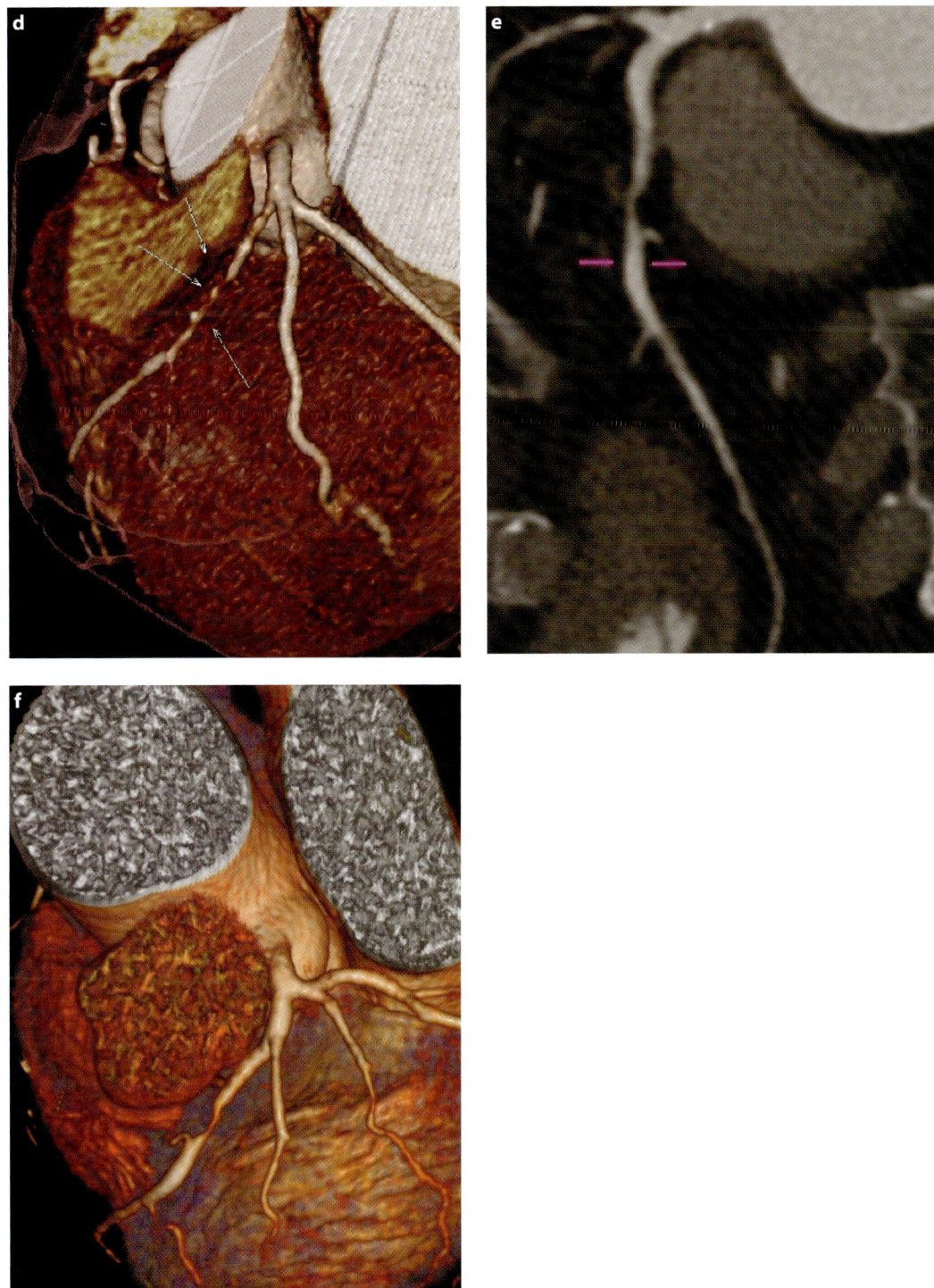

Fig. 1 a-f (continued)

Case 4
High Grade Stenoses in an Asymptomatic, High Performance Athlete

Patient: 38-year-old white male. Risk factors consisted in HTN, hypercholesterolemia, +FHX. The patient was asymptomatic, and a high-performance athlete.

Case Description

Figure 1a-c shows high-grade tandem RCA stenoses, LAD plaque, and normal LCX. Tandem RCA stenoses are depicted in Figure 2a,b.

This proves that asymptomatic high-performance athletes may harbor significant CAD. This raises the question of possibly using CCTA as a screening test in marathon runners, as an example.

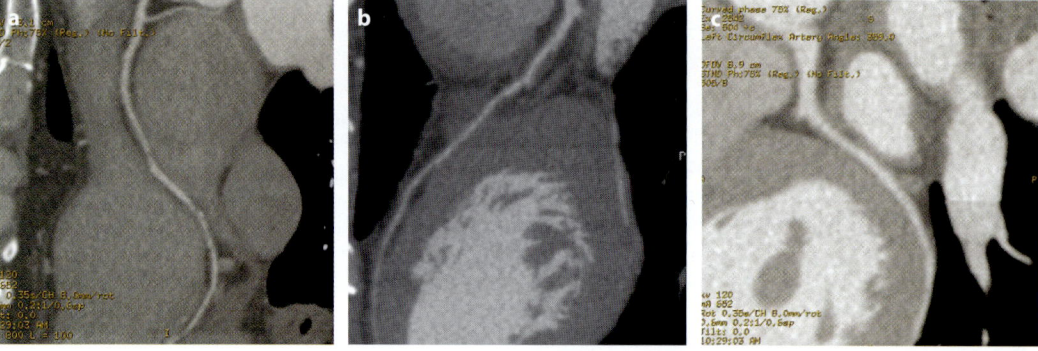

Fig. 1 a-c High-grade tandem RCA stenoses, LAD plaque, and normal LCX

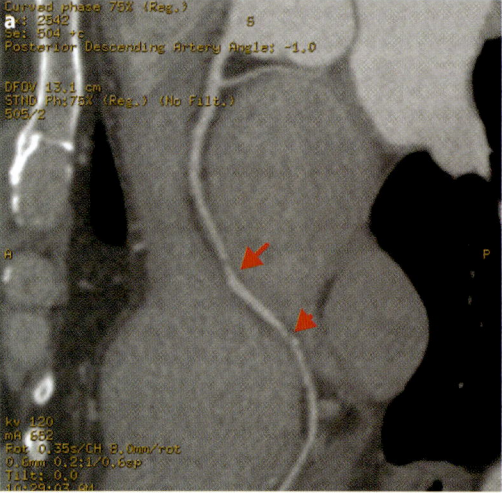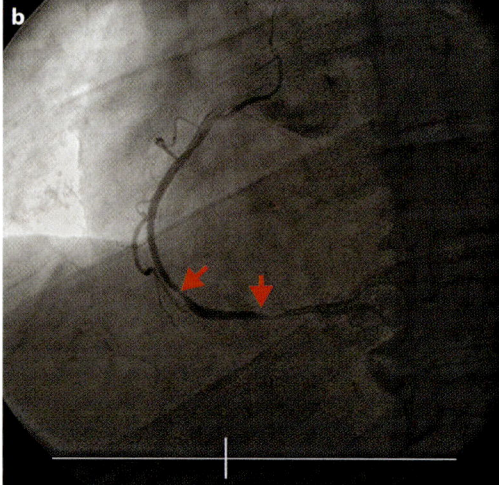

Fig. 2 a, b Tandem RCA stenoses

Case 5
High Grade Stenosis in an Asymptomatic, High Performance Athlete with No Risk Factors for Coronary Artery Disease and Silent Ischemia

Patient: 55-year-old male, asymptomatic, with no family history. Serum cholesterol = 205. Runs 3.5 miles per day (Fig. 1a-d). In particular, Figure 1d shows severe stenosis with vessel expansion, consistent with the presence of thrombus.

Case Description

Inferior wall ischemia was seen on myocardial perfusion imaging (Fig. 2).

High grade-stenosis was also present, with numerous small collateral vessels (Figs. 3, 4). Figure 5 shows no residual stenosis status after percutaneous coronary stent placement.

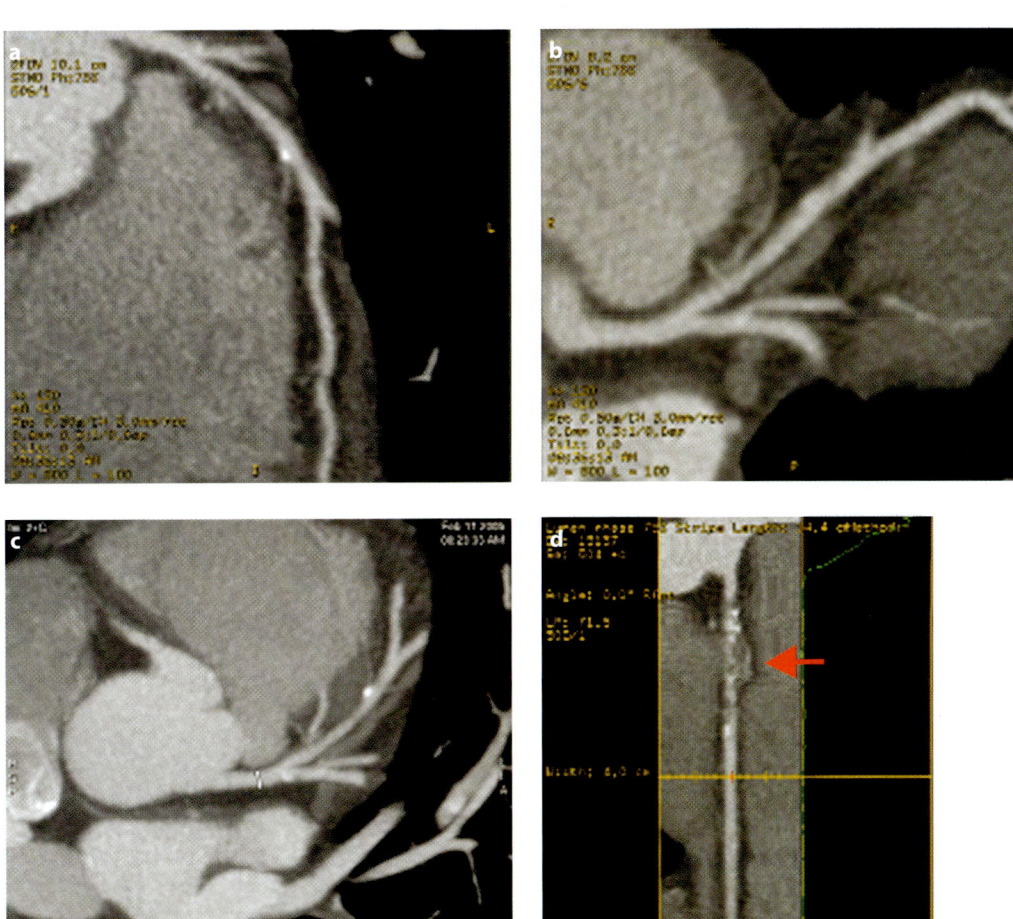

Fig. 1 a-d Severe stenosis with vessel expansion

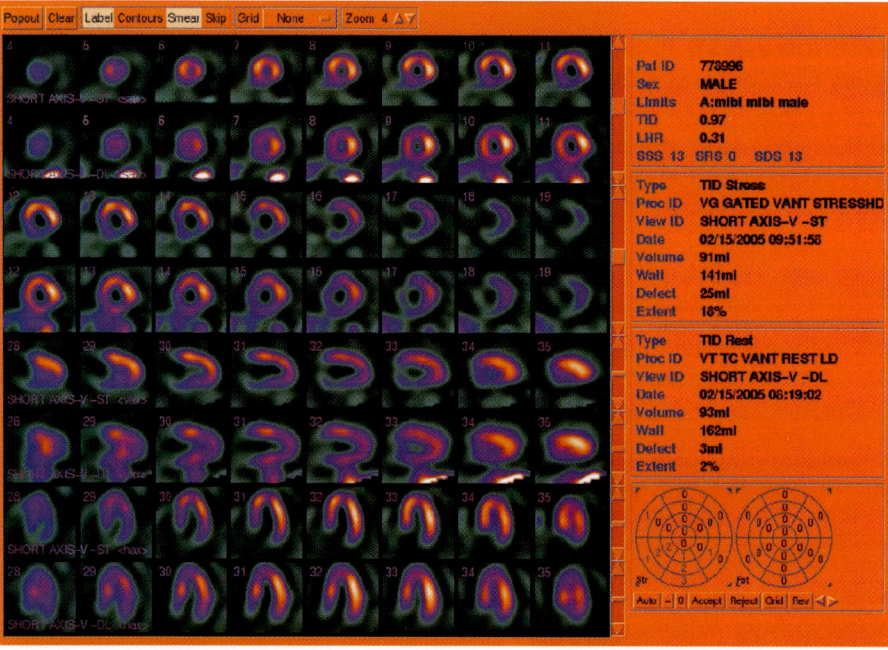

Fig. 2 Inferior wall ischemia as seen on myocardial perfusion imaging

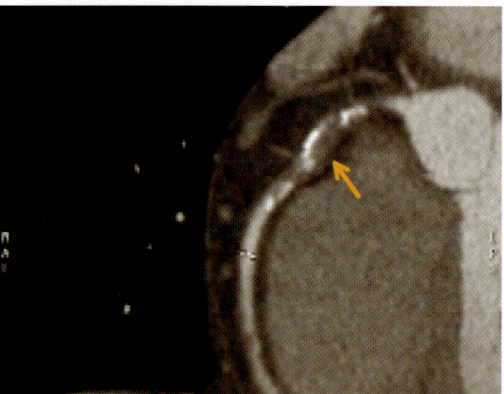

Fig. 3 High grade-stenosis with numerous small collateral vessels

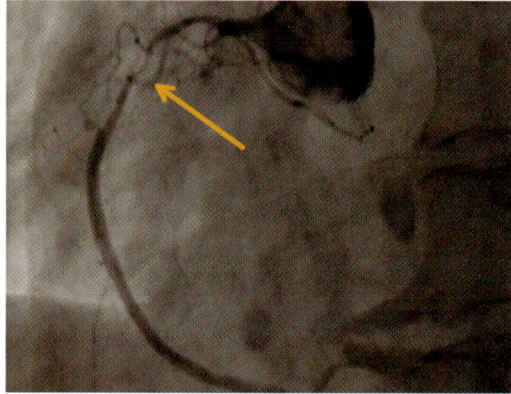

Fig. 4 High grade-stenosis with numerous small collateral vessels

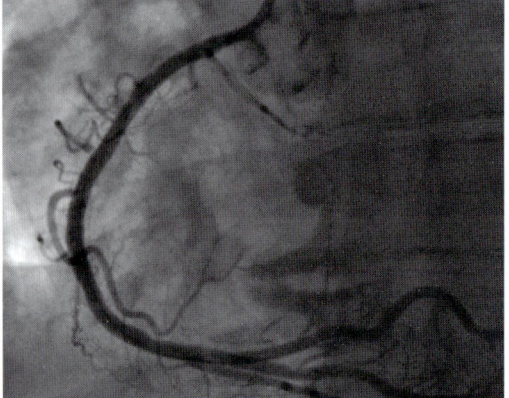

Fig. 5 No residual stenosis status after percutaneous coronary stent placement

Case 6
High Grade Stenosis in an Asymptomatic Helicopter Pilot

Patient: 39-year-old, asymptomatic white male, helicopter pilot. Risk factors consisted in +FHx and mild hypercholesterolemia.

Case Description

Figure 1a-c shows >70% stenosis at mid-RCA. The Figure 1a-c, displays symptomatic significant CAD in a patient with an occupation that could put others at risk. This raises the question of using CCTA as a screening exam.

Normal LCX and LAD were seen in this patient (Fig. 2a-c)

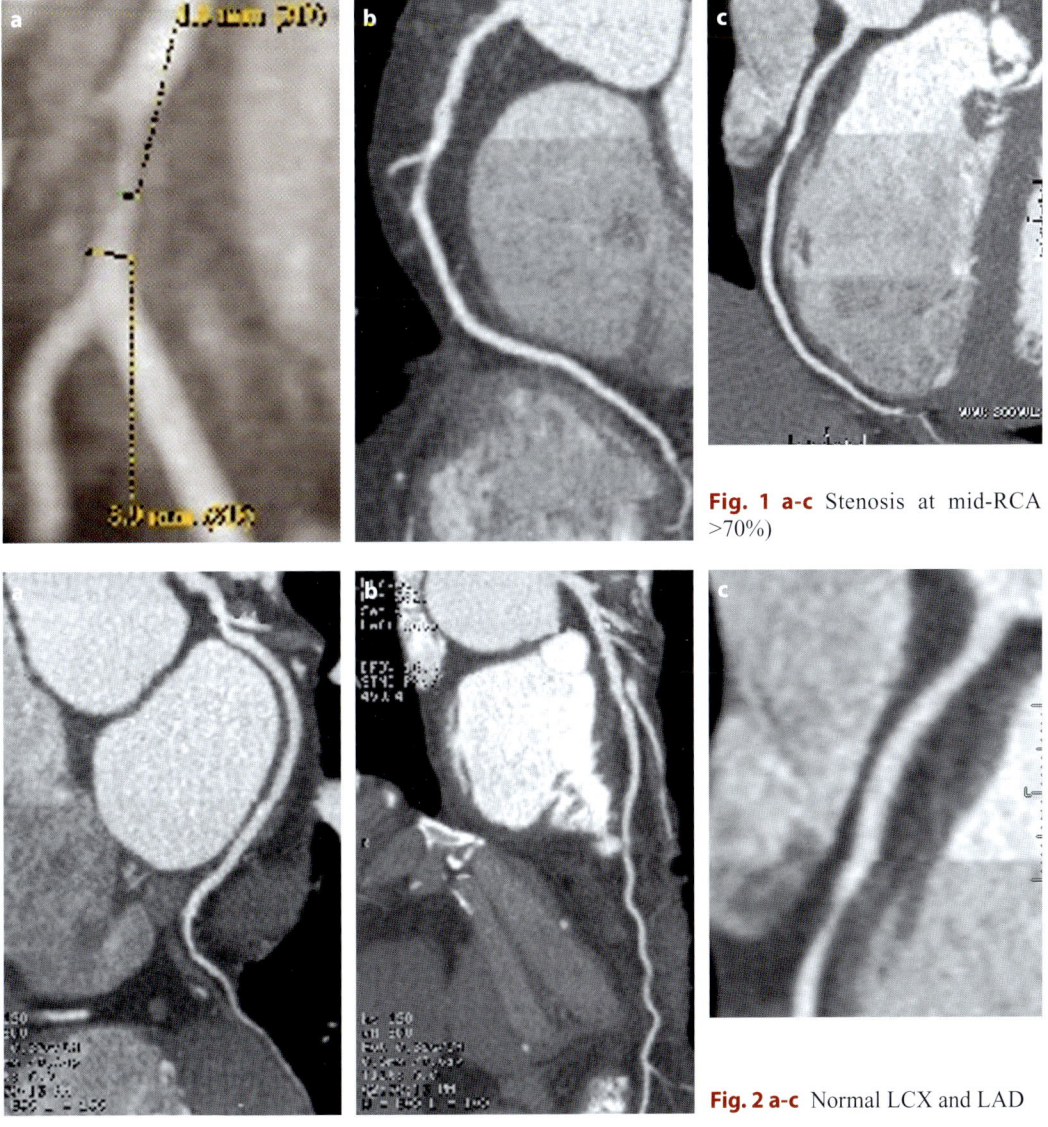

Fig. 1 a-c Stenosis at mid-RCA >70%)

Fig. 2 a-c Normal LCX and LAD

Case 7
Distal Stenosis of the Right Coronary Artery in Three Patients with Mild Symptoms During Intensive Exercise

Patients: Three relatively young patients (ages 48, 53, and 56) who experienced mild chest pain during intensive exercise (running). They had no risk factors, were non-smokers, and had normal cholesterol values. Their treadmill tests were negative.

Case Description

The MPR (Fig. 1a–c) and VRT (Fig.1d–f) images show very similar findings: a soft plaque in the distal segment of the right coronary artery. All other coronary artery segments are completely normal. In these patients, stenting was performed following coronary CTA. No residual symptoms occurred after stenting.

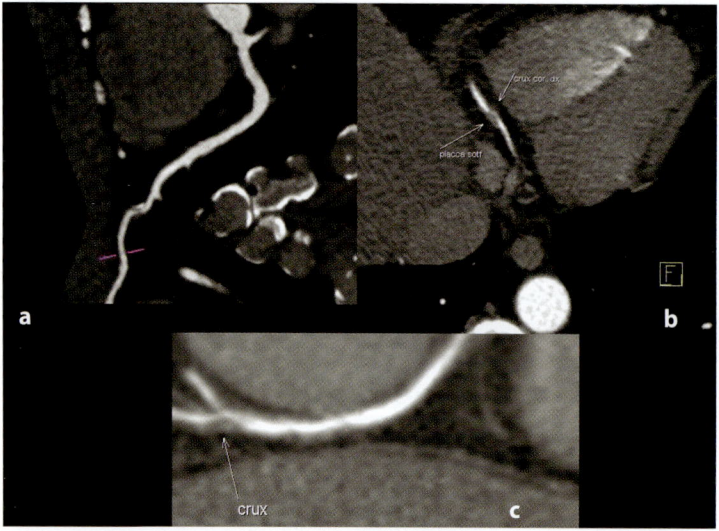

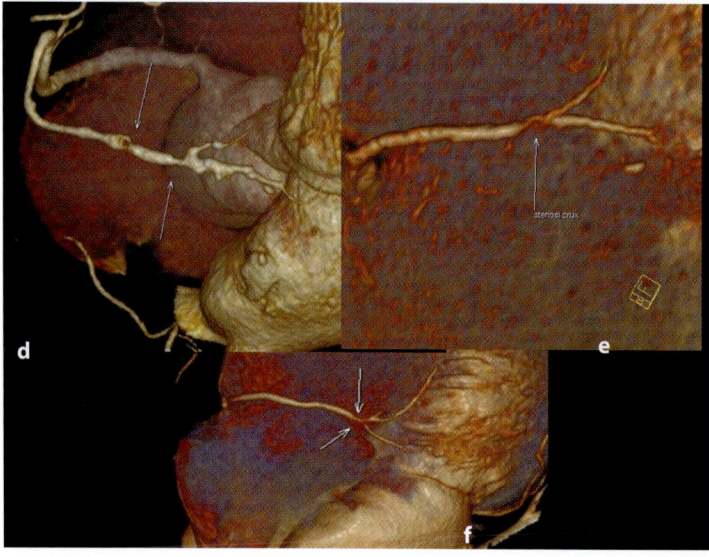

Fig. 1 a-f

Case 8
Incidental Finding of LAD Occlusion in a Patient with an Inconsistent History of Myocardial Infarction

Patient: 65-year-old male with intermediate risk factors, including high cholesterol, hypertension, family history. He had never been clinically diagnosed with myocardial infarction. Coronary CTA was performed as a screening procedure.

Case Description

Figure 1a, b shows an occlusion of the third proximal segment of the LAD. The diffuse atheromatous plaques of the right coronary artery did not cause significant stenosis (Fig. 1c). The large right coronary artery and the large circumflex artery account for the development of collateral circulation and the recanalization distal to the chronic occlusion of the LAD.

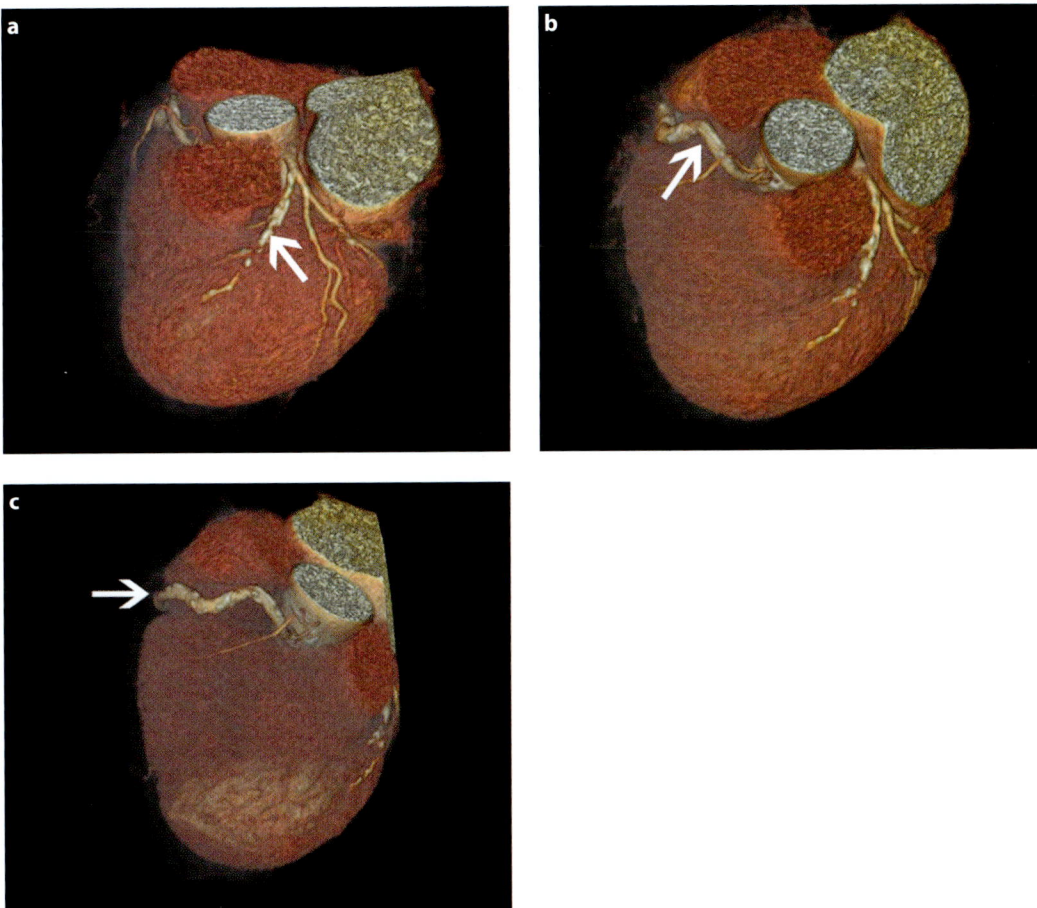

Fig. 1 a, b Occlusion of the third proximal segment of the LAD. **c** Diffuse atheromatous plaques of the right coronary artery: no significant stenosis

19.2 CAD Risk Factor Evaluation

Case 9
Unreliability of Framingham Risk Factors in Predicting Coronary Artery Disease

Patient: 44-year-old white female with chest pain and total cholesterol = 350.

Case Description

Figure 1a,b shows normal RCA and posterior descending artery (PDA). LAD and LCX also have a normal appearance (Fig. 2a,b). Framingham risk factors correlate poorly with plaque burden, as seen on CCTA.

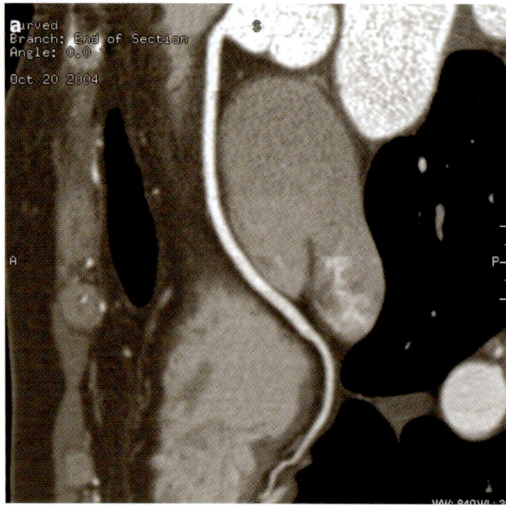
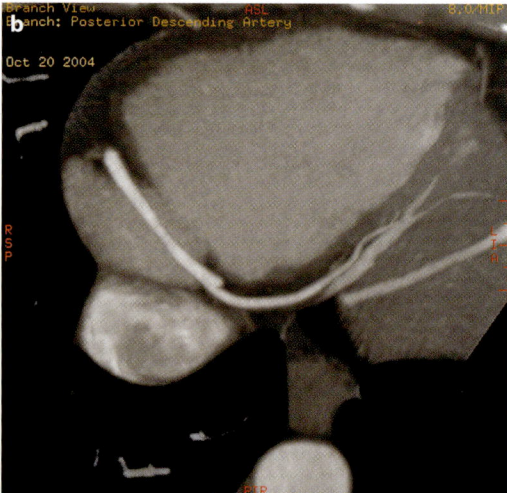

Fig. 1 a, b Normal RCA and PDA

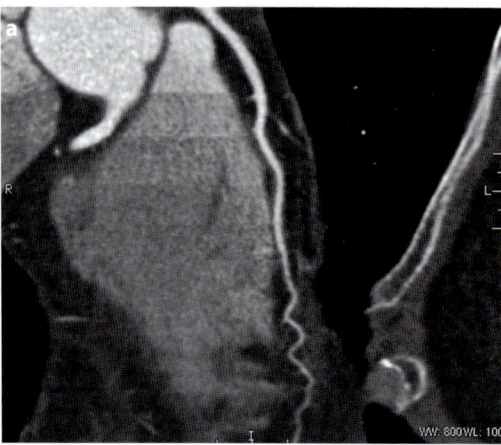
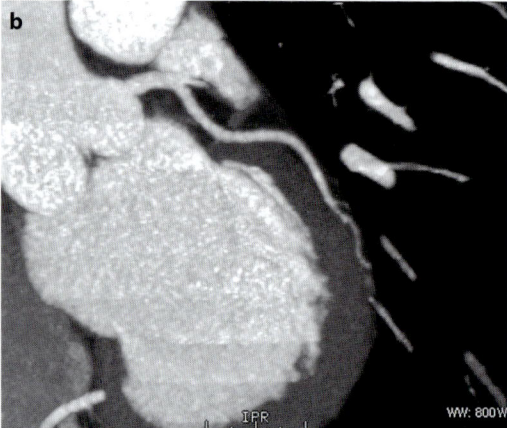

Fig. 2 a, b Normal LCX

Case 10
Unreliability of Framingham Risk Assessment

Patient: 50-year-old white female with familial hyperlipidemia. Total cholesterol has been >500 "for years", and has now decreased to 350 after one year of statins.

Case Description

Imaging shows minimal plaque burden (Fig. 1a-c), which means that there is poor correlation of plaque burden as seen on CCTA with Framingham Risk Factors.

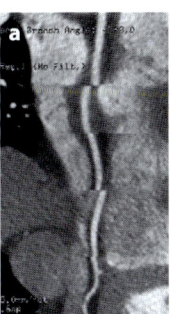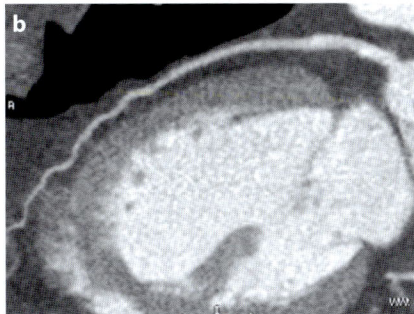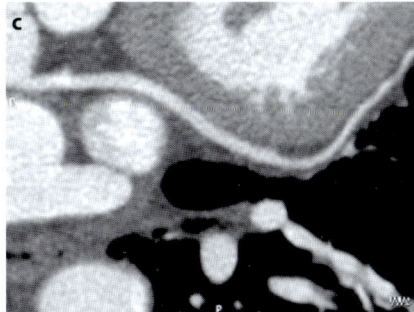

Fig. 1 a-c Minimal plaque burden

Case 11
Radiation Therapy as a Risk Factor for Coronary Artery Disease

Patient: 31-year-old white male with atypical chest pain. The patient is a smoker with a history of mediastinal radiation therapy (RT) for Hodgkin's lymphoma.

Case Description

Prior radiation therapy is a risk factor for ostial and proximal vessel CAD (Figs. 1a,b, 2a,b).

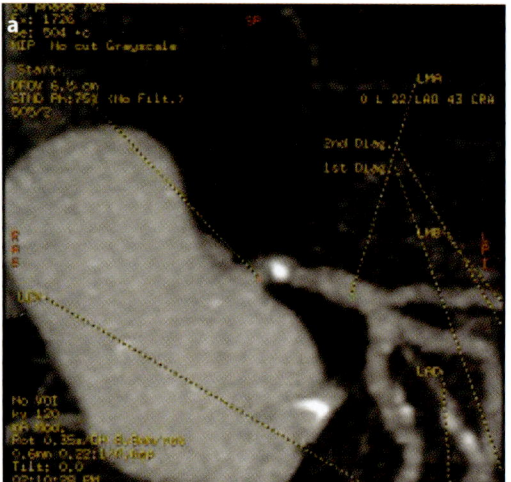 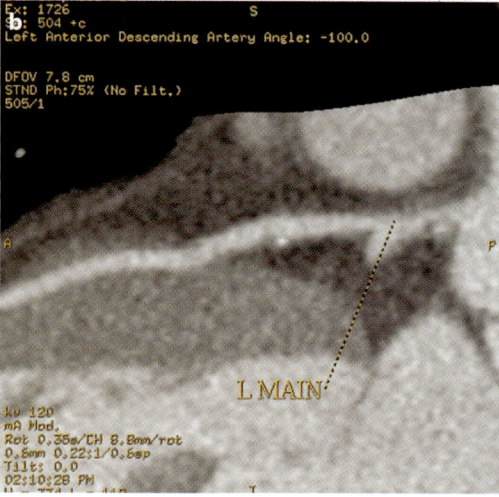

Fig. 1 a, b Prior radiation therapy as a risk factor for ostial and proximal vessel CAD

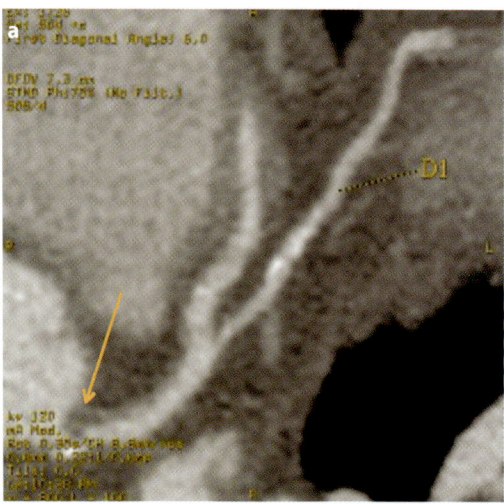 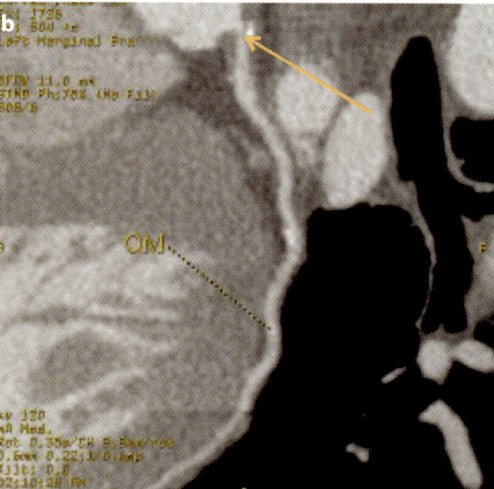

Fig. 2 a, b Prior radiation therapy as a risk factor for ostial and proximal vessel CAD

Case 12
Mixed Plaque in a Patient Undergoing Screening Coronary CTA

Patient: 49-year-old male with no symptoms of cardiac disease and negative EKG and treadmill tests. The only known risk factor was heavy smoking (up to 50 cigarettes a day).

Case Description

The MPR and VRT images of Fig. 1a, b show the mixed plaque, with a central calcium core and extended fibrolipidic content. There is a high degree of stenosis of the proximal LAD at the origin of a diagonal branch. Atheroma was not detected in the other coronary vessels.
One week after stenting of the coronary lesion, the patient experienced referred chest pain and thus again underwent coronary CTA. Figure 1c, d shows the optimal result, with patent stent, good distal flow, and patency of the diagonal branch.

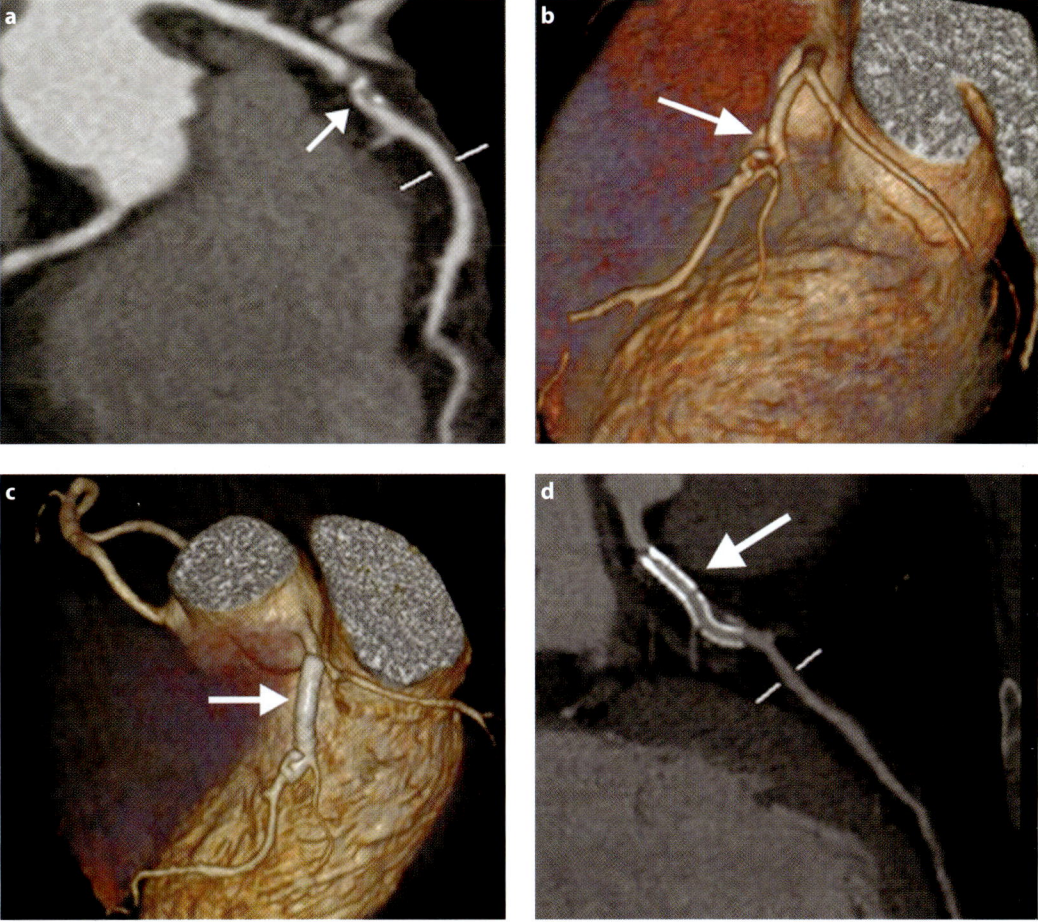

Fig. 1 a, b Atheromatous plaque: fibrolipidic with calcified core. 90%stenosis. **c, d** CT angiography control after stenting: no residual stenosis

Case 13
Calcified and Non-calcified Plaques: Relative Importance in Severe Stenotic Disease

Patient: 65-year-old male, heavy smoker but without symptoms. A routine CTA of the coronary arteries was performed as a screening procedure.

Case Description

Figure 1a, b shows the heavy atheromatous burden in the proximal LAD. Most of the plaques are calcified, causing significant "blooming" artifacts on the 2D images. The area of significant stenosis (>70%) of the LAD is related to the only non-calcified (soft) plaque. In most patients, both calcified and non-calcified plaques are present. As a rule, the radiologist should focus on the non-calcified plaque, which in most cases is the site of severe stenosis due to plaque growth.

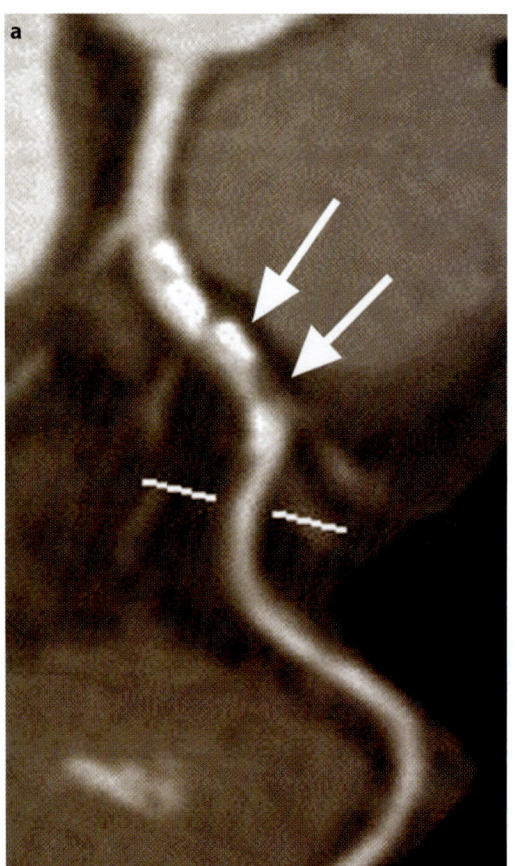 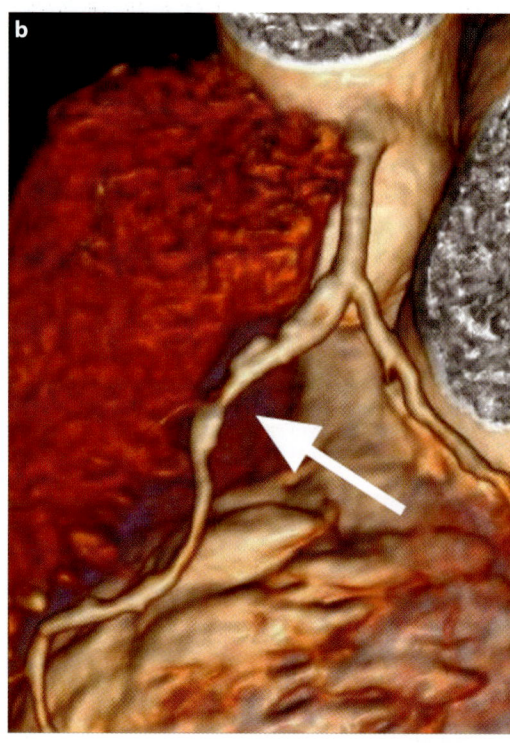

Fig. 1 a, b MIP and VRT images show diffuse LAD plaques. Blooming effects of calcified plaques. Vascular stenosis is only evident at site of the soft plaque (*arrows*)

Case 14
Female Smoker with Coronary Artery Disease

Patient: 64-year-old female, heavy smoker (up to 2 packs a day for over 30 years). She came to our attention during lung cancer screening and agreed to undergo a coronary CTA study as well. She had no cardiac symptoms and both her at-rest EKG and her treadmill test were negative.

Case Description

The MPR and VRT images of Fig. 1a, c show extensive atherosclerotic involvement of the left descending coronary artery. A concentric severe stenosis of the right coronary artery is seen in Fig. 1b, d. The severe stenotic involvement was due to a soft plaque, i.e., with a fibrolipidic content, which carries an increased risk of plaque complications (hemorrhage, dissection) and acute occlusion. The patient underwent stenting of both arteries, considered by the angiographist to be life-saving in this case.

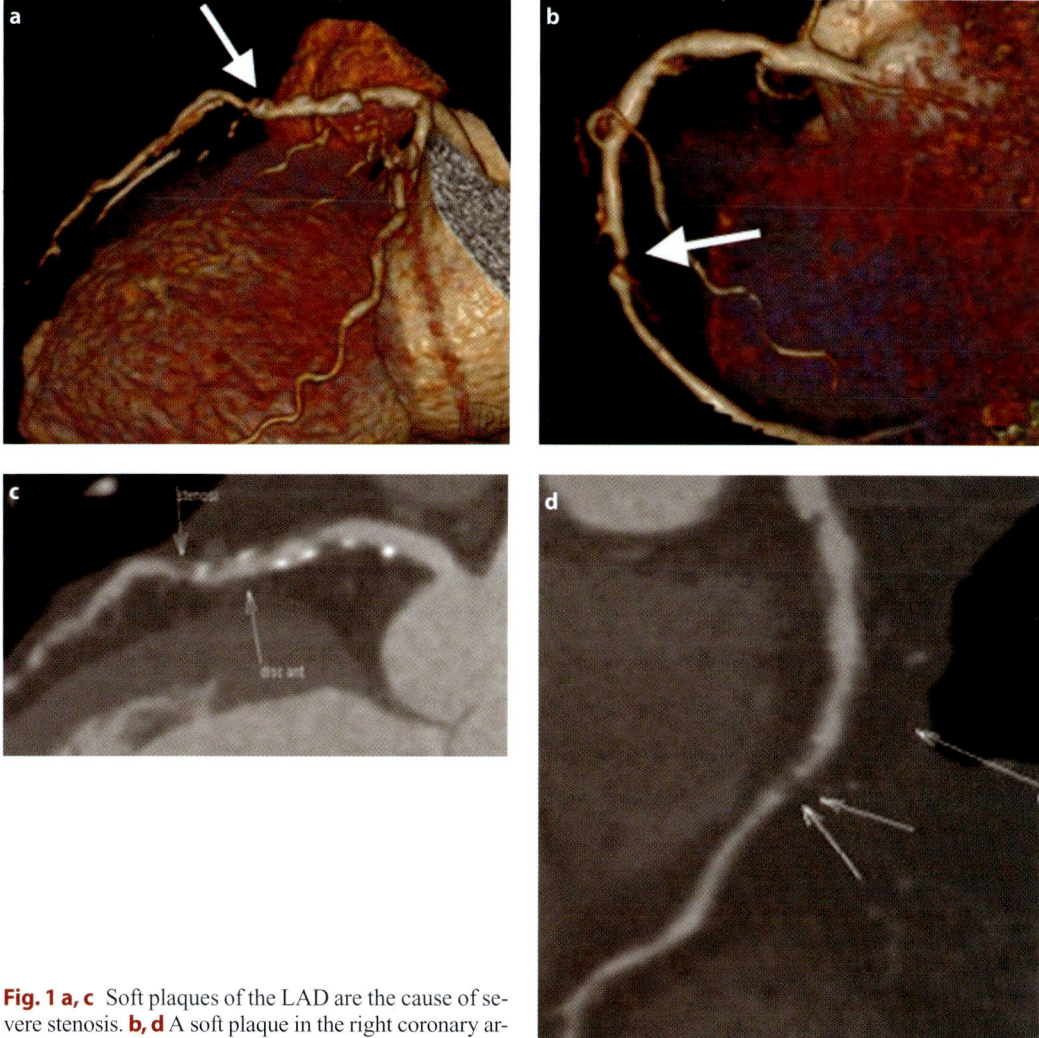

Fig. 1 a, c Soft plaques of the LAD are the cause of severe stenosis. **b, d** A soft plaque in the right coronary artery also caused severe stenosis

Case 15
Important Atherosclerotic Disease in a Heavy Smoker

Patient: 52-year-old male who smoked up to 50 cigarettes a day. He agreed to a screening CTA procedure.

Case Description

Important and diffuse atheromatous involvement of the proximal LAD is seen in Fig. 1b, d. Mixed plaque components (partially calcific, partially made up of soft plaques). As in most such cases, the calcific plaques are parietal, eccentric, and are usually not the cause of the stenosis. A severe reduction in vessel caliber, if present, in the distal part of a plaque can typically be attributed to a soft, non-calcific plaque. In the same patient, an anomalous, very angulated origin of the right coronary artery was also diagnosed (Fig. 1a, c). Usually, this type of vascular anomaly is not the cause of symptoms; however, it must be described in the coronary CTA report.

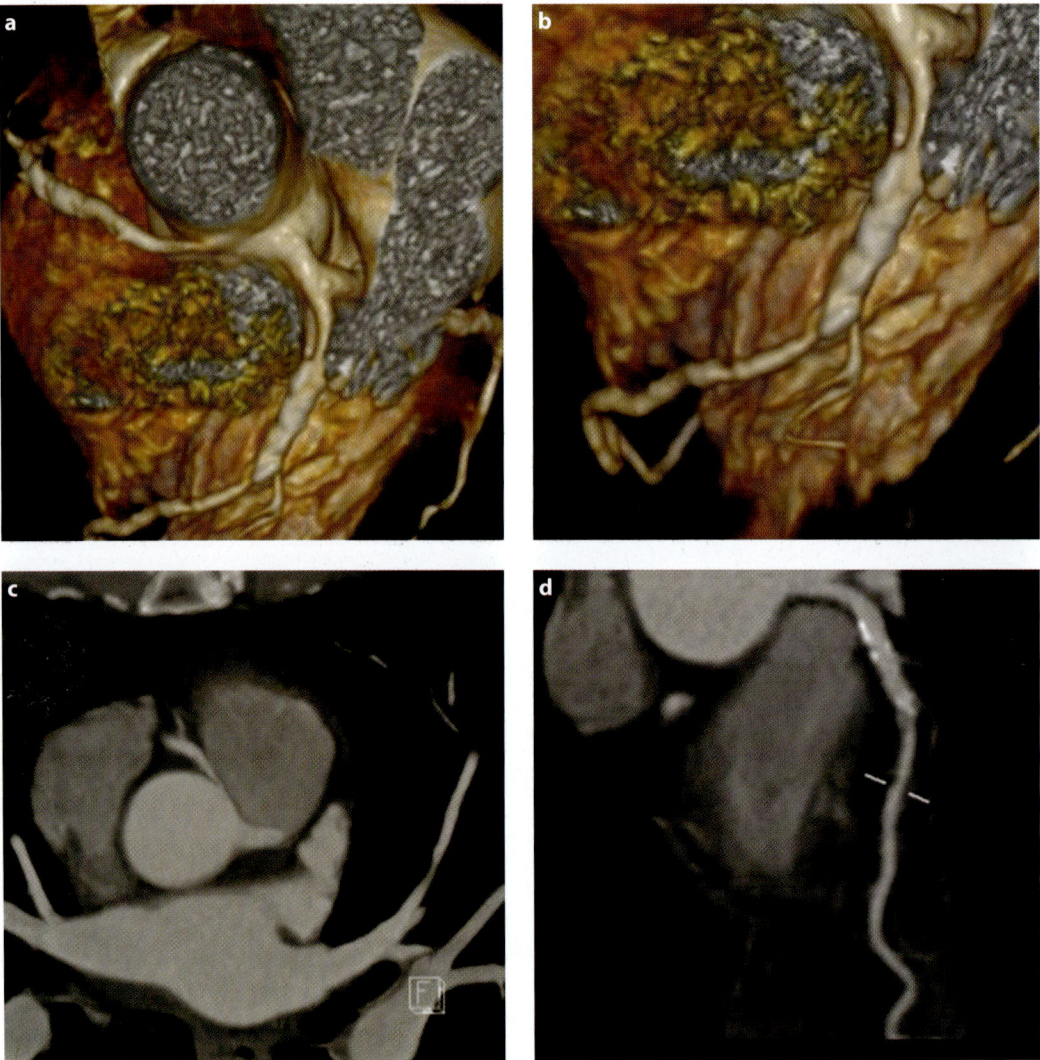

Fig. 1 a, c Angulated origin and stenosis of the right coronary artery. **b, d** Diffuse LAD plaques and severe stenosis

Case 16
Non-specific Chest Pain in a Female Heavy Smoker

Patient: 56-year-old female, heavy smoker (30 cigarettes a day). She complained of non-specific and periodic episodes of chest pain. Her EKG was normal.

Case Description

The MPR (Fig. 1a) and VRT (Fig. 1b) images show single-vessel involvement. The plaque in the middle LAD is characterized by a fibrolipidic component and a calcific internal core. Significant stenosis (over 60%) is evident.

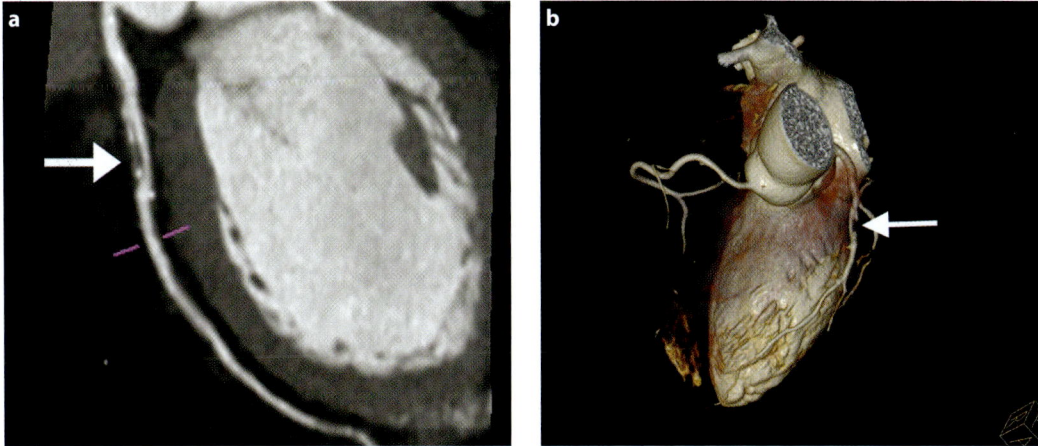

Fig. 1 a, b Fibrolipidic plaque with calcified core of the LAD resulting in 50% stenosis

Case 17
Minimal Coronary Artery Disease in a Patient with Severe Smoking History

Patient: 57-year-old white male with chest pain. The patient had a 120 pack-year history of smoking, hypercholesterolemia, and hypertension.

Case Description

Imaging shows a high-risk patient with minimal CAD (Fig. 1a-c).

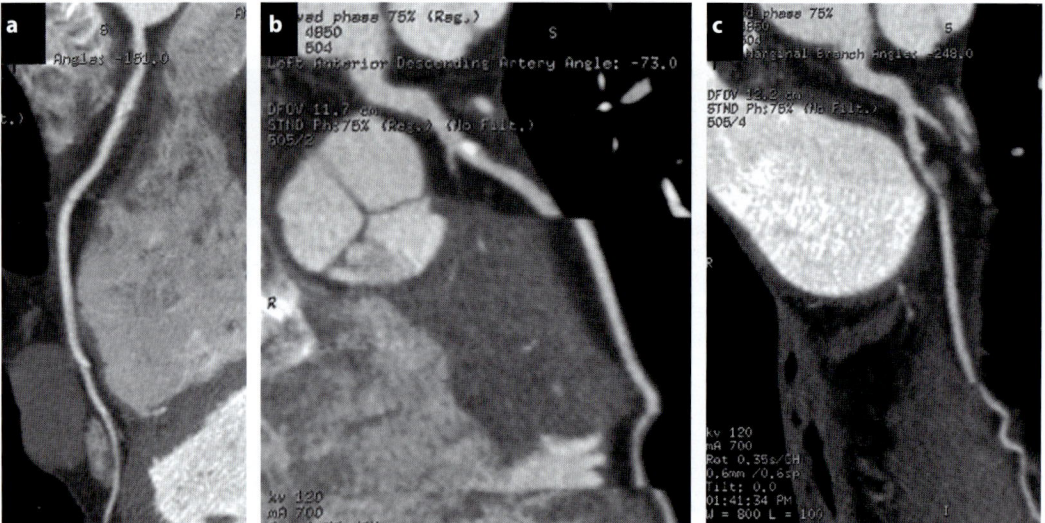

Fig. 1 a-c High-risk patient with minimal CAD

Case 18
Two Cases of Severe Coronary Disease and a Negative Calcium Score

Patient 1: 45-year-old asymptomatic male with negative EKG and treadmill tests. His father had died of myocardial infarction at age 43. The patient had never smoked and his cholesterol values were normal, as was his blood pressure. He came to us for routine screening due to his positive family history.

Case Description

Figure 1a–d shows a severe stenosis of the LAD caused by a concentric soft plaque. Minimal parietal calcification is also present.

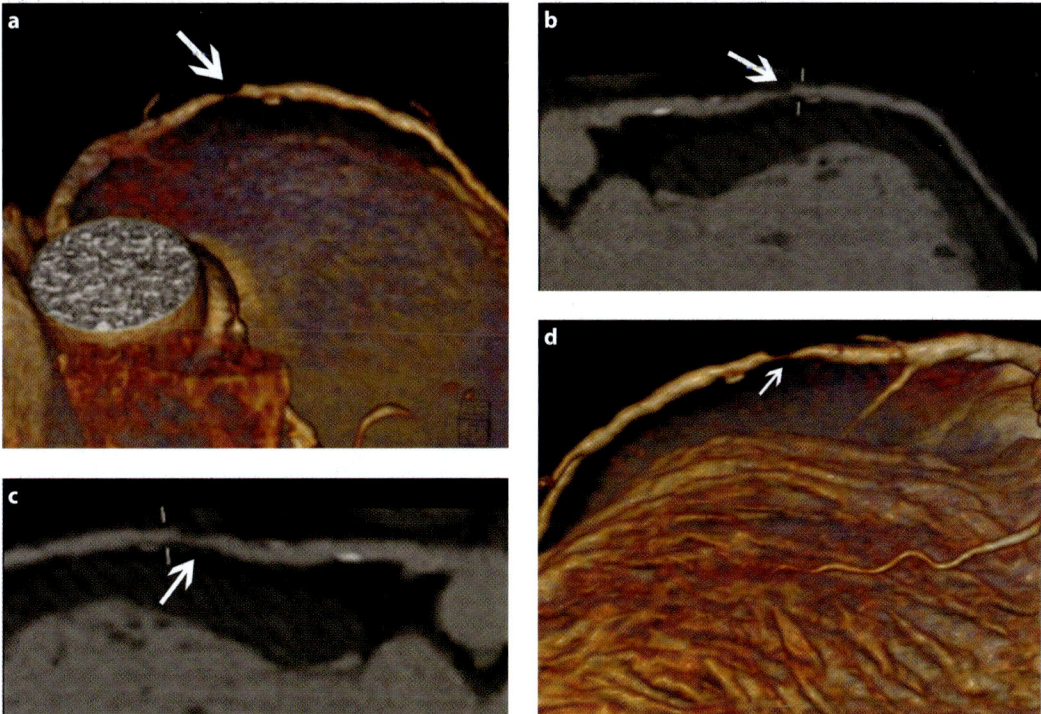

Fig. 1 a-d Multiple view of the LAD. *Arrow* shows a severe (> 85%) focal concentric stenosis due to a soft plaque

Patient 2: 67-year-old heavy smoker who agreed to undergo coronary CTA as a screening procedure.

Case Description

Figure 2a, b shows a concentric soft plaque with severe, subocclusive stenosis of the mid portion of the LAD. In the images, there is no evidence of parietal calcium. The other vessels were normal. The stenosis was stented (Fig. 2c, d).

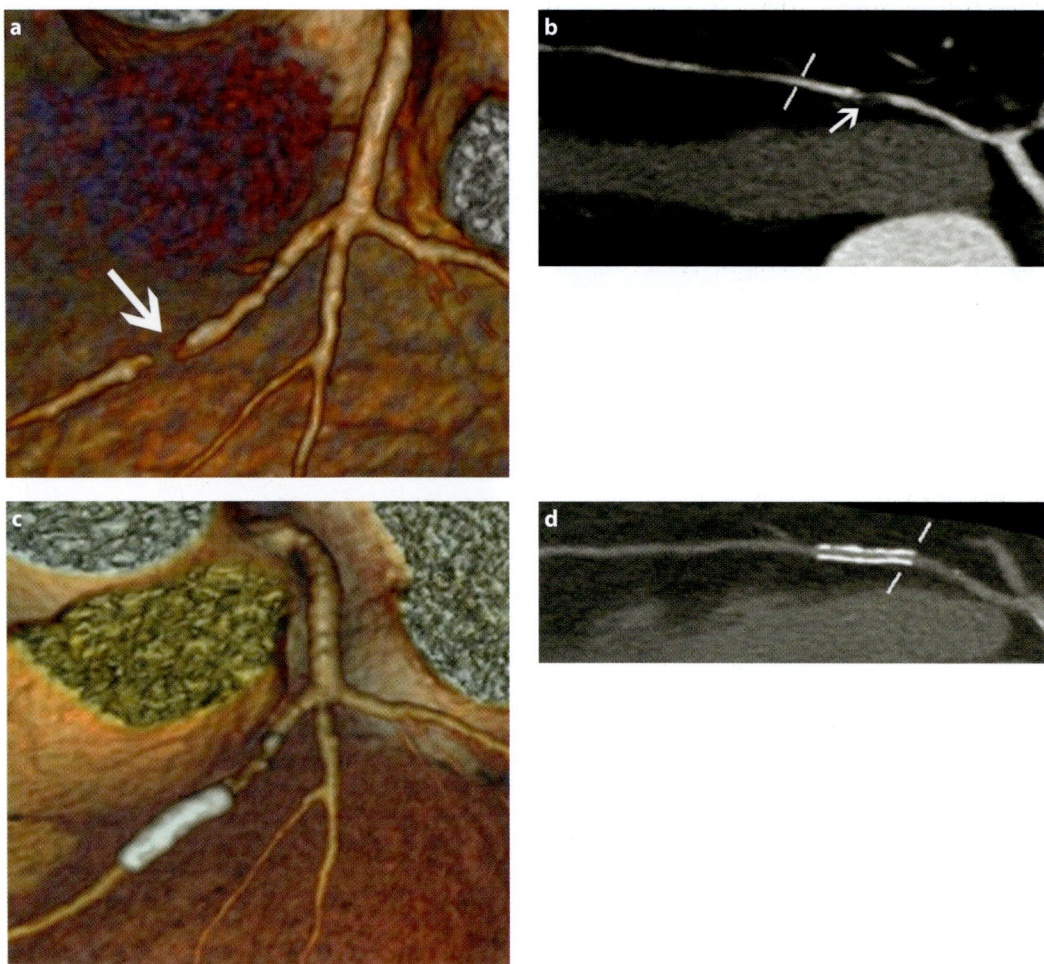

Fig. 2 a, b Severe concentric LAD stenosis; soft plaque (*arrow*). **c, d** Control follow-up 1 year after stenting

Comment

If these two patients had been evaluated on the basis of the calcium score, their results would have been normal. These two cases show the value of coronary CTA compared to calcium-score screening.

Case 19
Symptomatic, High Risk Patient with a Normal Coronary CTA

Patient: 55-year-old white female who had suffered from IDDM for 35 years. Risk factors consisted in HTN, hypercholesterolemia, and a weak family history with chest pain and shortness of breath.

Case Description

Figure 1a-c shows minimal (if any) plaque burden. It is common for high-risk, symptomatic patients to have no significant CAD on CCTA. Therefore, coronary catheterization should not be hastily performed in these patients unless the electrocardiogram (EKG) or troponin levels are abnormal.

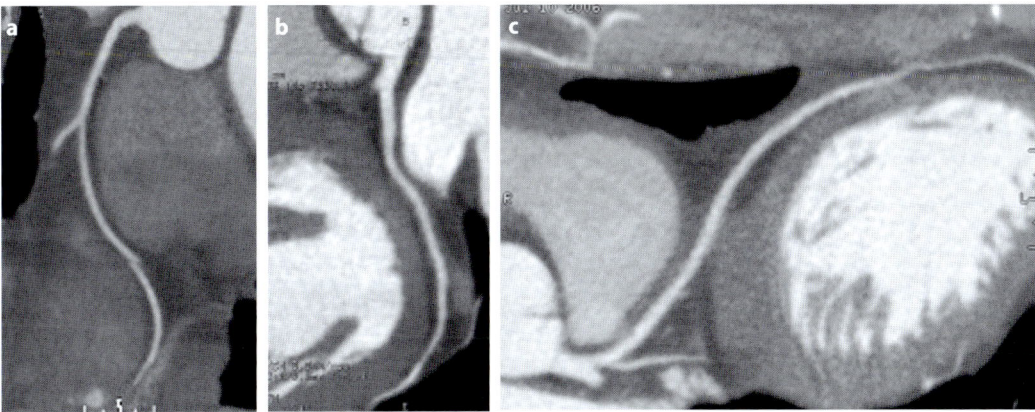

Fig. 1 a-c Minimal (if any) plaque burden

19.3 CAD and Associated Diseases

Case 20
Coronary Artery Disease Associated with an Early Presentation of Erectile Dysfunction

Patient: 41-year-old white male with erectile dysfunction. No risk factors for CAD were reported.

Case Description

Figure 1a-c shows single-vessel LAD disease. Early-onset erectile dysfunction may be on the basis of atherosclerosis. Patients with these dysfunctions may also be harboring asymptomatic CAD.

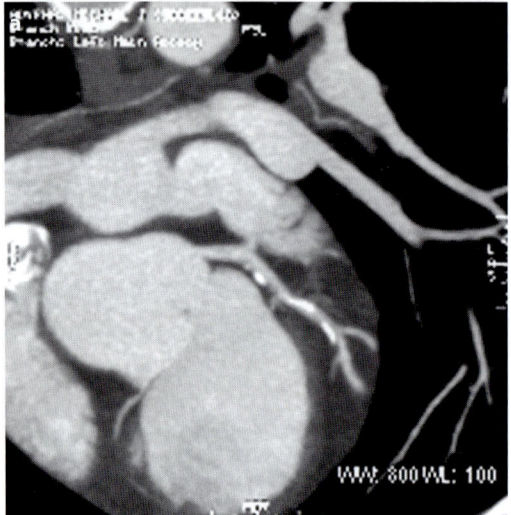
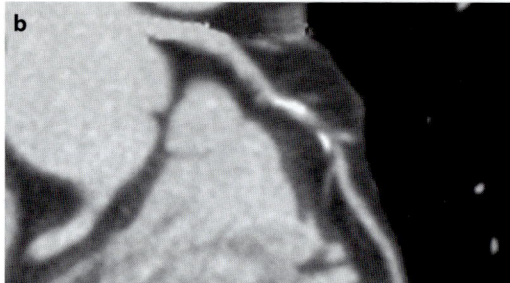
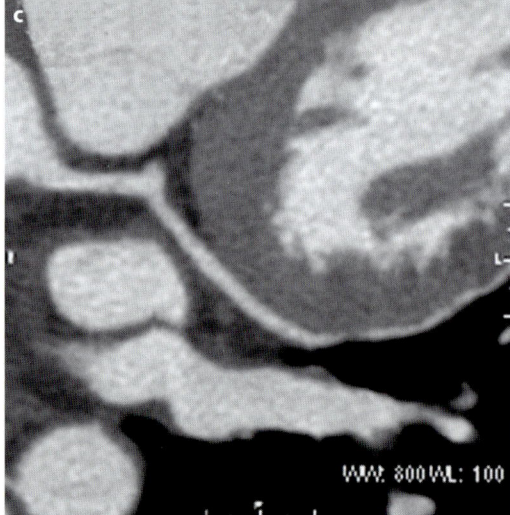

Fig. 1 a-c Single-vessel LAD disease

Case 21
Significant Coronary Artery Stenosis as an Incidental Finding Prior to Aortic Valve Surgery

Patient: 65-year-old male who underwent coronary CTA prior to surgery for aortic valve stenosis.

Case Description

The VRT (Fig. 1a) and MIP (Fig. 1b) images show a soft concentric plaque of the middle segment of the LAD causing a lumen stenosis of > 80%. Figure 1c,d shows the aortic valve, with a tight stenosis and significant thickening. The patient underwent aortic valve surgery. A bypass of the left mammary artery to the distal LAD was performed at the same time.

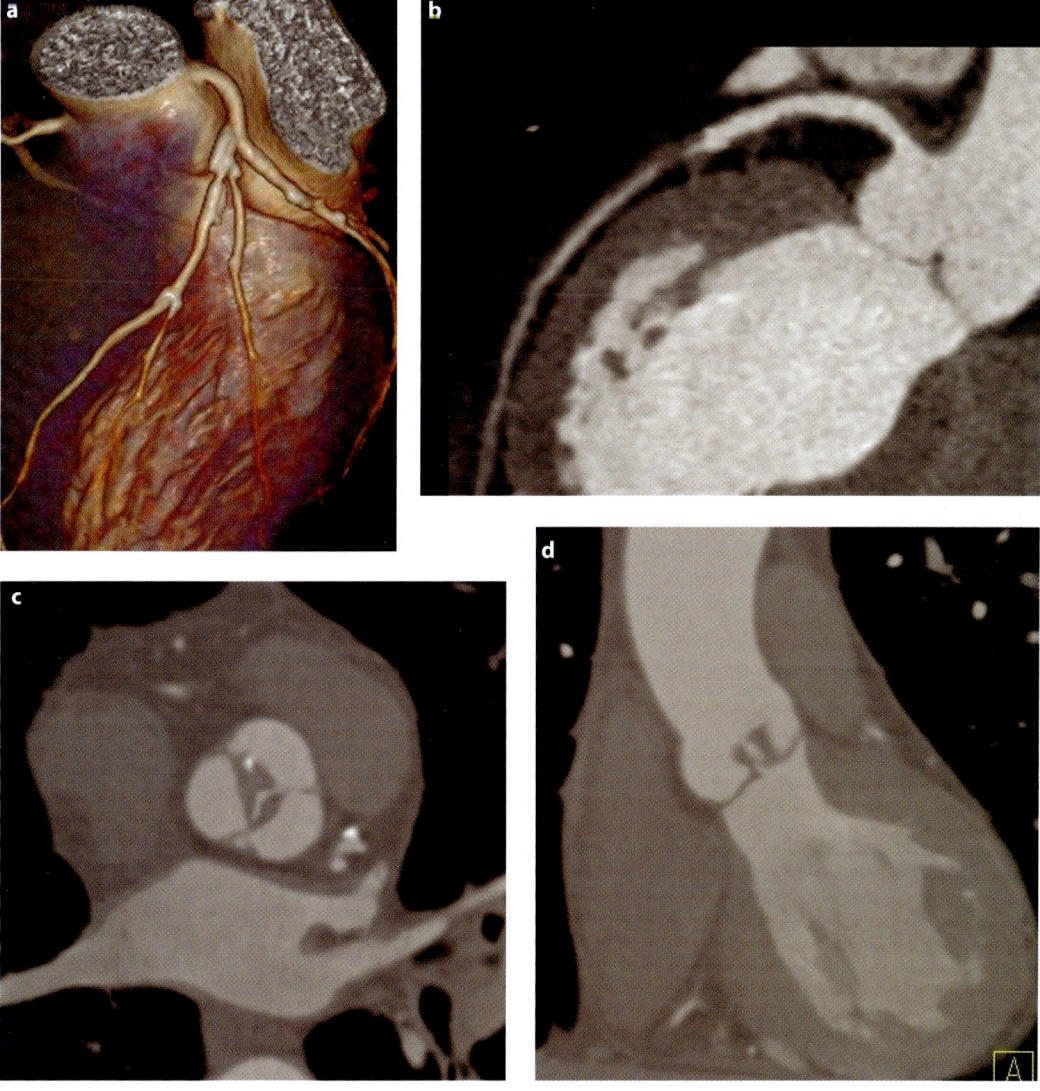

Fig. 1 a-d

Case 22
Incidental Finding of Severe Coronary Stenosis During a CT Evaluation of Abdominal Aortic Aneurysm (AAA)

Patient: 71-year-old male admitted to the hospital for scheduled AAA surgery. A final CT of the aneurysm prior to surgery had been planned. The radiologist decided to include a coronary angiographic study using the same CTA settings. The patient had multiple risk factors, including previous smoking, high cholesterol, and hypertension.

Case Description

The MPR and VRT coronary CTA images of Fig. 1a–d show severe and diffuse plaque involvement of the LAD. Subocclusive stenosis of the mid portion of the artery is evident. AAA surgery was rescheduled and coronary angiography was immediately planned. Extending a vascular CTA study to include an evaluation of the coronary arteries is possible and should be performed in high-risk patients. In older patients, the increased radiation dose of the extended examination should not be considered as problematic.

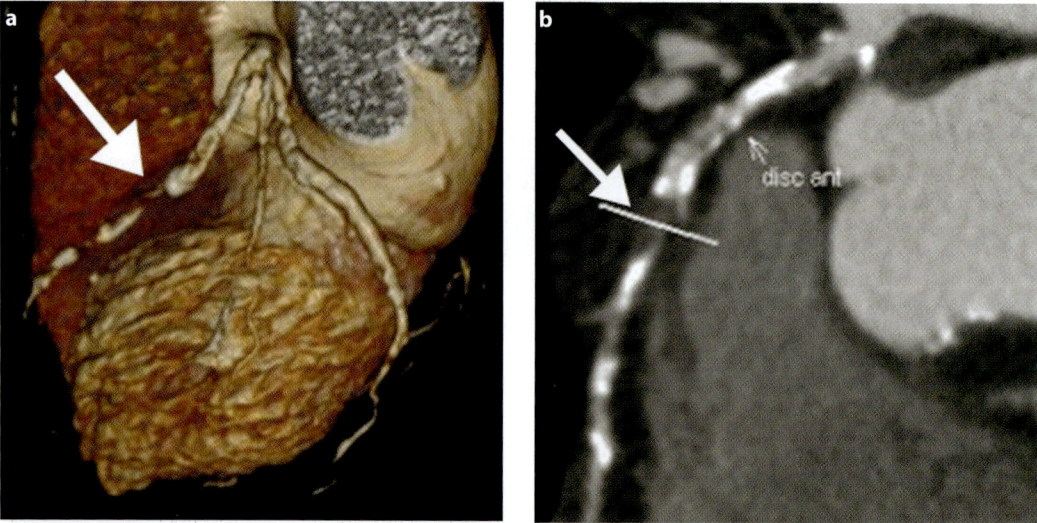

Fig. 1 a-d Diffuse plaques. Severe (90%) stenosis is caused by a large soft plaque. The stenosis was successfully treated with stenting (*cont.* →)

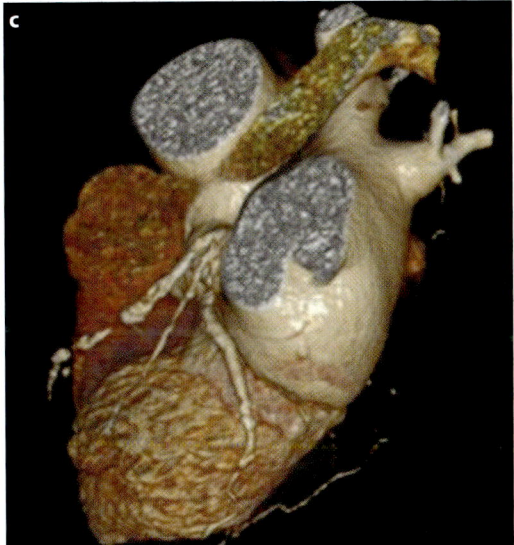 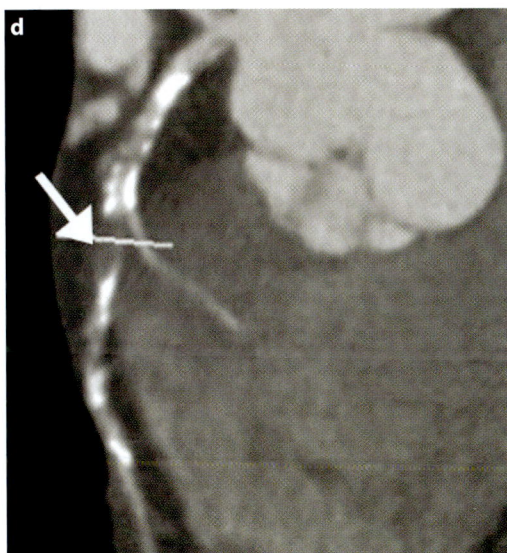

Fig. 1 a-d (continued)

19.4 Severity of Atherosclerotic Plaque and Coronary Stenosis

Case 23
Early Presentation of Coronary Artery Disease

Patient: 27-year-old white male with chest pain at rest radiating to the left arm, dyspnea at rest. Risk factors consisted in hypercholemia, positive family history (+FHx), smoking and hypertension (HTN).

Case Description

Figure 1 shows diffuse LAD plaque without stenosis. A mild plaque is displayed in the right coronary artery (RCA) and left circumflex artery (LCX) (Fig. 2).

The patient's 30-year-old asymptomatic brother, ex-smoker, presented with the same +FHx. CCTA results were normal (Fig. 3). Framingham risk factors had a variable expression and did not correlate. Figure 3 shows plaque burden as seen on CCTA.

Fig. 1 a, b Diffuse LAD plaque without stenosis

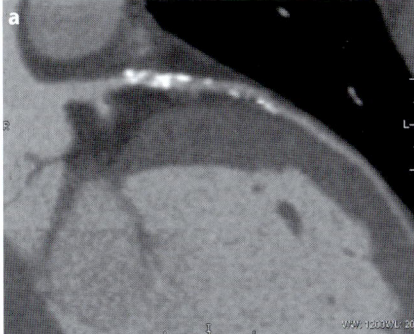 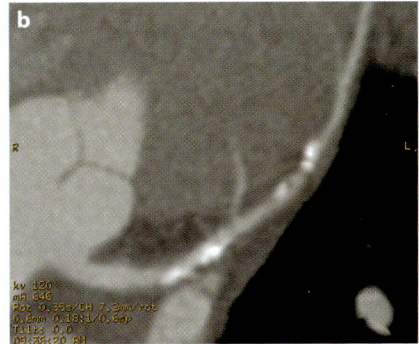

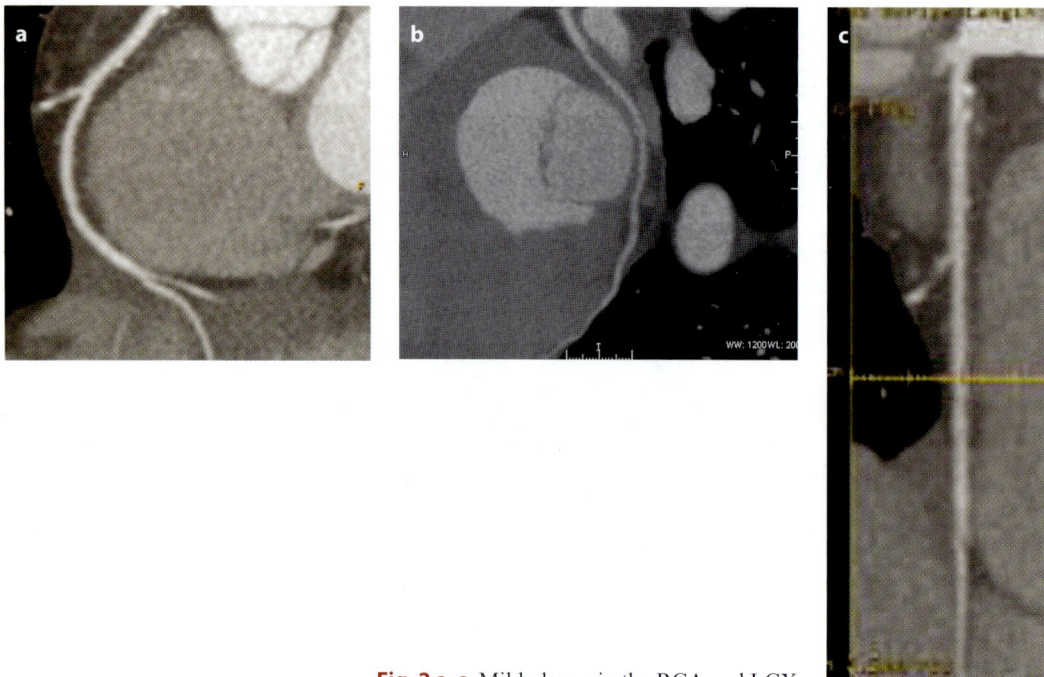

Fig. 2 a-c Mild plaque in the RCA and LCX

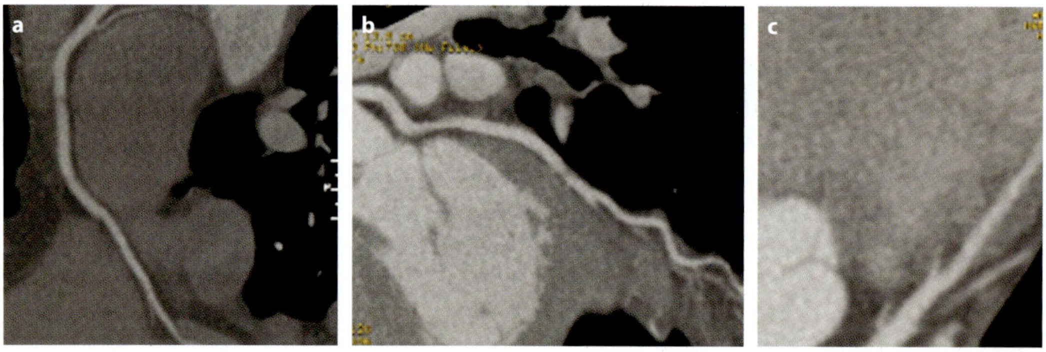

Fig. 3 a-c Normal CCTA

Case 24
Single-Vessel Involvement and Soft Plaque

Patient: 54-year-old male who underwent a screening procedure based on the presence of general intermediate risk factors.

Case Description

Figure 1a, b and Figure 1c, d show, respectively, the MPR and 3D VRT images, which evidence single-vessel involvement with a soft plaque. There is no calcium, a finding supported by a calcium score equal to zero. The other vessels were completely normal.

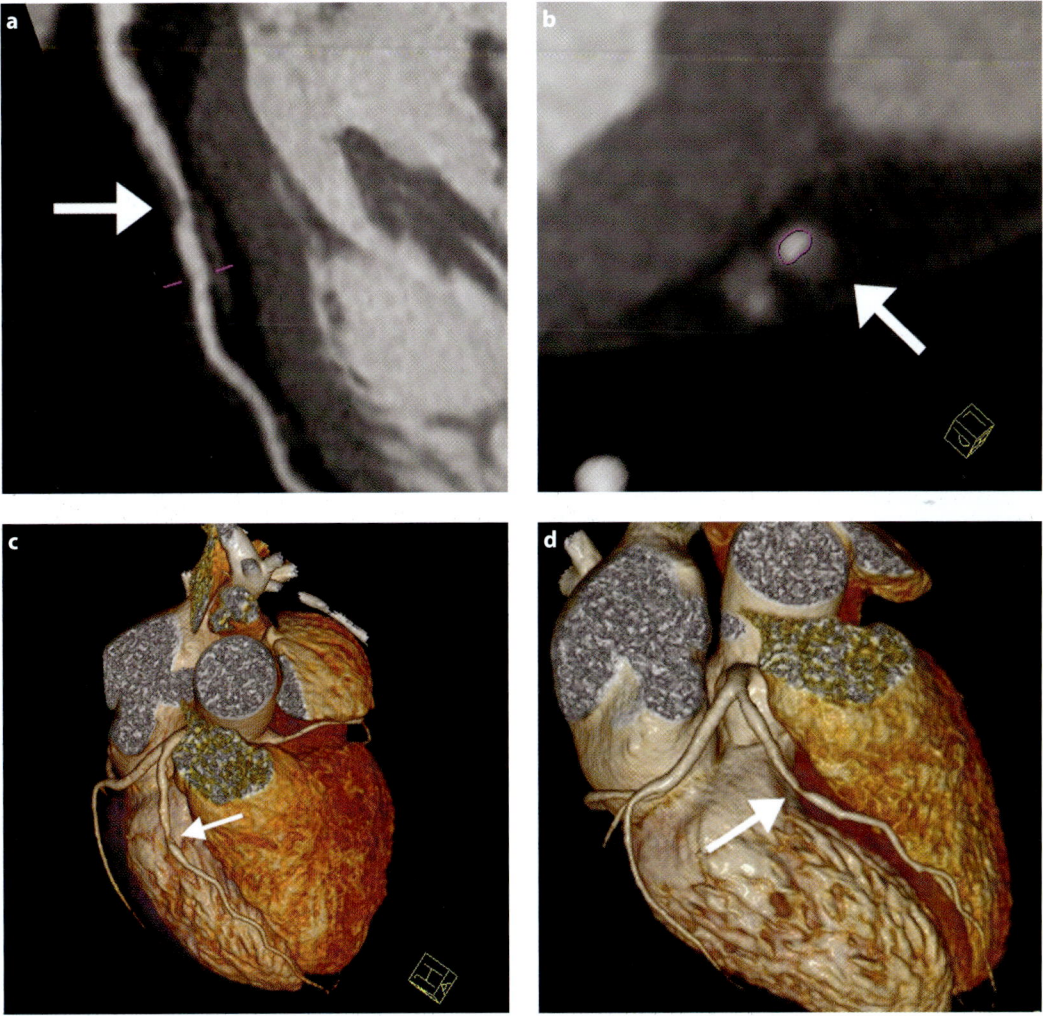

Fig. 1 a, b Fibrolipidic plaque of the third proximal segment of the LAD resulting in 70% stenosis. **c, d** VRT images show the stenosis

Case 25
Mixed Atheromatous Involvement: Focal Stenosis Due to a Soft Plaque

Patient: 65-year-old male with generic risk factors (including previous smoking habit, hypertension). A screening coronary CTA was performed.

Case Description

Figure 1a, b shows diffuse plaque involvement of the proximal LAD, with a predominant calcific component. The single focal stenotic segment is related to the presence of a soft plaque (arrow). An anomalous origin of the right coronary artery was also observed (arrow in Fig. 1c).

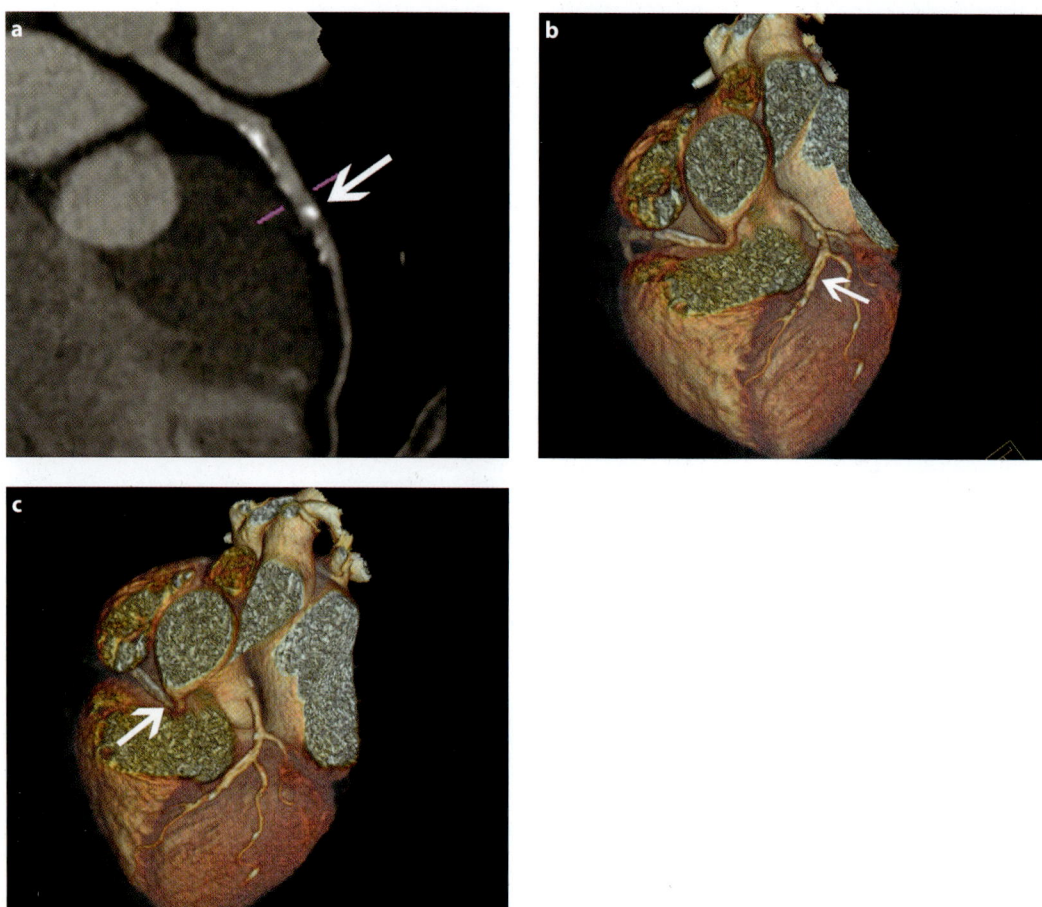

Fig. 1 a, b Atheromatous plaques of the LAD cause 50% stenosis. **c** Anomalous origin of the right coronary artery

Case 26
Severe and Diffuse Mixed Plaque of the Coronary Arteries in a Patient with Non-specific Chest Pain

Patient: 75-year-old male with multiple risk factors, including previous smoking, hypertension, and hypercholesterolemia. He complained of non-specific chest pain. As a clinical diagnosis of cardiac pain was not possible, he underwent CTA instead of coronary angiography (in case of definite cardiac chest pain, direct access to coronary angiography should be suggested).

Case Description

Figure 1a-e shows diffuse vascular atherosclerotic disease. Mixed plaques, with calcific and non-calcific components, are present. A CTA-based diagnosis is limited by the blooming effect of the diffuse calcific component of the plaque. However, a CTA diagnosis of multiple and diffuse vascular involvement is possible. The patient underwent coronary angiography, which confirmed the diagnosis. Stenting was not possible due to the diffuse involvement; instead, a coronary artery bypass was performed.

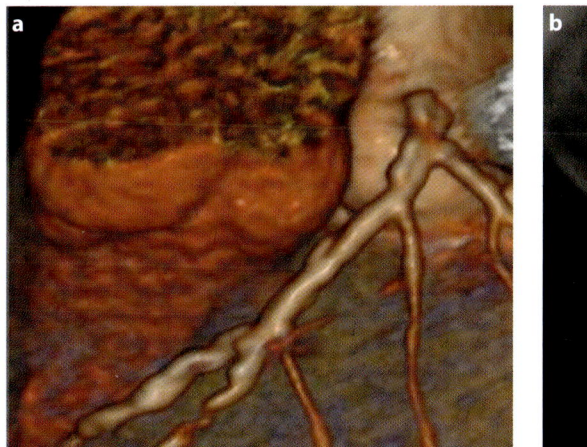 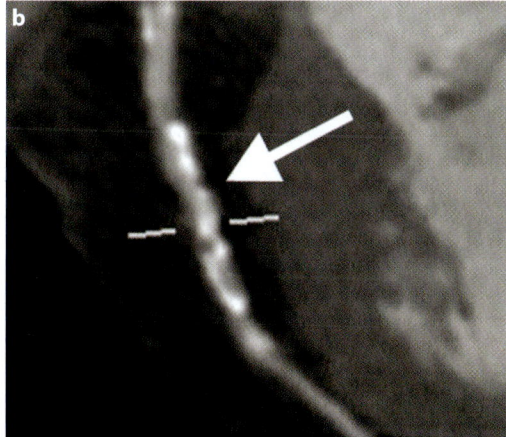

Fig. 1 a-e Multiple diffuse stenotic lesions of the coronary arteries. **b** Severe main left coronary artery stenosis. The patient underwent a bypass operation (*cont.* →)

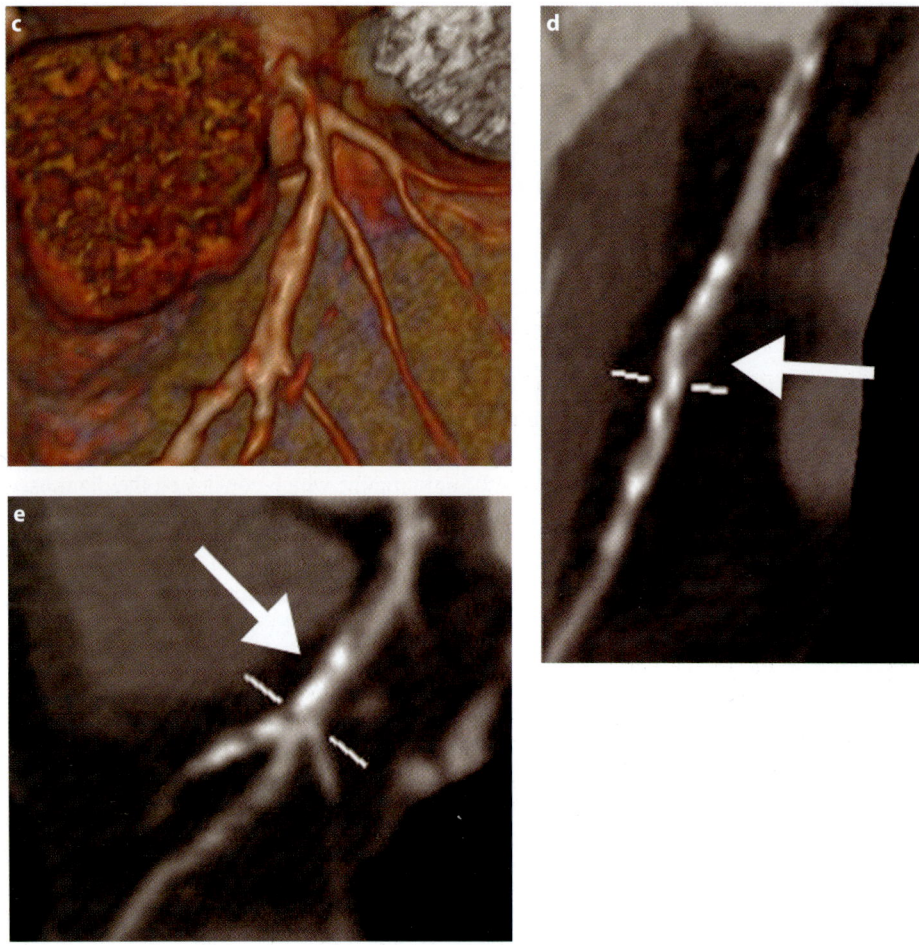

Fig. 1 a-e (continued)

Case 27
Diffuse Plaque Involvement Without Significant Stenosis

Patient: 56-year-old male with a family history of coronary disease (his older brother had undergone a coronary bypass).

Case Description

Figure 1a, b shows diffuse atheromatous plaques of the right coronary artery but without significant stenosis. The VRT images in Fig. 1d, e show an intermediate branch of the artery. In this patient, no further angiographic procedure was performed; instead, follow-up was initiated.

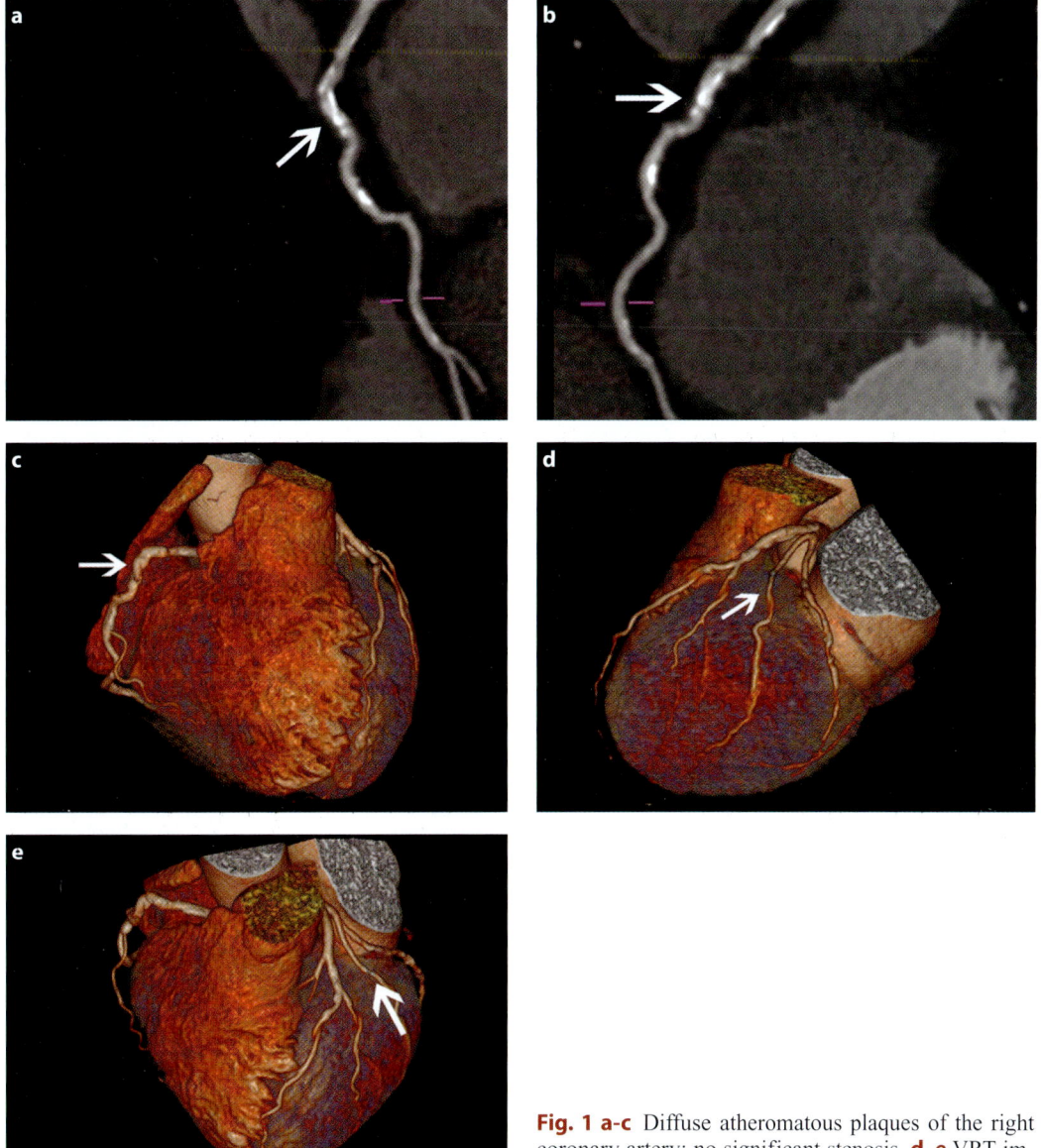

Fig. 1 a-c Diffuse atheromatous plaques of the right coronary artery: no significant stenosis. **d, e** VRT images show an intermediate branch of the artery

Case 28
Diffuse Plaques and Single-Vessel Stenosis

Patient: 71-year-old male with no specific cardiac symptoms.

Case Description

Atheromatous involvement of the right coronary artery is seen in Figure 1a, b. There is a large calcified plaque, causing a blooming effect. Significant stenosis is evident just proximal to the calcified plaque and is caused by a soft, fibrolipidic plaque. The VRT image (Fig. 1c) shows diffuse atheromas of the LAD, with prevalent calcific components. No stenosis of this vessel is evident.

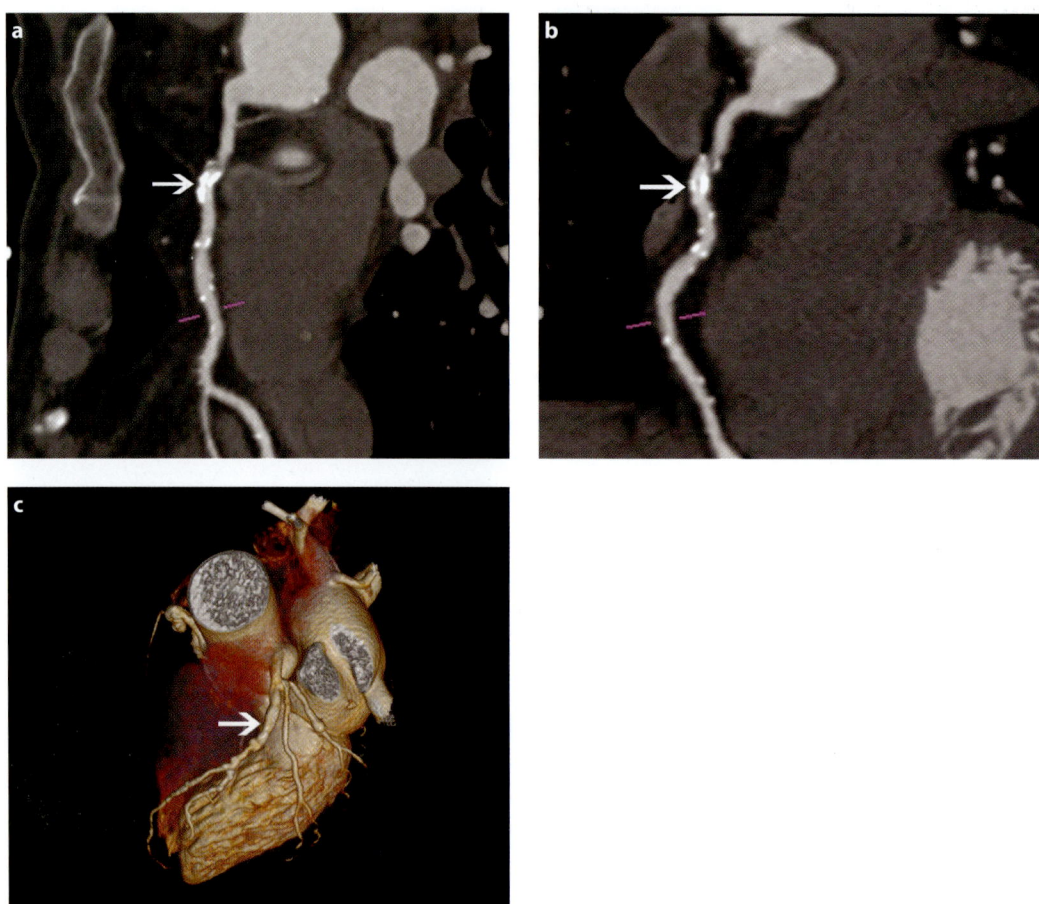

Fig. 1 a, b Patent stent of the right coronary artery. **c** Diffuse atheromatous plaques of the LAD: no significant stenosis

Case 29
Color Characterization of Plaques

Patient: 62-year-old white female presents with chest pain and heartburn. The patient had a family history of HTN and CAD.

Case Description

Imaging shows critical LAD stenosis (Fig. 1a,b). Color coding of the plaque based on Hounsfield Units can increase diagnostic certainty.

Normal RCA and LCX were depicted (Fig. 2a,b).

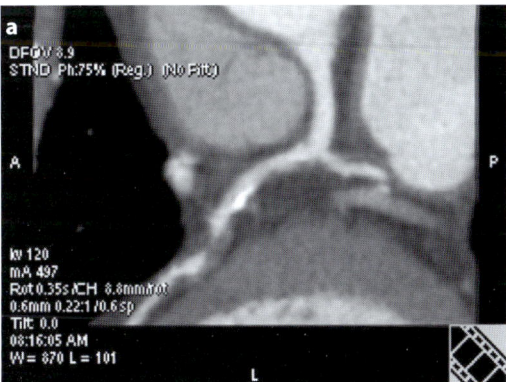 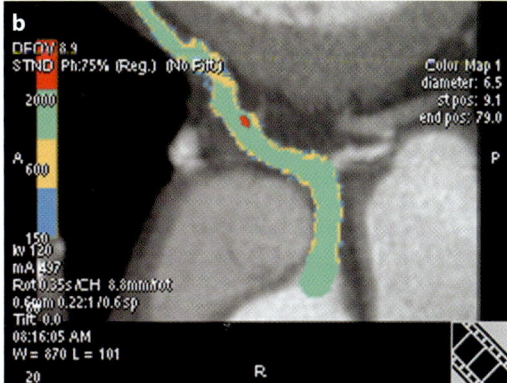

Fig. 1 a, b Critical LAD stenosis

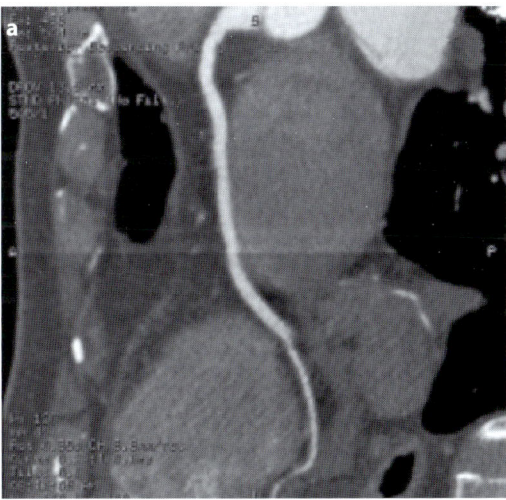 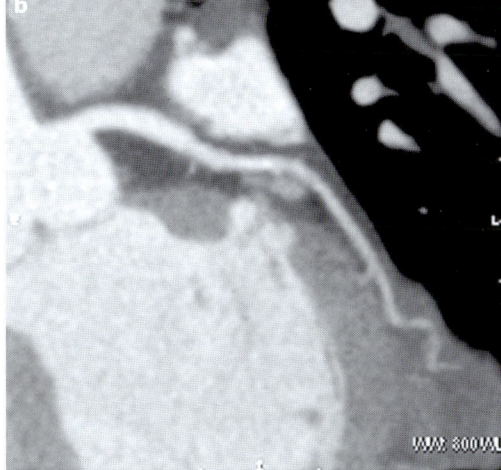

Fig. 2 a, b Normal RCA and LCX

Case 30
Color Characterization of Plaques

Patient: 65-year-old white female with atypical chest pain.

Case Description

LAD stenosis was produced by an eccentric, irregular soft plaque (Fig. 1a,b). Color coding added confidence in the diagnosis (Fig. 2a,b).

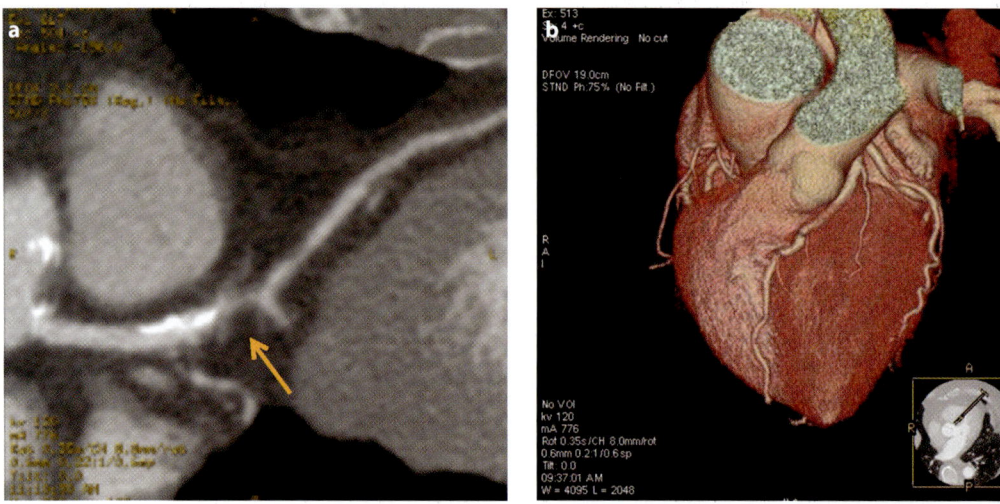

Fig. 1 a, b LAD stenosis was by eccentric, irregular soft plaque

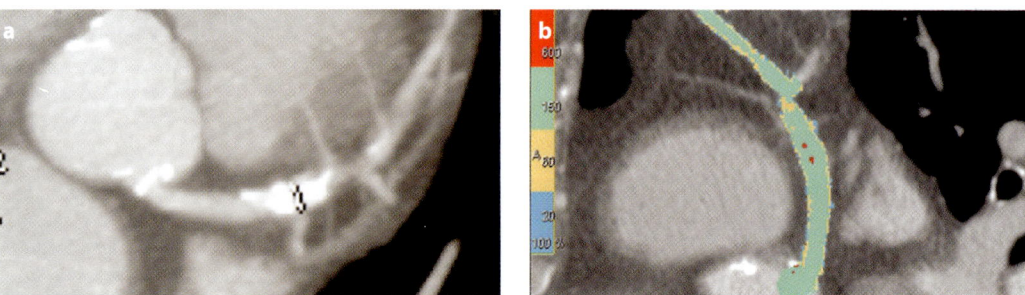

Fig. 12 a, b Color coding adding confidence in diagnosis

Case 31
Chronic Angina and Left Main Stenosis

Patient: 74-year-old male who had suffered repeated and persistent chest pain over the previous 2 years. His EKG was negative; a treadmill test was not performed. Prior to quitting 10 years earlier, he had been an heavy smoker. His cholesterol was normal under 4 years of statin control.

Case Description

Figure 1b–f shows the results of coronary CTA, revealing significant concentric stenosis of the origin of the left main trunk. Other atheromatous lesions are present along the anterior descending coronary artery (Fig. 1d, arrow), but remodeling of the artery has limited the stenotic involvement. Diffuse stenoses of the right coronary artery are also evident (Fig. 1e, f).
Angiography (Fig. 1a, g) confirmed the results of coronary CTA. The patient underwent a surgical bypass procedure.

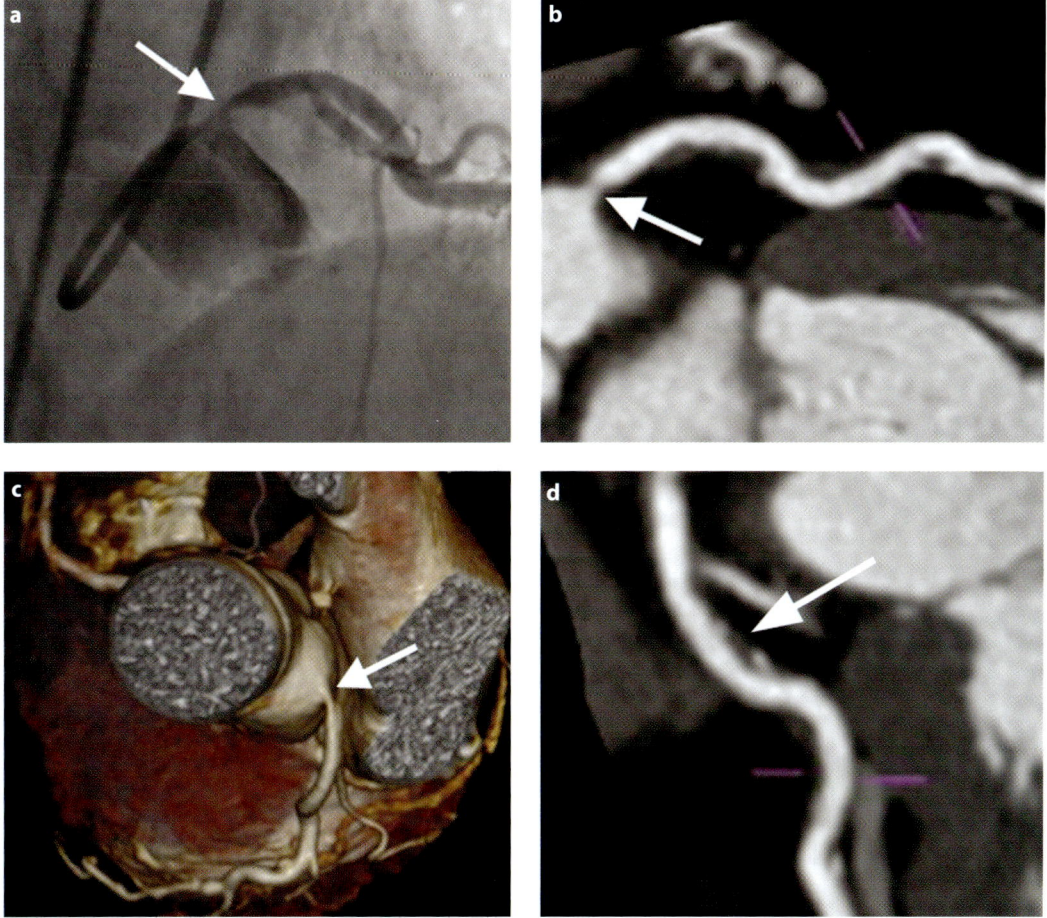

Fig. 1 Angiography (**a**) and CT angiography (**b-e**) show a stenosis of the left main trunk. CT angipgraphy (**f**) and angiography (**g**) show multiple stenotic lesions of the right coronary artery (*cont.* →)

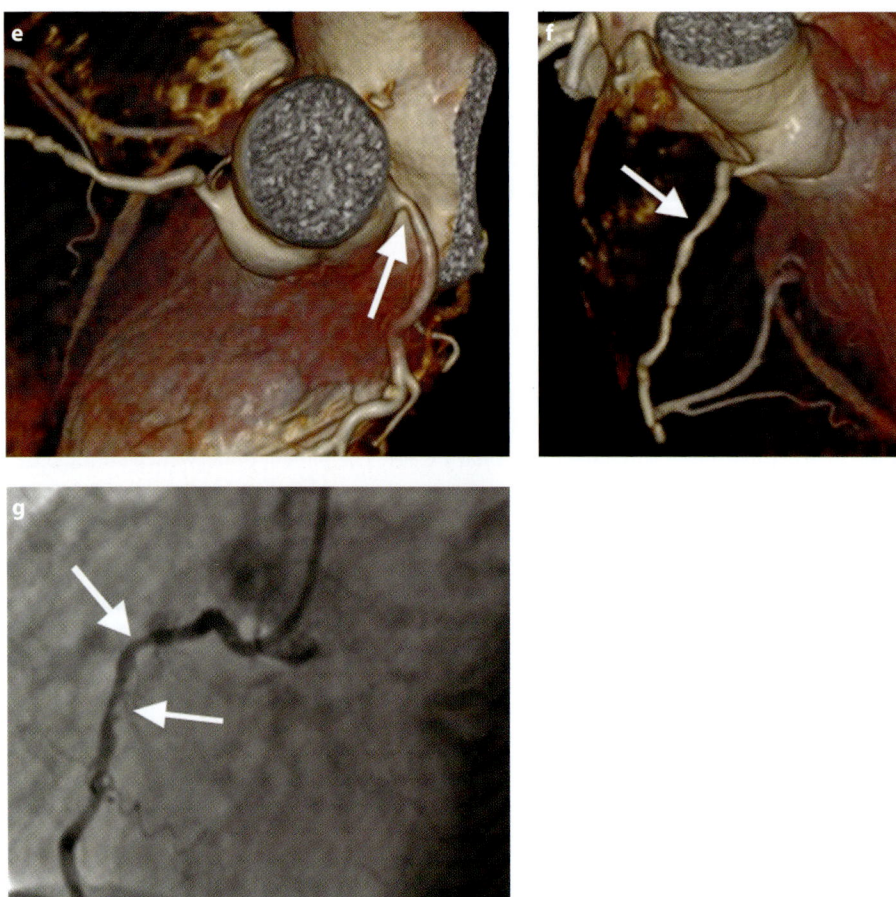

Fig. 1 (continued)

Case 32
Severe Stenosis of the Right Coronary Artery

Patient: 66 year-old male with risk factors of hypertension, smoking, and high cholesterol. Symptoms related to chronic cardiac disease and suspected angina were present. As his EKG results were normal, he underwent coronary CTA.

Case Description

The MPR and VRT images of Figure 1a–d show the right coronary artery, with diffuse involvement by chronic, mostly calcified plaques. In the mid segment, a soft plaque is seen to be the cause of a sub-occlusive stenosis of the right coronary artery. The patent lumen cannot properly be imaged. In some cases, coronary CTA is unable to differentiate between chronic occlusion and severe stenosis.

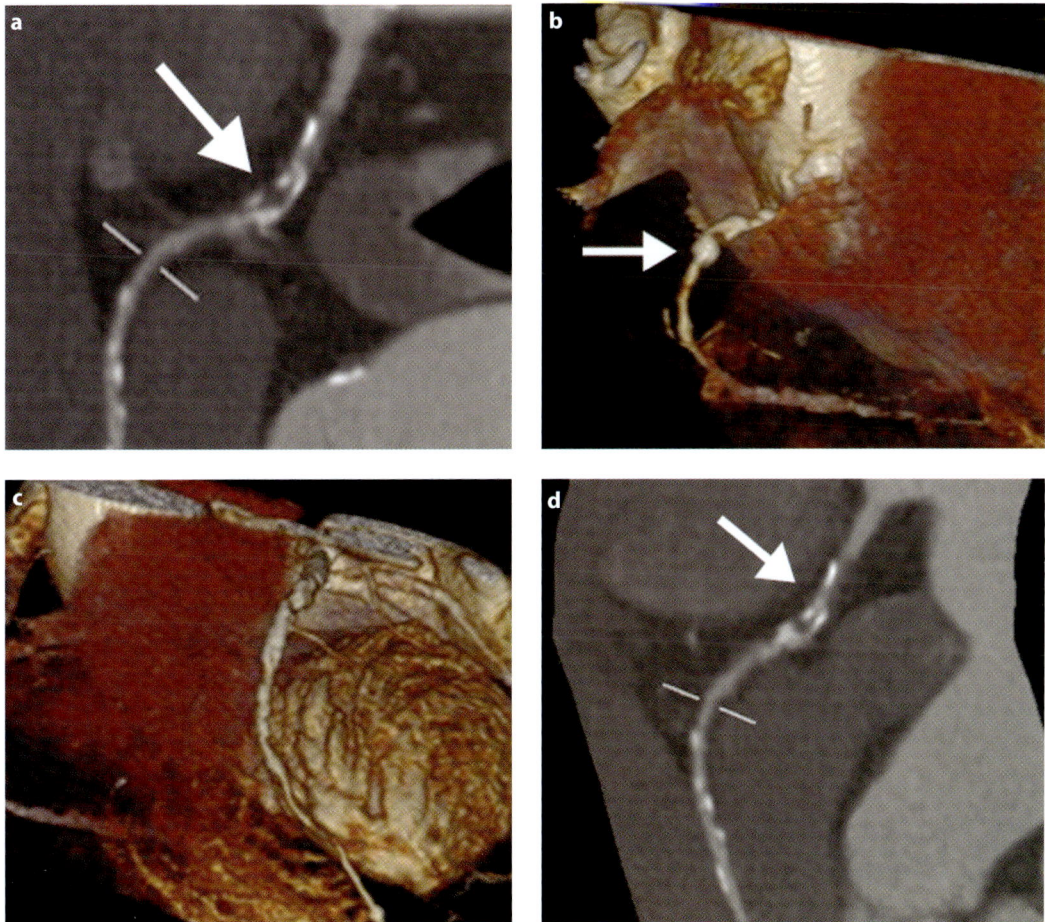

Fig. 1 a-d Diffuse atherosclerotic involvement of the right coronary artery

Case 33
CTA Diagnosis of Severe Stenosis of the LAD, with LAD Occlusion and Myocardial Infarction During Follow-Up

Patient: 72-year-old male with relevant risk factors (previous smoker, hypertension, hypercholesterolemia). No symptoms and negative treadmill test. CTA was performed as part of a routine check-up.

Case Description

The 3D images of the LAD (Fig. 1a, b) evidence multiple atheromas. There is a high-grade stenosis (>70%), attributable to a non-calcific soft plaque. The diagnosis of severe stenosis was confirmed by evaluation of the 2D images. However, due to the lack of symptoms, the patient's personal cardiologist decided to delay an angiographic procedure, instead opting for monitoring. After 6 months, the patient developed severe acute cardiac symptoms and an acute myocardial infarction was diagnosed. He underwent coronary angiography, which confirmed complete occlusion of the LAD (stenting was no longer possible). A CTA control was performed at 10 months, just prior to the bypass procedure. Figure 1c, d shows the level of the LAD occlusion.

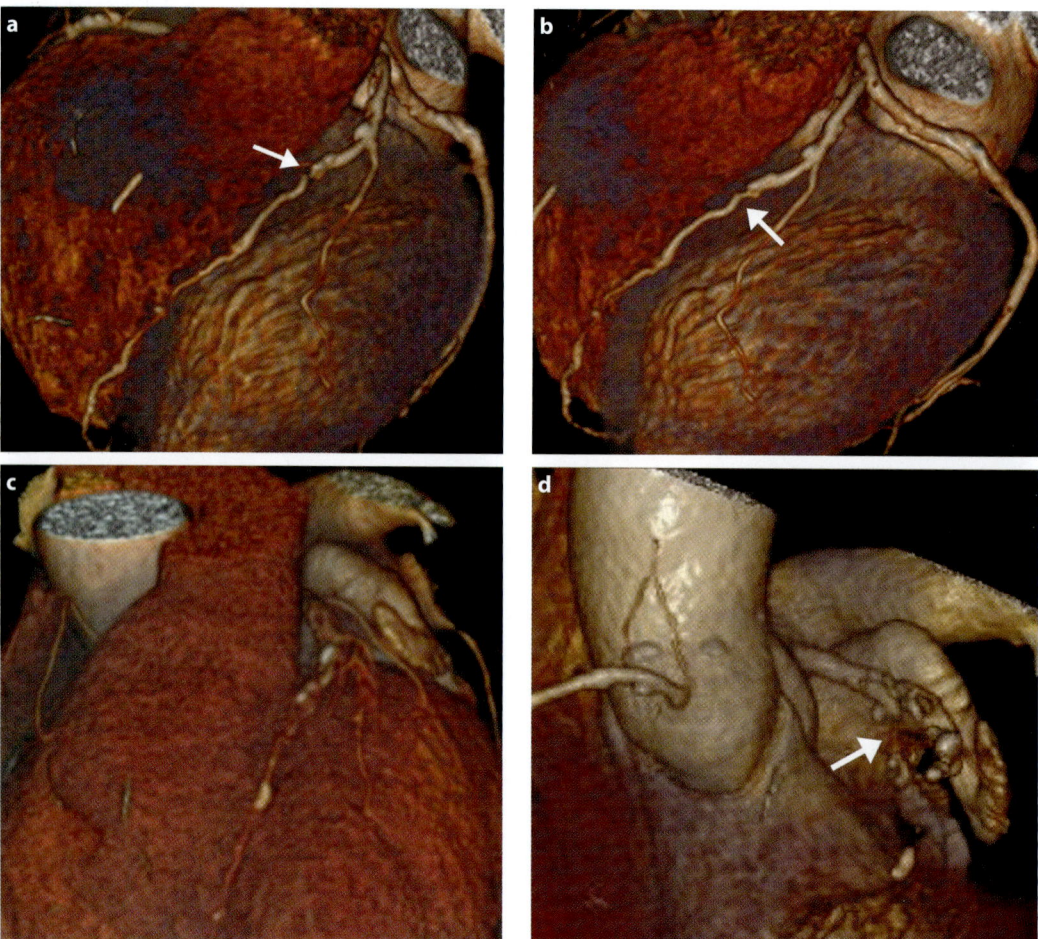

Fig. 1 a, b Severe (> 70%) focal concentric stenosis in the LAD. Soft plaque, no calcium. Stenting was not performed. **c, d** The patient had an acute myocardial infarction 6 months later: occlusion of LAD was diagnosed at angiography. CT angiography control at 10 months shows complete LAD occlusion

Case 34
Stenosis Evaluation of Noncalcified, Mixed and Calcified Plaques

Patient: 50-year-old, white female with chest pain. SPECT imaging results were within normal limits. Risk factors consisted in non-insulin-dependent diabetes mellitus (NIDDM), HCO and HTN.

Case Description

Figure 1a-c shows 80% LAD stenosis by non-calcified plaque in a patient with a calcium score of 0.

High remodeling index levels were measured, and high grade stenosis was observed (Fig. 2a-d).

Beam hardening artifacts can appear adjacent to dense structures such as calcium (Fig. 3a,b). A helpful hint is that it may be the same shape and size as the dense object. It may also vanish when the vessel is rotated on curved multiplanar images.

Stenosis Evaluation

For stenosis evaluation, the North American Symptomatic Carotid Endarterectomy Trial (NASCET) criteria should be used:
- stenosis must be detected;
- the lumen must be measured at its smallest diameter. Any plane may be used to find the lumen; and
- the lumen should be measured of the most adjacent, normal vessel diameter distal to the stenosis.

Figure 4 depicts examples of non-calcified plaque: mild stenosis (Fig. 4a), moderate stenosis with plaque erosion (Fig. 4b), and severe stenosis (Fig. 4c).

In Figure 5 we see examples of a mixed plaque: mild stenosis (Fig. 5a), moderate stenosis (Fig. 5b), and severe stenosis (Fig. 5c).

Lastly, Figure 6 shows examples of a calcified plaque: mild stenosis (Fig. 6a), moderate stenosis (Fig. 6b), and severe stenosis (Fig. 6c).

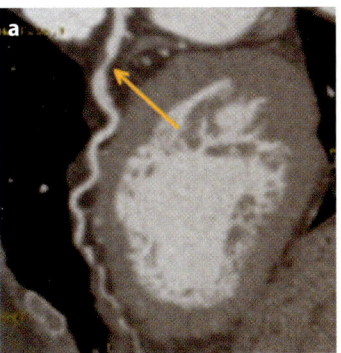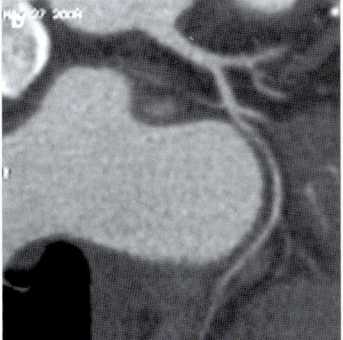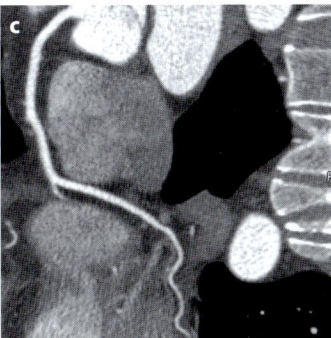

Fig. 1 a-c LAD stenosis (80%)

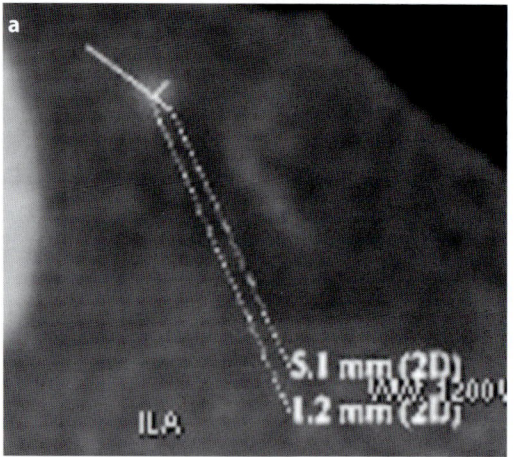
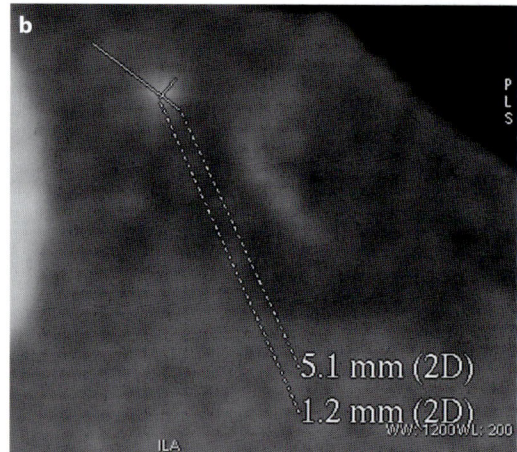
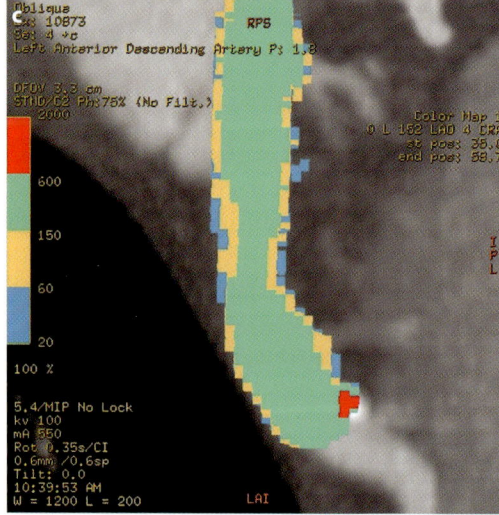
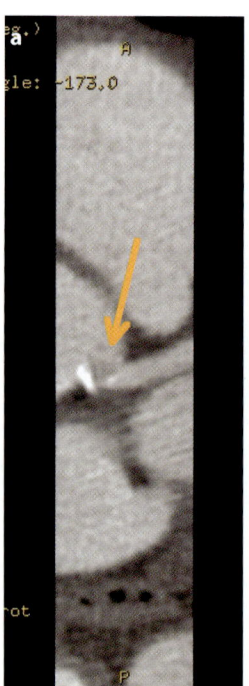
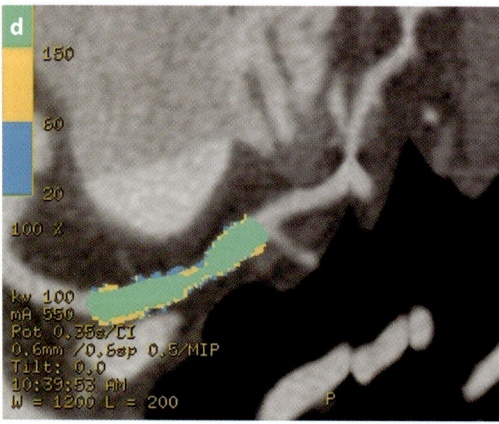
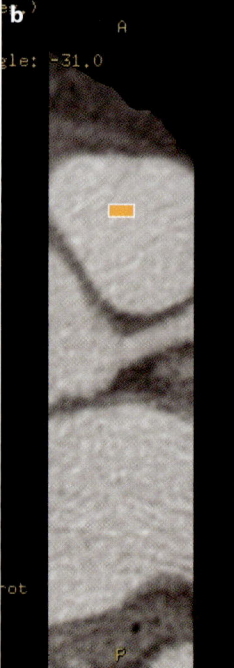

Fig. 2 a-d High remodeling index levels and high-grade stenosis

Fig. 3 a, b Beam hardening artifacts

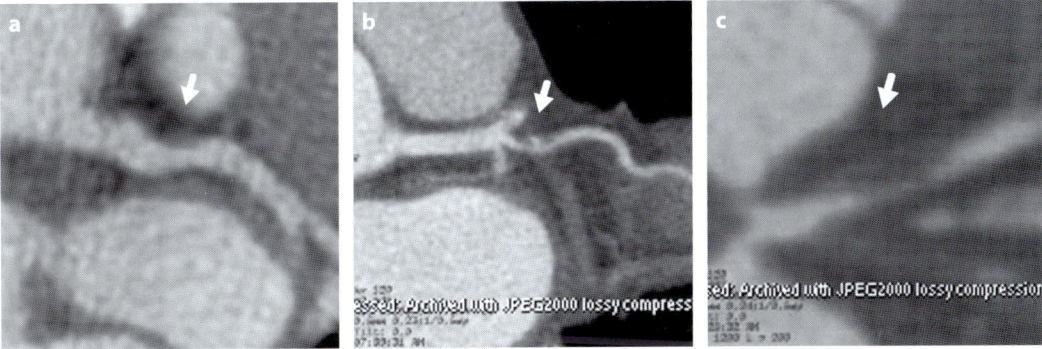

Fig. 4 Examples of non-calcified plaque. **a** Mild stenosis; **b** moderate stenosis with plaque erosion; **c** severe stenosis

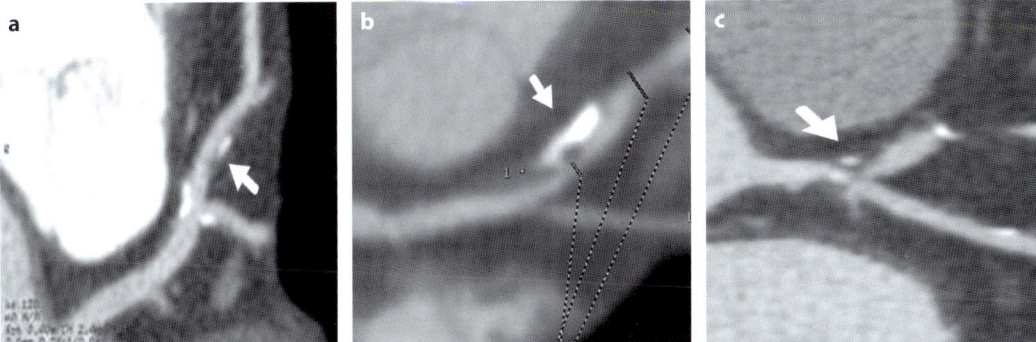

Fig. 5 Examples of mixed plaque. **a** Mild stenosis; **b** moderate stenosis; **c** severe stenosis

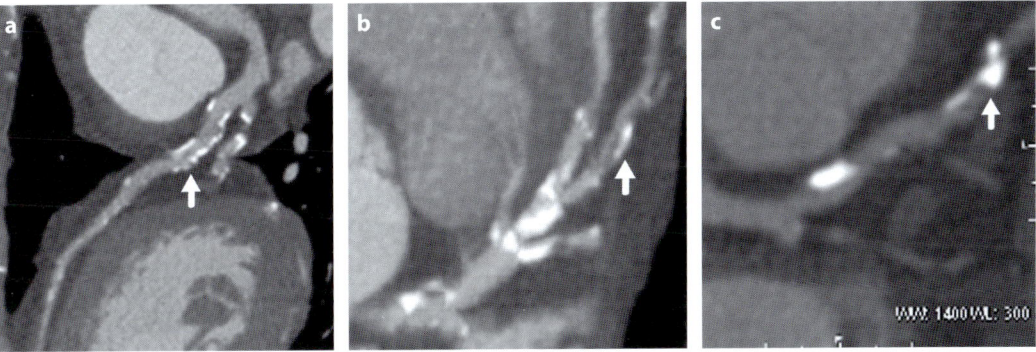

Fig. 6 Examples of calcified plaque. **a** Mild stenosis; **b** moderate stenosis; **c** severe stenosis

Case 35
High Grade Stenosis in Symptomatic Patient with a Negative Stress Test and a Calcium Score of Zero

Patient: 49-year-old white female complaining of chest pain at 13 metabolic equivalents (METS) of exercise.

Case Description

A high-grade soft plaque stenosis is observed in a patient with a calcium score of 0 (Fig. 1a,b).

Only an 85% positive predictive value may be achieved when comparing CCTA with quantitative coronary angiography (QCA) (Fig. 2a,b), as this depends on the acquisition plane (as seen in Fig. 3a, showing a 90% stenosis, and Fig. 3b, which displays a 50% stenosis).

The degree of stenosis may vary greatly depending on subtle changes in the plane in which one is imaging. The advantage for CCTA is that each vessel is viewed in 360 degrees, where coronary catheterization uses limited numbers of orthogonal image planes.

The question is what do we want to see, just like what does a RBC see? The answer is that we should make like an RBC, by adjusting the center tracking line, as shown in Figures 4a (pre-adjustment) and 4b (post-adjustment), and again in Figure 5a (pre-adjustment), and 5b (post-adjustment).

Vessel tracking software may indicate false positive stenoses by tracking material more dense than the contrast agent, such as calcium. It is important to recognize this and adjust the tracing line.

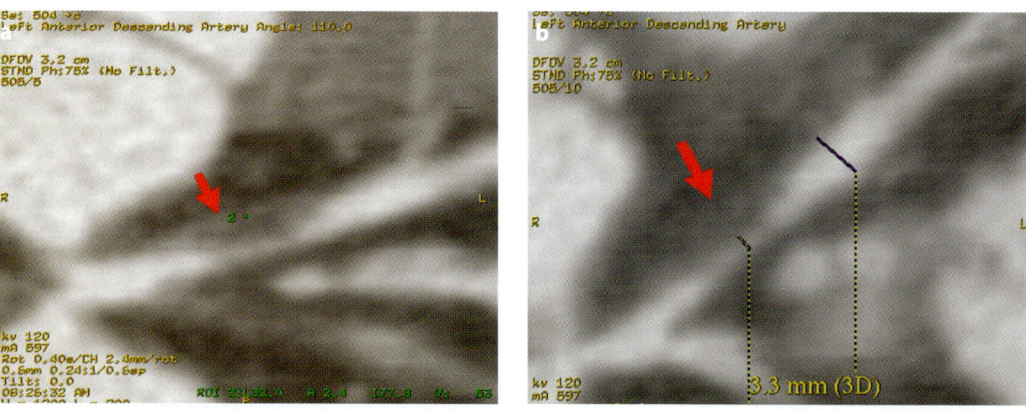

Fig. 1 a, b High-grade soft plaque stenosis in patient with calcium score = 0

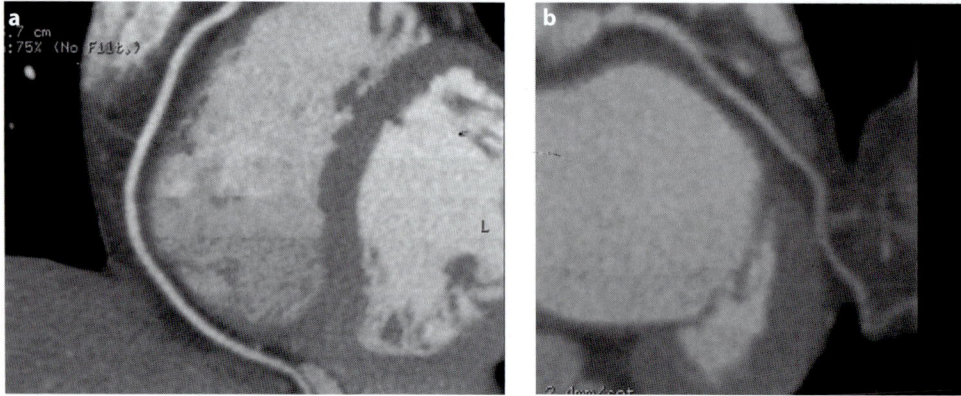

Fig. 2 a, b Positive predictive value achieved when comparing CCTA with QCA (85%)

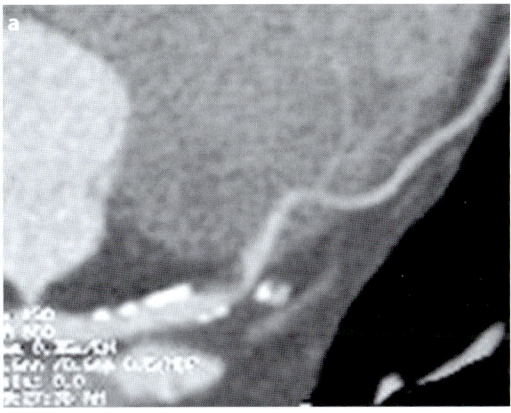
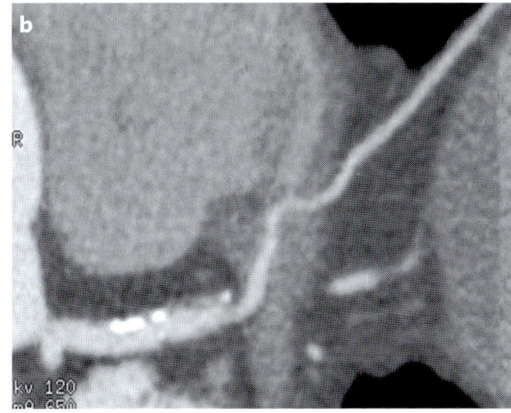

Fig. 3 a 90% stenosis; **b** 50% stenosis

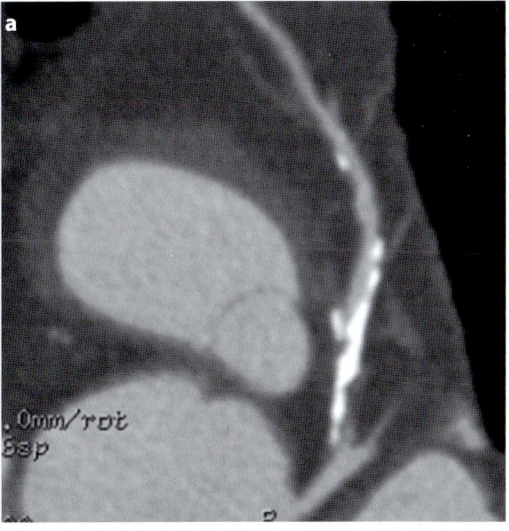
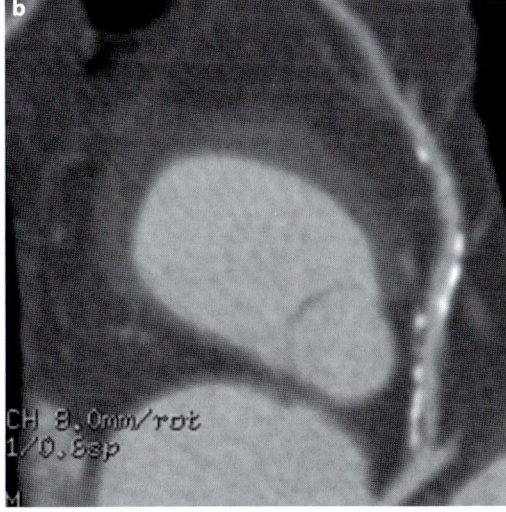

Fig. 4 Center tracking line adjustment. **a** Pre-adjustment; **b** post-adjustment

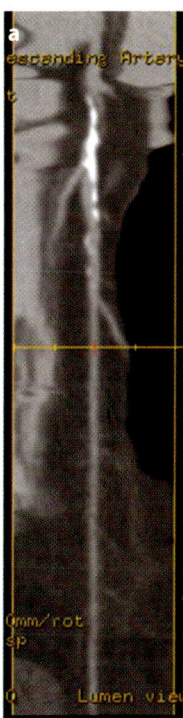
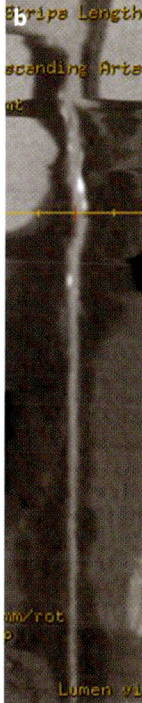

Fig. 5 Center tracking line adjustment. **a** Pre-adjustment; **b** post-adjustment

Case 36
High Grade Stenosis in a Symptomatic Patient with Two Risk Factors

Patient: 57-year-old asymptomatic white male, smoker. Risk factors consisted in: hypercholesterolemia and HTN.

Case Description

Figure 1a,b shows RCA occlusion, a mild LCX plaque (Fig. 2a,b), and only one LAD stenosis (Fig. 3a,b). Once the lumen was completely obscured by calcium it was difficult to determine the degree of stenosis. In this case, we observed a low-grade stenosis.

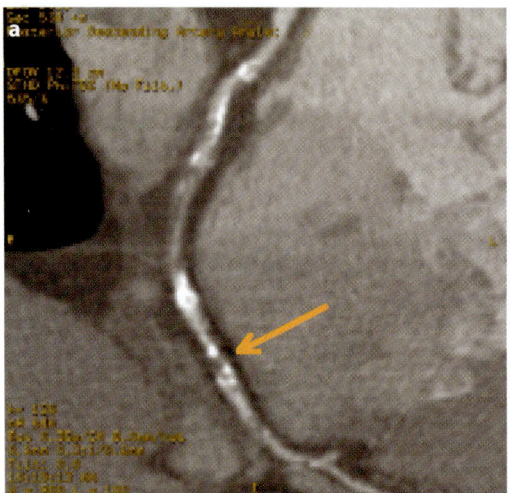
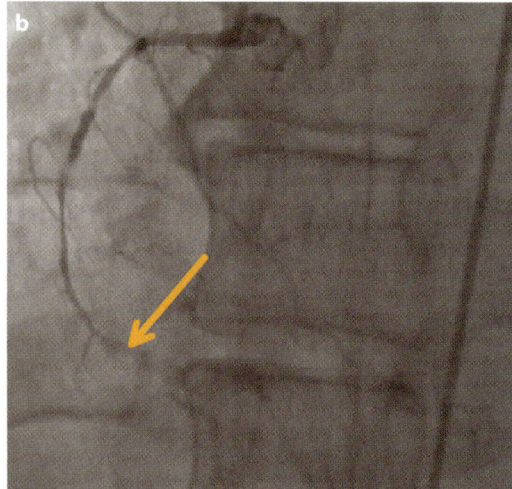

Fig. 1 a, b RCA occlusion

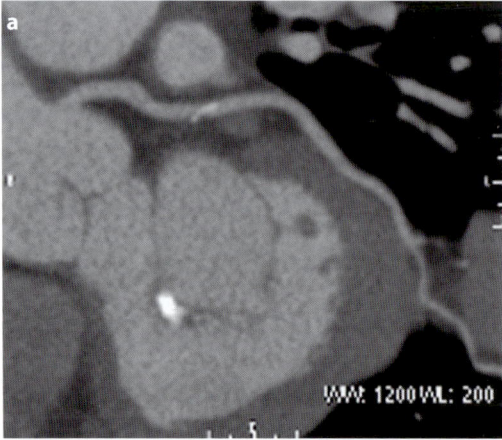
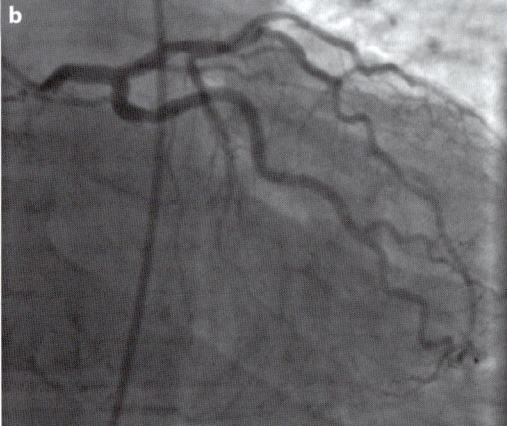

Fig. 2 a, b Mild LCX plaque

19 Clinical Cases

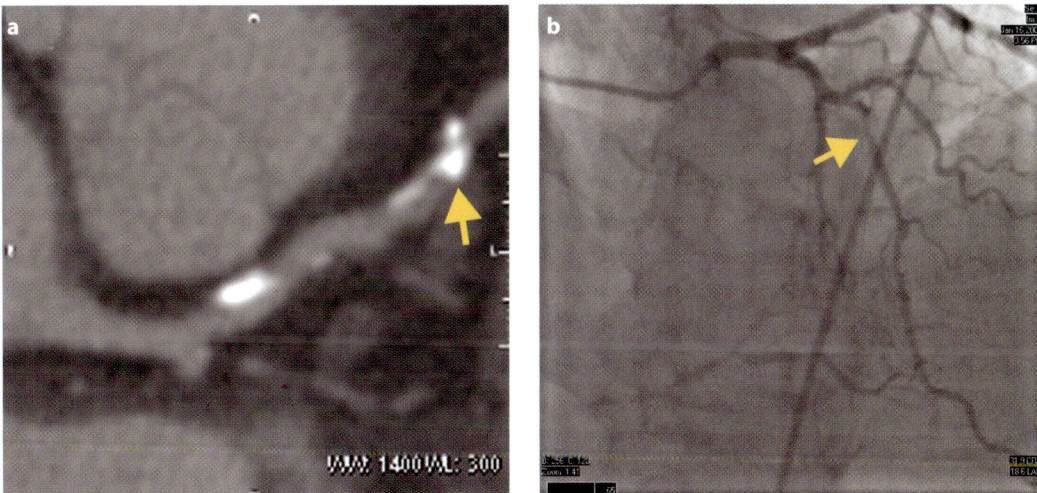

Fig. 3 a, b Single LAD stenosis

Case 37
High Grade Stenosis in a Symptomatic Patient with a Normal EKG and Negative Troponins

Patient: 59-year-old white male carpenter. The patient had presented with classic chest pain to the ER five days earlier, and at present is nearly asymptomatic; however, he does not want to wait three weeks to see a cardiologist.

Case Description

Imaging shows: RCA stenoses (Fig. 1a,b), normal LCX (Fig. 2a,b), and LAD stenosis (Figs. 3a,b, 4a,b).
 Luckily, no residual stenosis status is evidenced after percutaneous coronary intervention (PCI) (Fig. 5a,b).

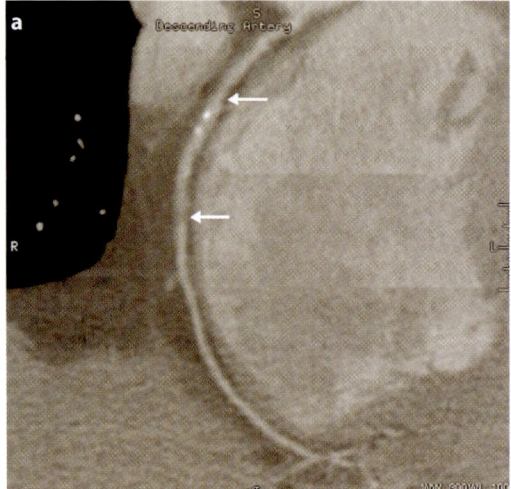
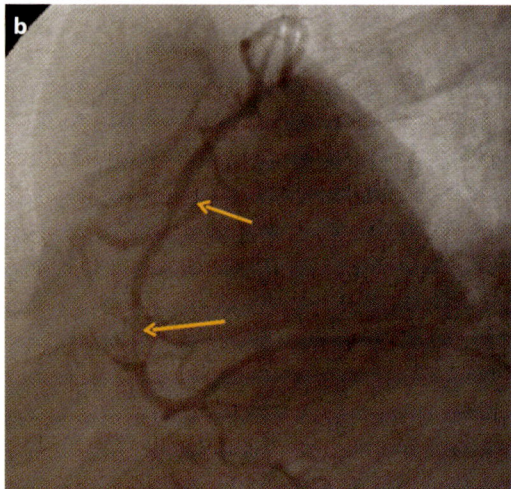

Fig. 1 a, b RCA stenoses

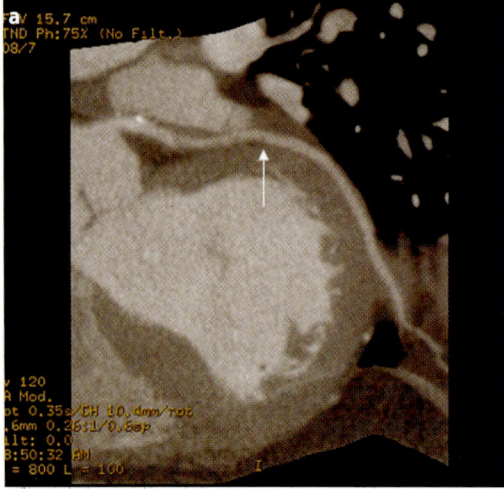
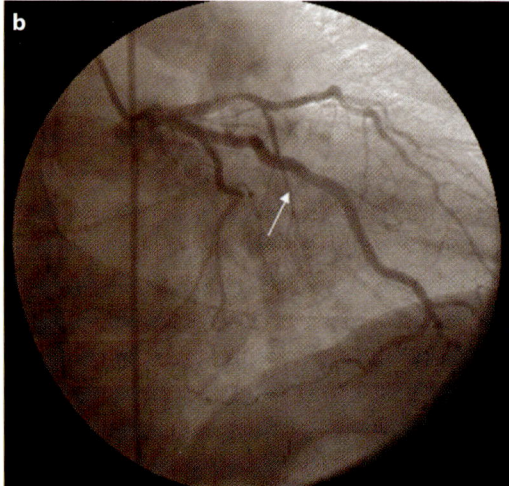

Fig. 2 a, b Normal LCX

19 Clinical Cases

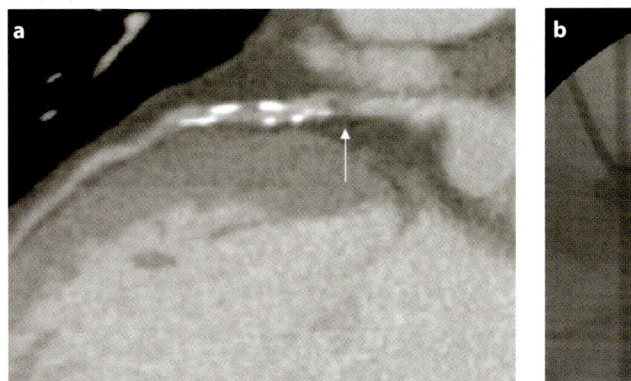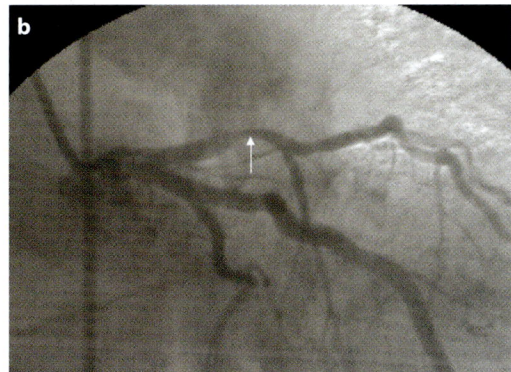

Figs. 3 a, b LAD stenosis

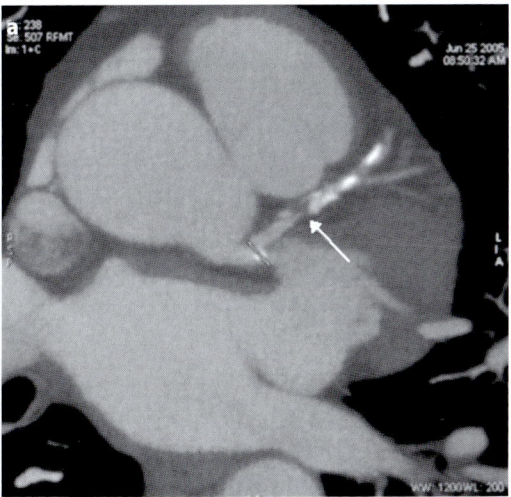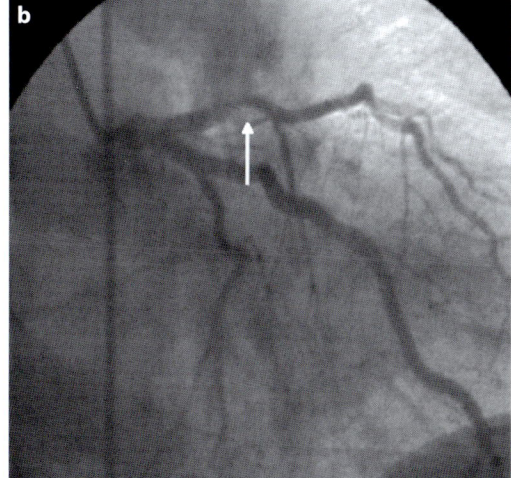

Fig. 4 LAD stenosis

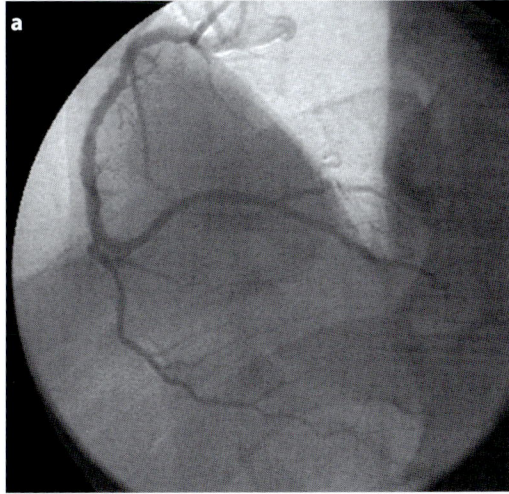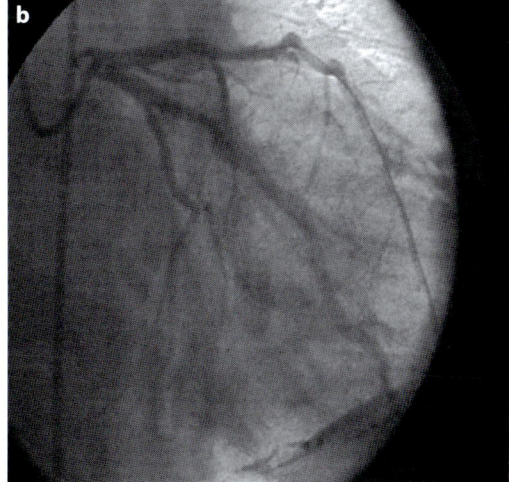

Fig. 5 a, b No residual stenosis after PCI

Case 38
Chronic Angina and Diffuse LAD Atherosclerosis

Patient: 73-year-old male, heavy smoker with a cholesterol of 240 and hypertension. He reported chest pain after long walks but his EKG was negative. As the chest pain was not clearly of cardiac origin, he instead underwent coronary CTA.

Case Description

Figure 1a–d shows diffuse atherosclerotic disease of the LAD. There are mixed plaques, with peripheral calcium and fibrolipidic involvement. In the mid-segment of the LAD, a clear stenosis (70%) is present. The patient underwent coronary angiography with stenting of the stenosed area. Diffuse parietal thickening and calcification were seen in the other coronary arteries but there was no sign of stenosis.

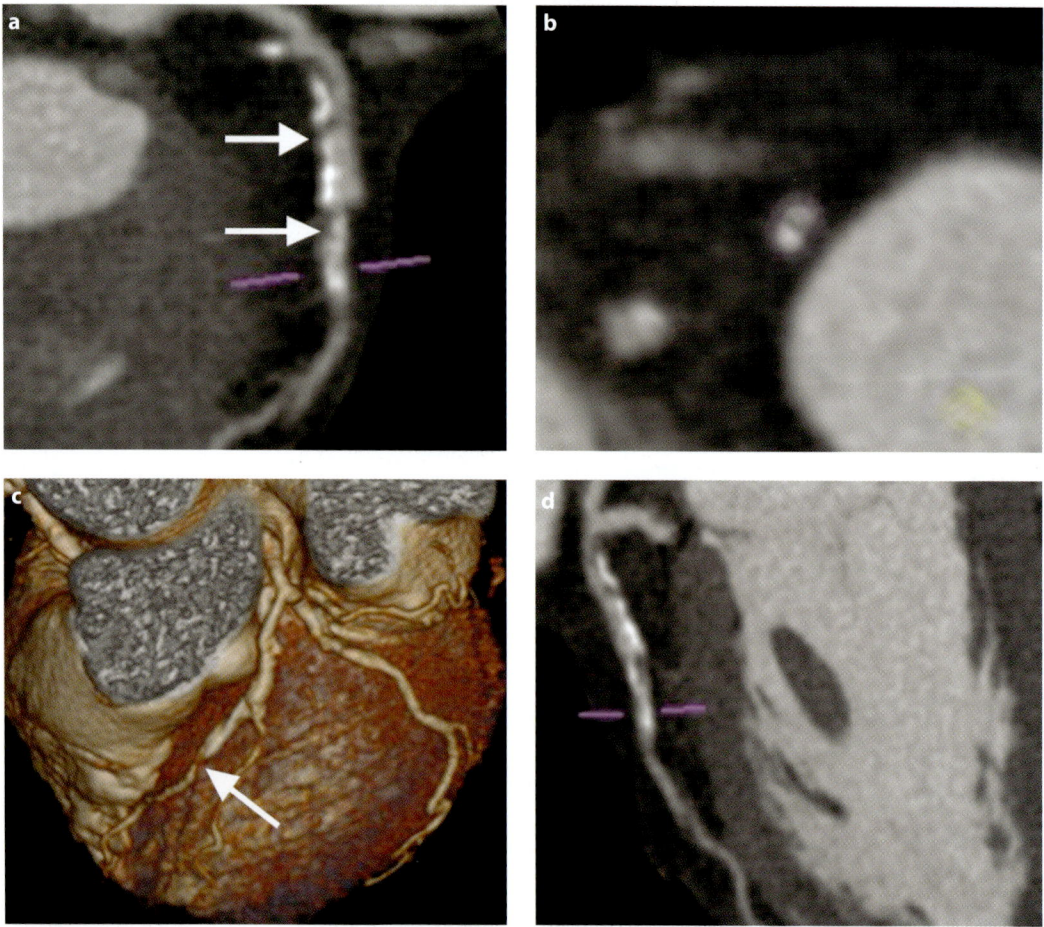

Fig. 1 **a-c** Multiple atheromatous lesions, peripheral calcium, and internal fibrolipid. **d** Maximum intensity projection (MIP) image shows diffuse atheromas with severe stenoses

Case 39
Chronic, Calcified Total Occlusion

Patient: 52-year-old white female with a history of a prior myocardial infarction (MI) presents now with chest pain.

Case Description

Figure 1a,b shows occlusion of a non-dominant RCA. Normal LAD and dominant LCX are depicted (Fig. 2a,b).

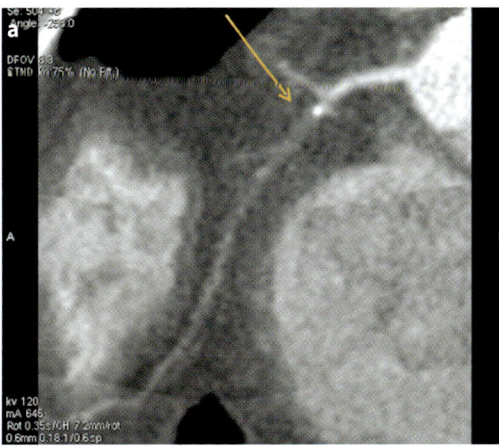
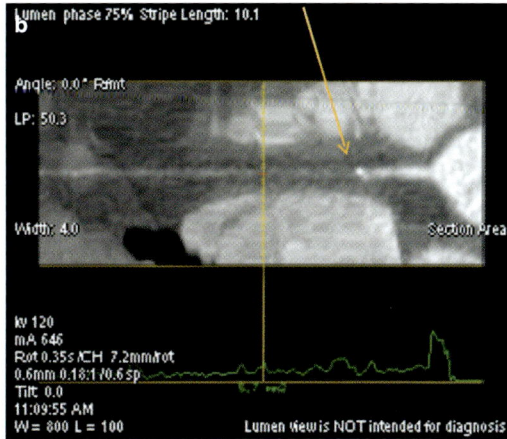

Fig. 1 a, b Occlusion of non-dominant RCA

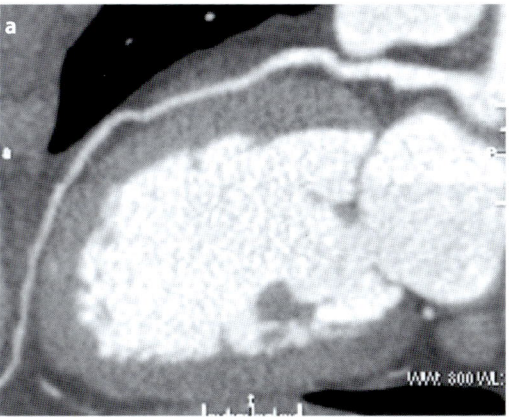
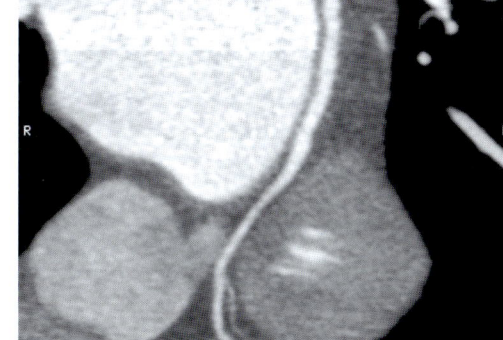

Fig. 2 a, b Normal LAD and dominant LCX

Case 40
Imaging Characteristics of a Vulnerable Plaque

Patient: 53-year-old white male with insulin-dependent diabetes mellitus (IDDM), HTN; the patient was an active smoker and complained of chest pain.

Case Description

Remodeling index >1.4 was calculated in this case (Fig. 1a-c). The remodeling index is a ratio of the external vessel diameter divided by the lumen diameter. When this ratio is greater than 1.4 it signifies a plaque with an increased risk of rupturing.

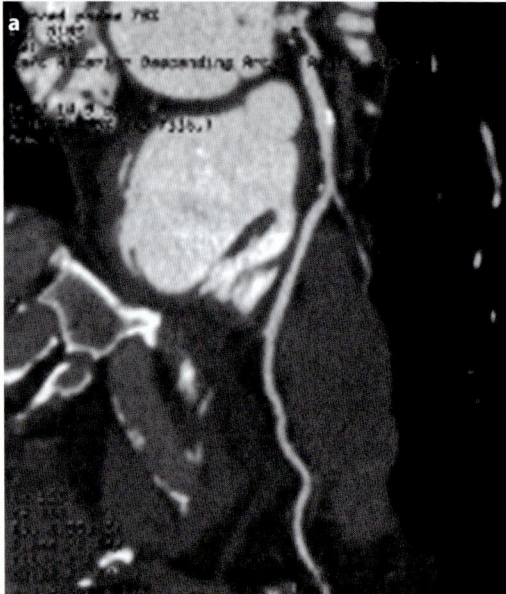
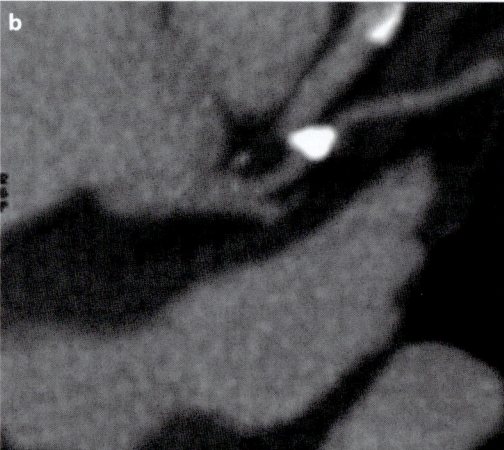
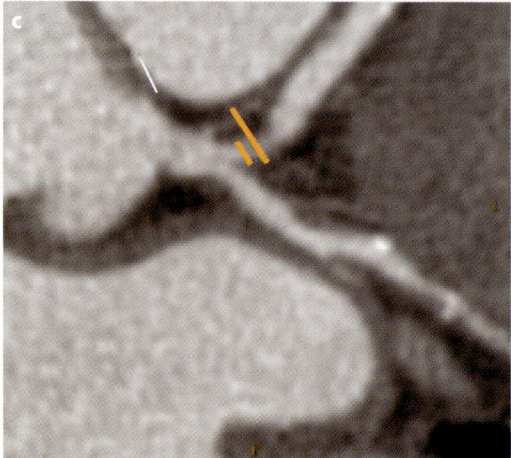

Fig. 1 a-c Remodeling index >1.4

Case 41
False Positive Coronary CTA by Calcified Plaques and the Venous Pseudoplaque Sign

Patient: 75-year-old white male with labile HTN and exertional angina.

Case Description

Severe mid LAD disease with mild LCX disease were highlighted (Fig. 1a,b). Once the lumen was completely obscured by calcium, it was difficult to determine the degree of stenosis. In this case, there was a low-grade stenosis.

Venous Pseudoplaque Sign

Figure 2 shows a large eccentric soft plaque, while in Figure 3 an eccentric soft plaque is depicted at the level of the LAD.

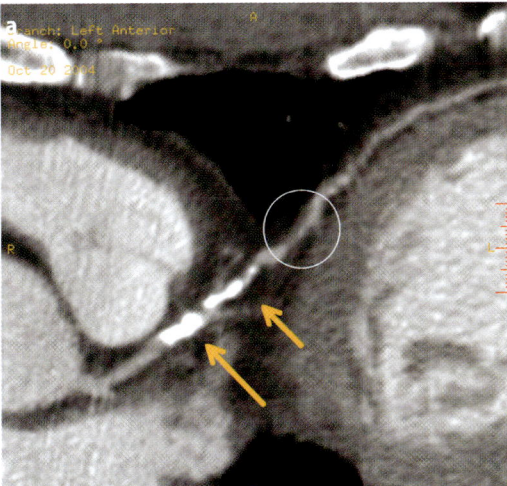
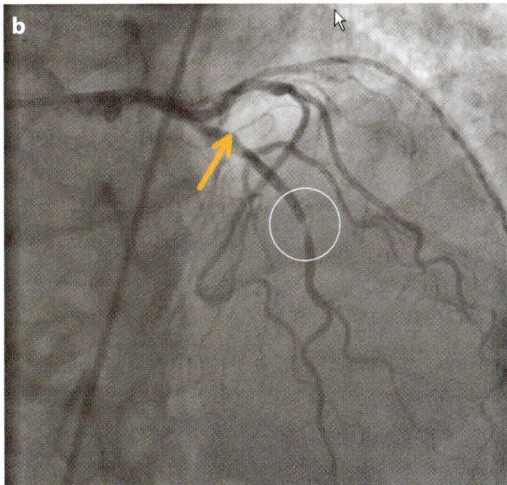

Fig. 1 a, b Severe mid LAD disease with mild LCX disease

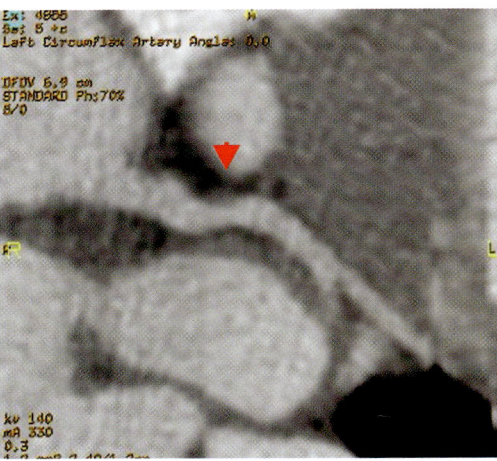
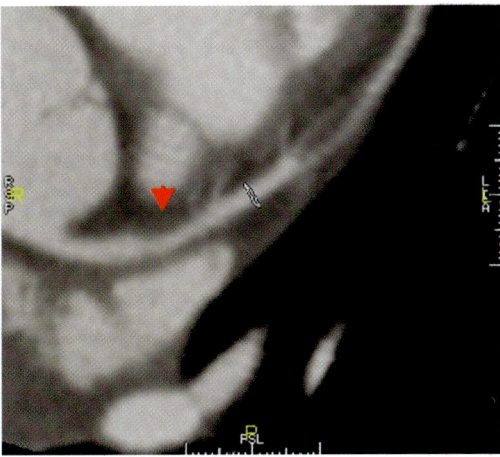

Fig. 2 Large eccentric soft plaque

Fig. 3 Eccentric soft plaque at the level of the LAD

Sometimes, it is not easy to identify the presence of a soft plaque (Fig. 4), in that adjacent unopacified veins may mimic soft plaques (Fig. 5). Adjacent unopacified venous pseudoplaques may be seen in Figure 6.

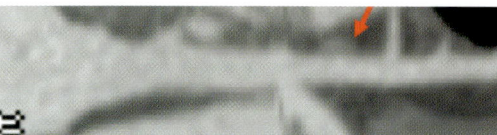

Fig. 4 Possible soft plaque

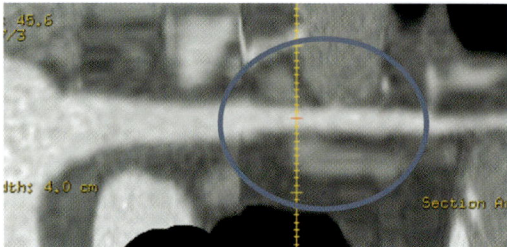

Fig. 6 Unopacified venous pseudoplaques

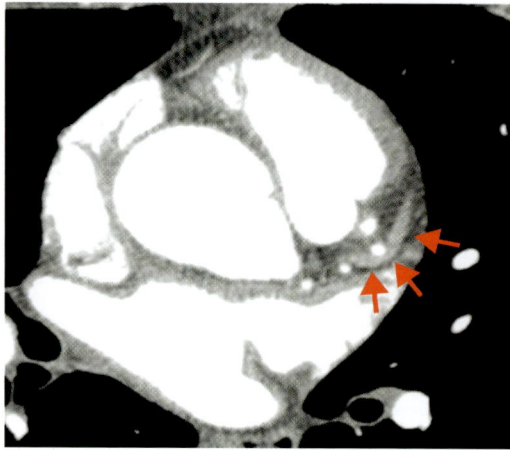

Fig. 5 Adjacent unopacified veins mimicking soft plaques

Case 42
Meniscus Sign in Acute Thrombosis

Patient: 64-year-old white male with recent onset of chest pain.

Case Description

Thrombosed LCX with "positive meniscus sign" was detected (Fig. 1a,b). Expansion of the vessel indicates the presence of a thrombus.

Mild CAD of LAD and RCA was identified (Fig. 2a,b).

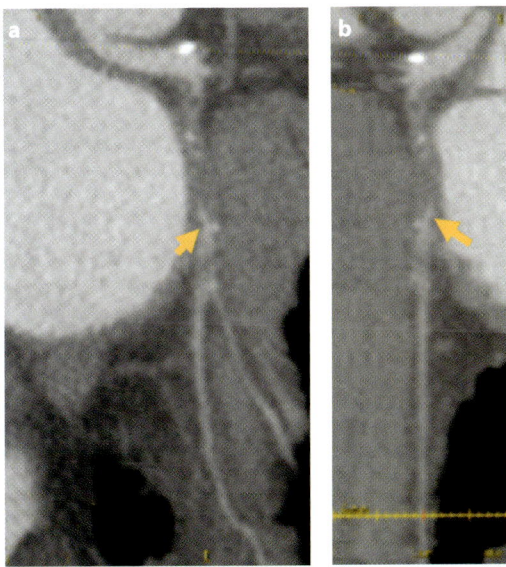

Fig. 1 a, b Thrombosed LCX with "positive meniscus sign"

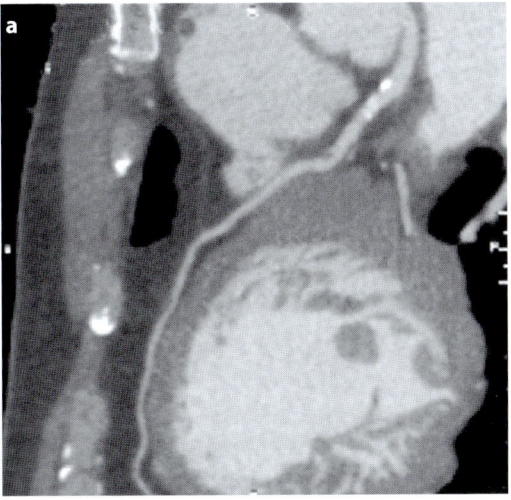
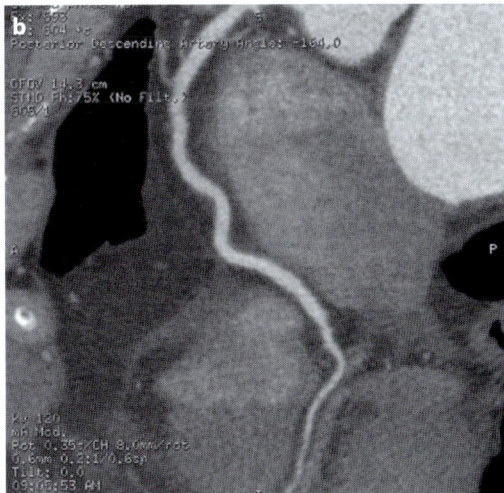

Fig. 2 a, b Mild CAD of LAD and RCA

Case 43
Healing of a Vulnerable Plaque

Patient: 53-year old asymptomatic male with hypercholesterolemia and a family history of coronary artery disease (CAD).

Case Description

Figure 1 shows an ulcerated proximal left anterior descending (LAD) artery plaque.

Follow-up examination performed 14 months later shows ulcerated LAD plaque (Fig. 2a,b). It is important to assess plaque size, plaque area, HU at relevant plaque components and degree of stenosis. Table 1 shows different measurements at baseline and first follow-up examination.

Measurements taken at follow-up show that the plaque has decreased in size. The soft plaque exhibits increasing HU, indicative of healing.

The same patient developed "angina like" chest pain and underwent his third cardiac computed tomography angiography (CCTA) on 26 June 2004, which highlighted the presence of an ulcerated LAD plaque (Fig. 3a-c). Table 2 shows measurements at baseline, first and second follow-up examinations.

Measurements showed that the plaque had calcified and continued to decrease in size. There was a false positive increase in plaque area in the transverse plane related to blooming of the calcified plaque.

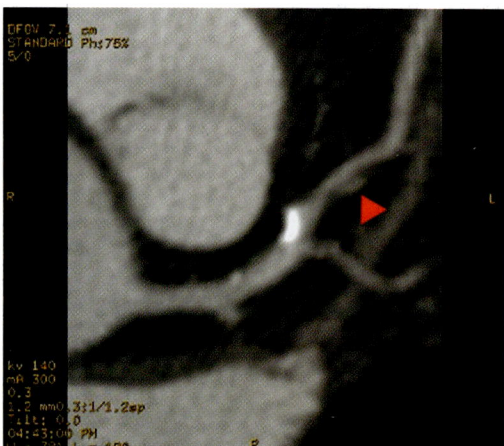

Fig. 1 Ulcerated proximal LAD plaque

Table 1 Measurements at baseline and first follow-up examination

30 April 2002	9 June 2003
Plaque = 13.6 mm long	Plaque = 13.2 mm long
Long area = 19.8 mm^2	Long area = 13.7 mm^2
Transverse area = 5.0 mm^2	Transverse area = 4.5 mm^2
Proximal fornix = 79 HU	Proximal fornix = 91 HU
Distal fornix = 73 HU	Distal fornix = 87 HU
Proximal crater = 221 HU	Proximal crater = 218 HU
Distal crater = 403 HU	Distal crater = 413 HU

19 Clinical Cases

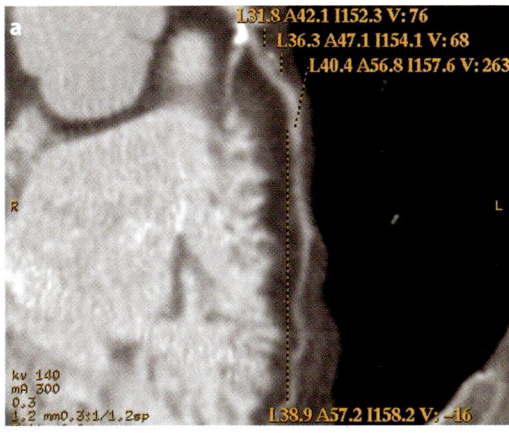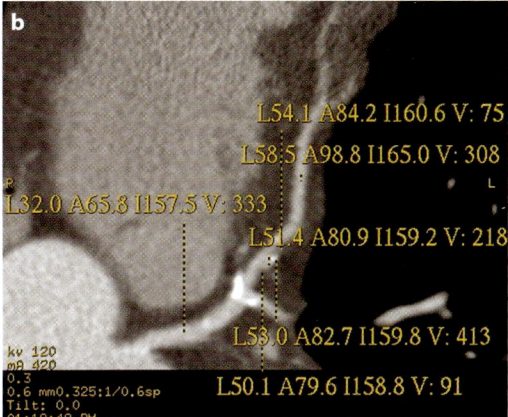

Fig. 2 a, b Ulcerated LAD plaque

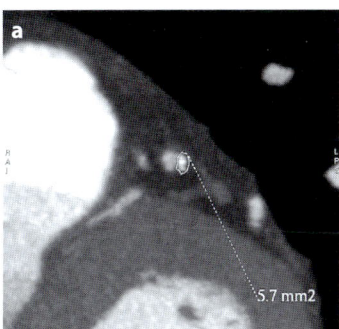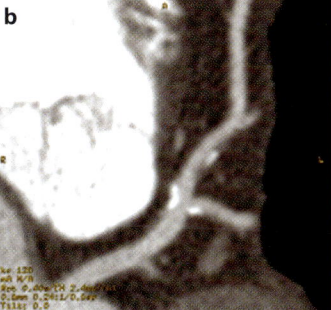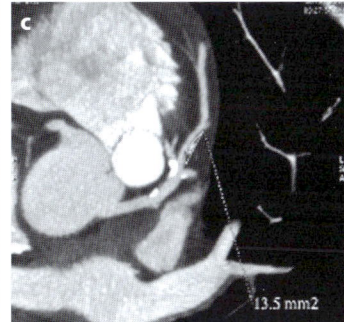

Fig. 3 a-c Ulcerated LAD plaque

Table 2 Measurements at baseline, first and second follow-up examinations

30 April 2002	9 June 2003	26 June 2004
MPlaque = 13.6 mm long	Plaque = 13.2 mm long	Plaque = 13.2 mm long
Long area = 19.8 mm^2	Long area = 13.7 mm^2	Long area = 10.8 mm^2
Transverse area = 5.0 mm^2	Transverse area = 4.5 mm^2	Transverse area = 5.4 mm^2
Proximal fornix = 79 HU	Proximal fornix = 91 HU	Proximal fornix = 98 HU
Distal fornix = 73 HU	Distal fornix = 87 HU	Distal fornix = 99 HU
Proximal crater = 221 HU	Proximal crater = 218 HU	Proximal crater = 606 HU
Distal crater = 403 HU	Distal crater = 413 HU	Distal crater = 578 HU

19.5 Pulmonary Embolism

Case 44
Single-Vessel Coronary Disease and Pulmonary Embolism

Patient: 73-year-old female with shortness of breath but no other specific cardiac symptoms. Her cholesterol was normal and no EKG changes were present.

Case Description

The MPR and VRT images of Fig. 1a–e show a severe stenosis of the circumflex artery due to a concentric fibrolipidic plaque. Plaque calcium is absent, consistent with the negative calcium score. Figure 1f, g shows the presence of pulmonary emboli in distal vessels of the lower left lobe, for which the patient was treated. Following her recovery, she was scheduled for coronary stenting.

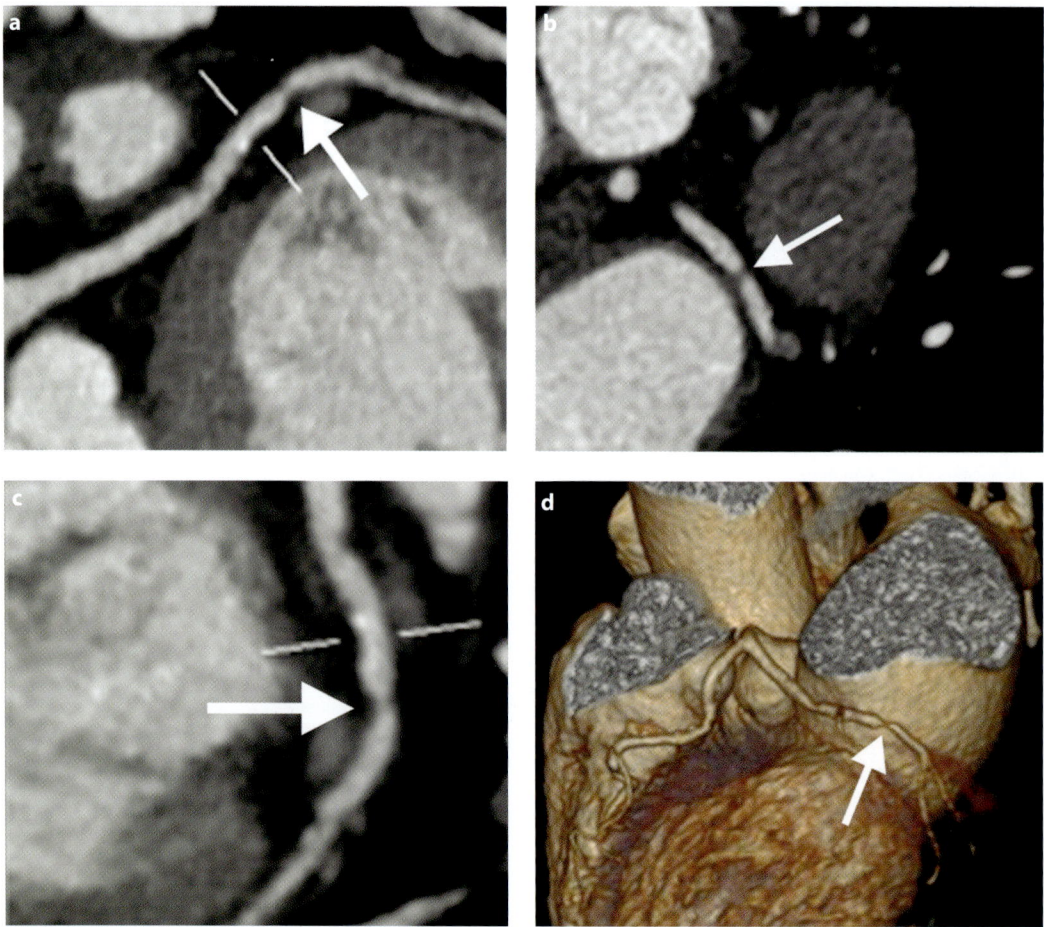

Fig.1 a-e Significant stenosis of the circumflex artery. **f, g** Pulmonary embolism of the lower left lobe arteries (*cont.* →)

19 Clinical Cases

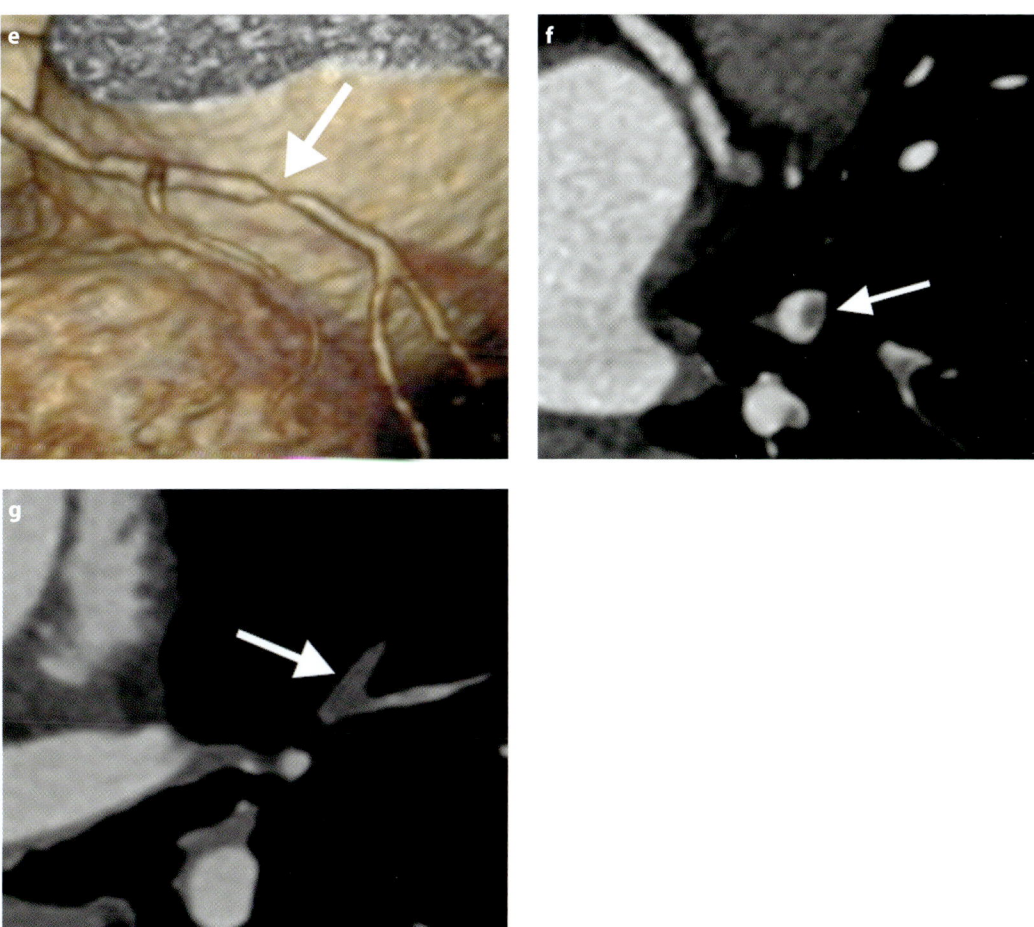

Fig. 1 a-e (continued)

Case 45
Chest Pain in a Patient with Normal Coronary Arteries and a Diagnosis of Pulmonary Embolism

Patient: 72-year-old with recent dyspnea and chest pain who was admitted to the hospital with a clinical suspicion of coronary artery disease.

Case Description

Figure 1a shows the completely normal coronary arteries. There are no plaques and the arterial lumens are normal. Figure 1b shows the evaluation of the axial slices obtained during the coronary artery acquisition. Pulmonary emboli are present in the right pulmonary artery and the anterior segment of the left upper lobe. Complete recovery was achieved following therapy.

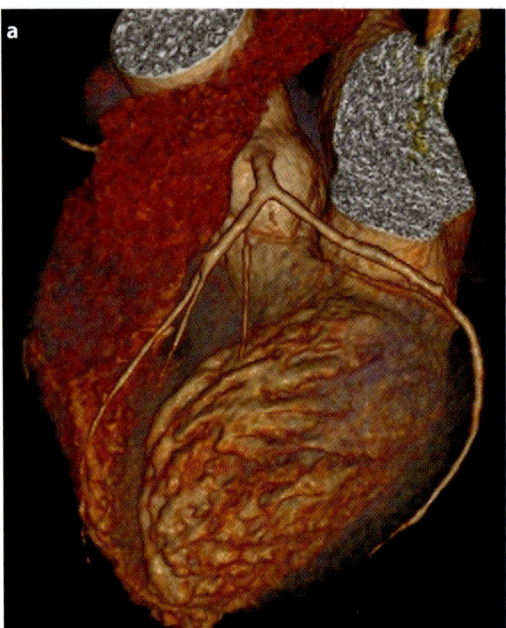
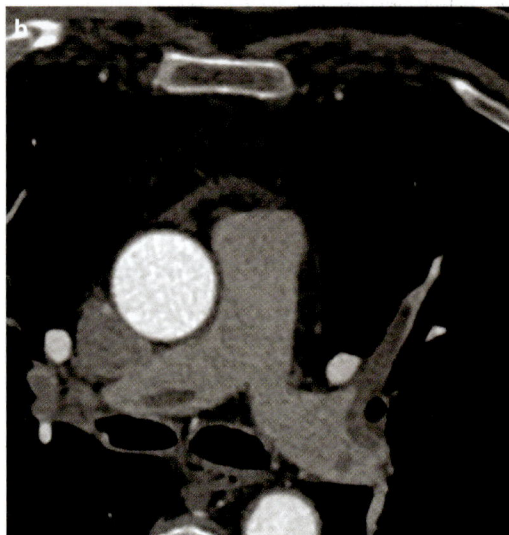

Fig. 1 a, b

19.6 Stent and CABG

Case 46
Coronary CTA Diagnosis of Severe Stenosis, with Stenting and Follow-Up

Patient: 67 year-old male with generic risk factors but no symptoms who underwent a screening coronary CTA.

Case Description

Figure 1a, b shows the diffuse plaques in the proximal and middle segment of the LAD. Multiple calcific plaques are evident in addition to two fibrolipidic soft plaques, with the latter causing significant stenosis. The control after stenting is shown in Fig. 1c, d. The proximal soft plaque (on the main left trunk) was not submitted to stenting as it was shown on coronary angiography to cause only a mild (30–40%) stenosis.

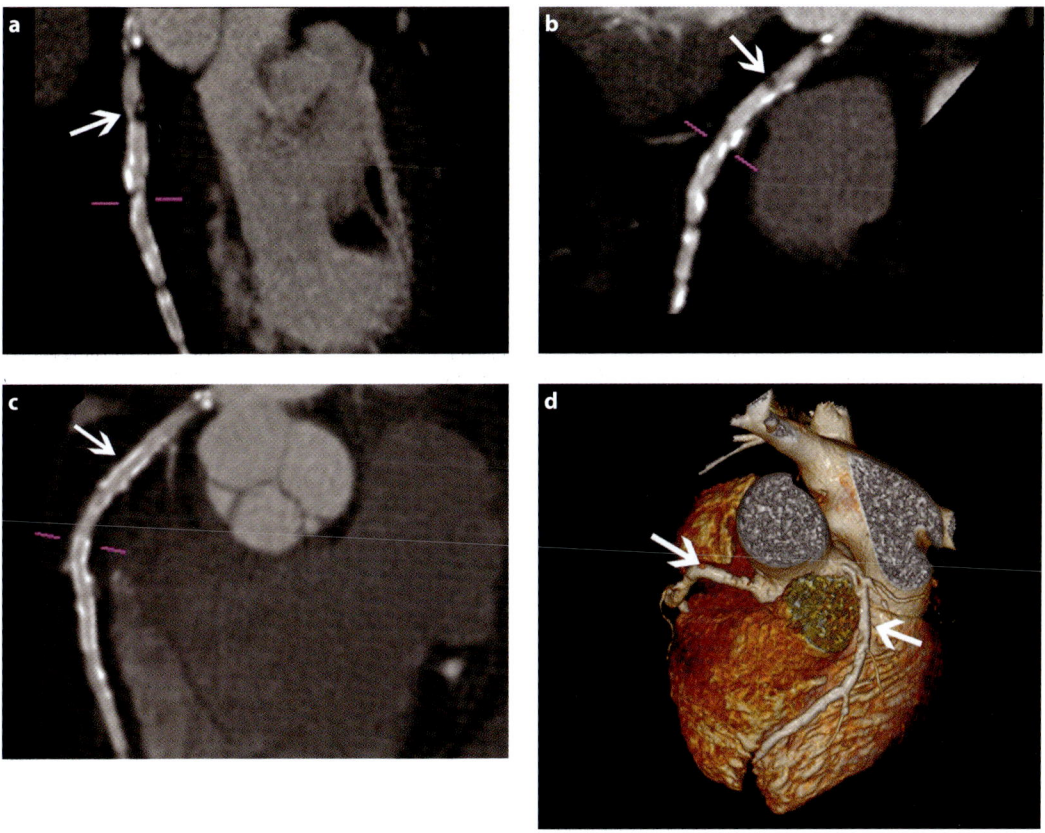

Fig. 1 a, b Fibrolipidic plaque of the third proximal segment of the LAD resulting in 70% stenosis. **c, d** CT angiography control after stenting: no residual stenosis

Case 47
Pre-stent Stenosis

Patient: 63-year-old male in whom one year previously a stent had been placed in the proximal LAD due to severe focal stenosis. He underwent routine stent control.

Case Description

MPR and VRT coronary CTA images of the stent are shown in Figure 1a–d. The stent is patent and there is distal flow. There are no signs of intra-stent disease. The clear plaque burden of the LAD wall just prior to the stent may be due to inappropriate stent placement and extensive disease above the stent. Nowadays, cardiologists suggest the routine use of intravascular ultrasound prior to stent placement in order to ensure complete coverage of the full extension of the plaque. Turbulent flow at the edge of the stent may also be the cause for the pre-stent stenosis.

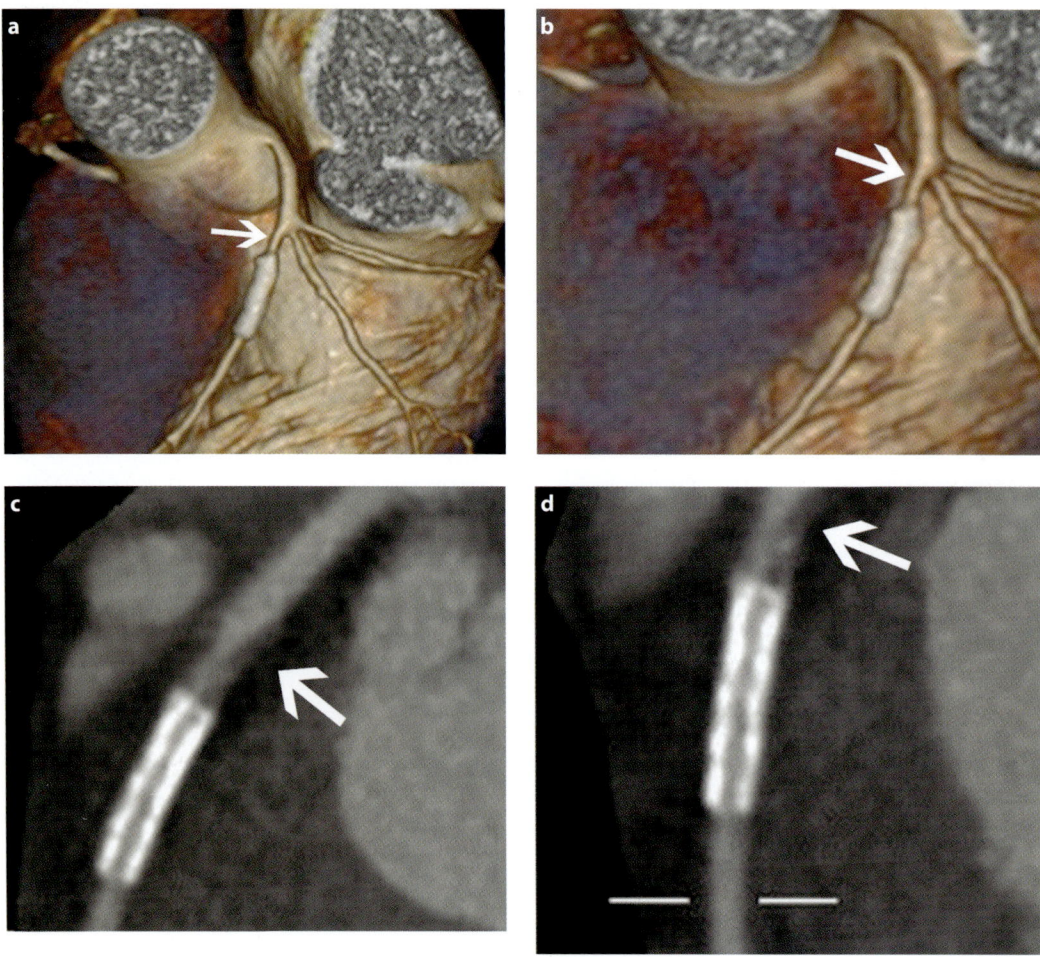

Fig. 1 a-d Multiple views of the LAD stent. *Arrow* shows a recurrent stenosis proximal to the stent (soft plaque)

Case 48
Subclavian Artery Stenosis Jeopardizing a LIMA Bypass Graft

Patient: 73-year-old asymptomatic white male with a history of three CABG interventions.

Case Description

Subclavian artery stenosis jeopardizing LIMA to LAD graft is evidenced (Fig. 1a,b). Subclavian artery disease is the most common cause of failure of internal mammary artery bypass conduits.

Figure 2a,b shows intact SVG to D1 and first obtuse marginal (OM1) branches.

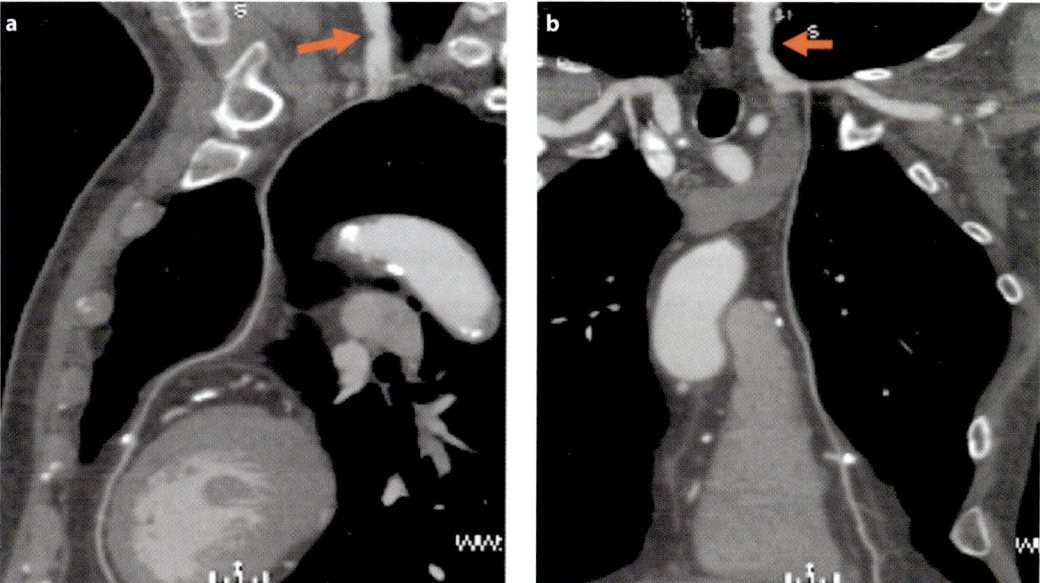

Fig. 1 a, b Subclavian artery stenosis jeopardizing LIMA to LAD graft

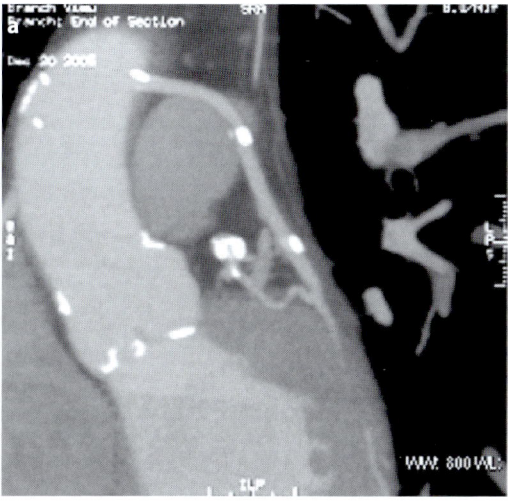
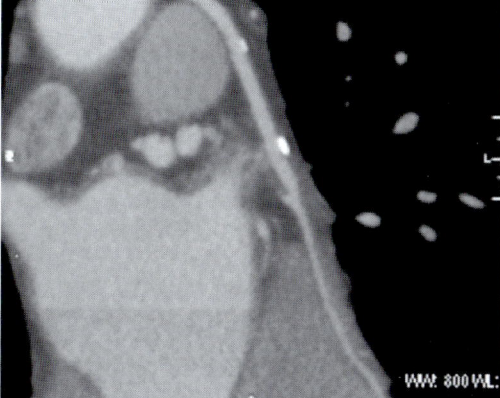

Fig. 2 a, b Intact SVG to D1 and OM1 branches

Case 49
Internal Mammary Arteries Bypass: Follow-Up

Patient: 75-year-old patient who underwent a surgical bypass procedure 6 years before.

Case Description

The VRT images in Figure 1a–c show the patent internal mammary arteries. Both adequate flow and the distal anastomosis are well documented in this coronary CTA.

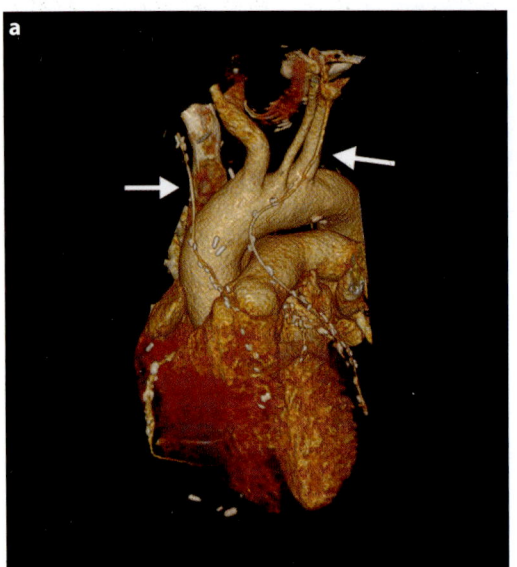
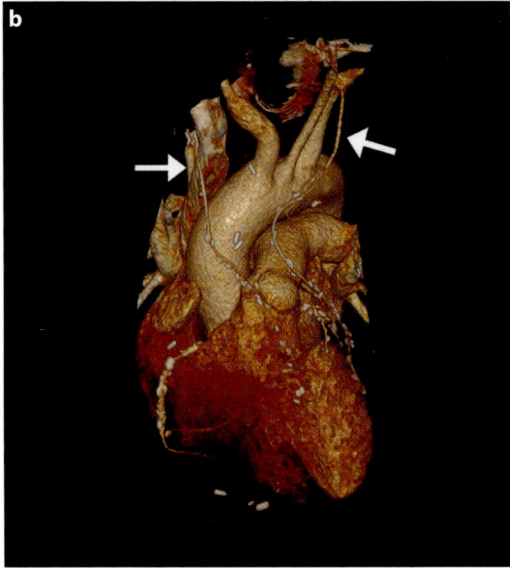
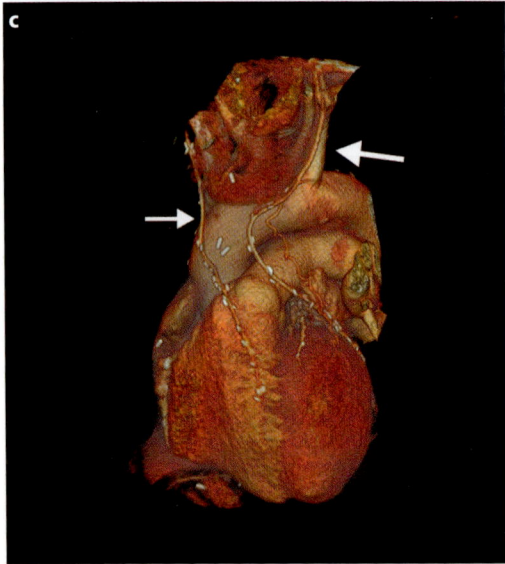

Fig. 1 Images show patent bypasses

Case 50
CABG Evaluation

Patient: 58-year-old internist with chest pain.

Case Description

A high-grade LAD stenosis was present in this case. Mild disease of LCX and RCA are depicted in Figure 1a-c.

The patient undergoes four successful coronary artery bypass grafting (CABG) interventions, followed by routine postoperative SPECT study that revealed anterior ischemia.

High-grade stenosis of the left internal mammary artery (LIMA) and LAD anastomosis is depicted in Figure 2a-c.

Figure 3a-c shows saphenous vein graft (SVG)-LCX patency and thrombosed SVG-RCA and SVG-first diagonal (D1). Bypassing uncompromised vessels may lead to acute graft thrombosis secondary to competing flow in the native vessels.

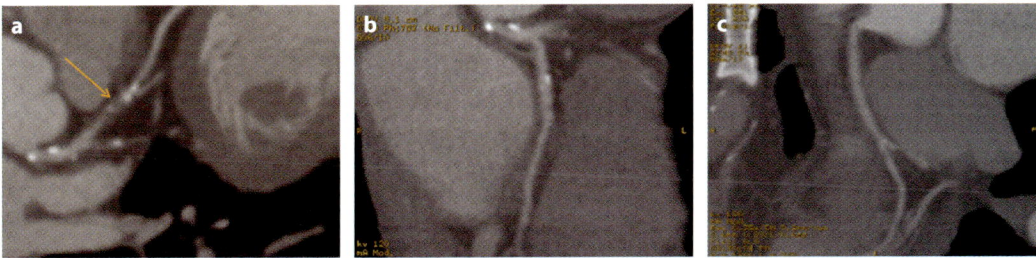

Fig. 1 a-c Mild disease of LCX and RCA

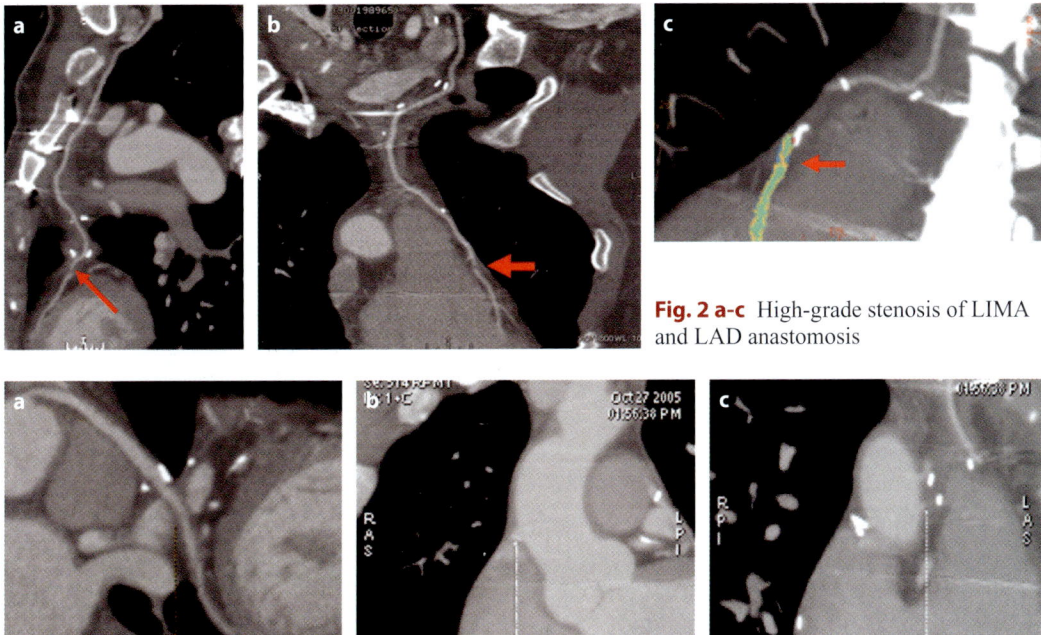

Fig. 2 a-c High-grade stenosis of LIMA and LAD anastomosis

Fig. 3 a-c SVG-LCX patency and thrombosed SVG-RCA and SVG-D1

Case 51
Stent Evaluation with Coronary CTA

Patient: 49-year-old white female with chest pain, presents with ST elevation at 13 METS of exercise. SPECT images are normal.

Case Description

False negative myocardial perfusion imaging may be unreliable (Fig. 1a,b). Conversely, CCTA has a negative predictive value of 100% (Fig. 2a,b).

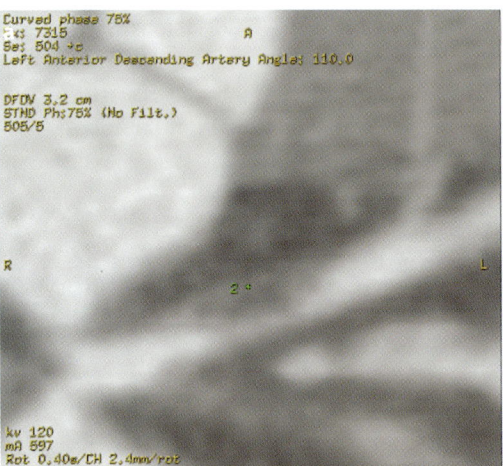
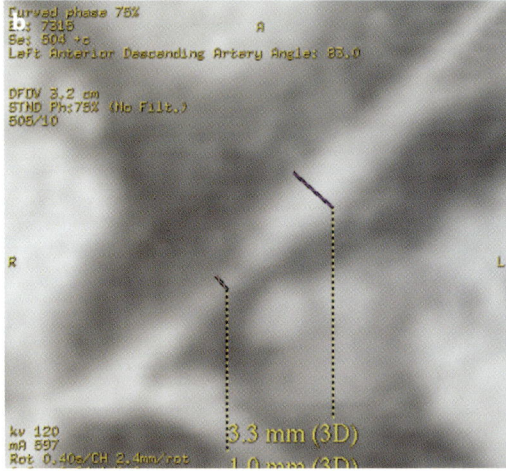

Fig. 1 a, b False negative myocardial perfusion imaging may be unreliable

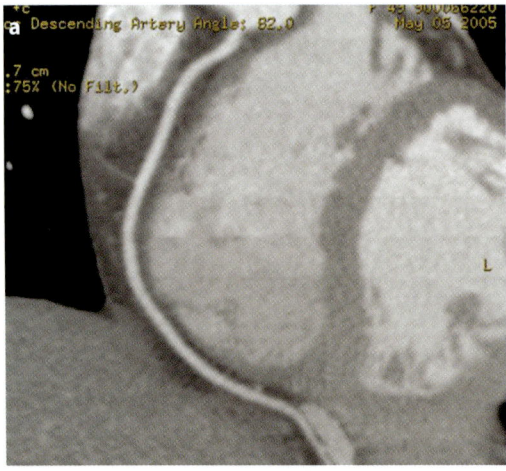
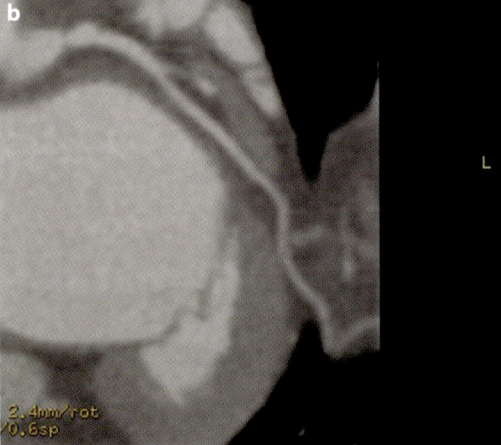

Fig. 2 a, b CCTA 100% negative predictive value

The same patient complained of chest pain one week later. CCTA is a good test to evaluate stents greater than 3 mm in size, as may be seen in Figure 3a,b, where there is no evidence of in-stent restenosis

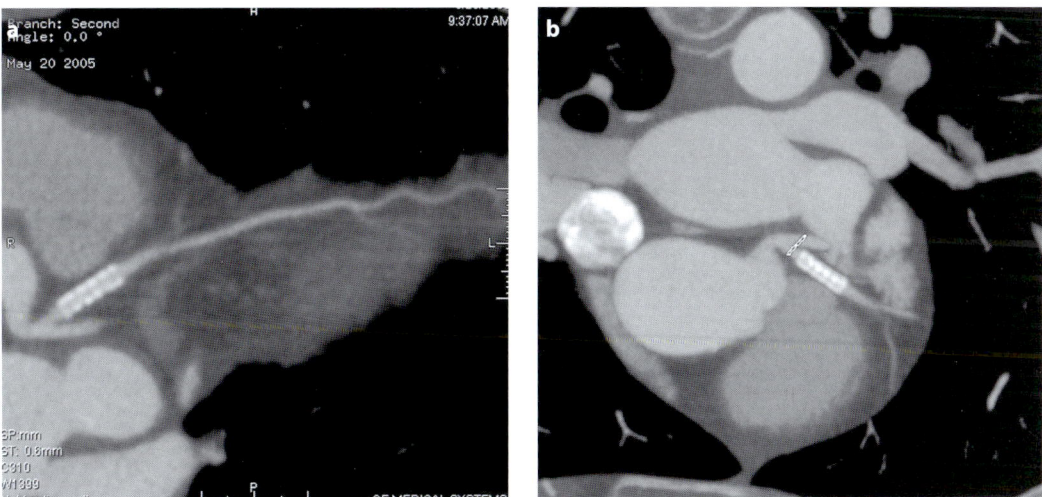

Fig. 3 a, b CCTA as a reliable test to evaluate stents greater than 3 mm in size

19.7 Stress Test

Case 52
Dangerous False Negative Stress Test Results

Patient: 39-year-old white male with chest pain. Stress testing provided normal results. Risk factors consisted in +FHx, hypercholesterolemia and HTN.

Case Description

Figure 1 shows high-grade LAD stenosis. Again, high-grade LAD stenosis is depicted, with normal LCX and RCA (Fig. 2a-c). CCTA has a negative predictive value of 100%, whereas stress tests do not reach the same levels. The results could have been tragic in this case if CCTA had not been performed.

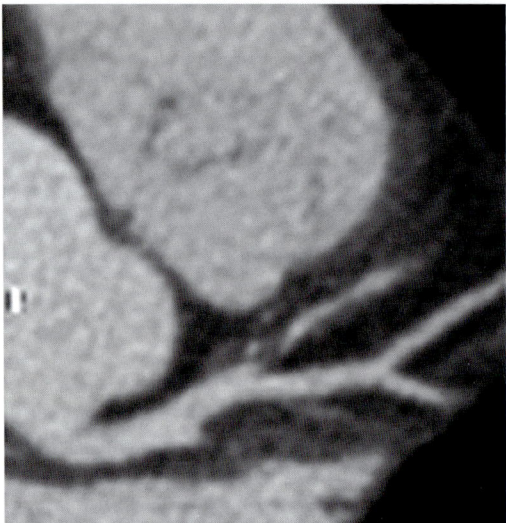

Fig. 1 High-grade LAD stenosis

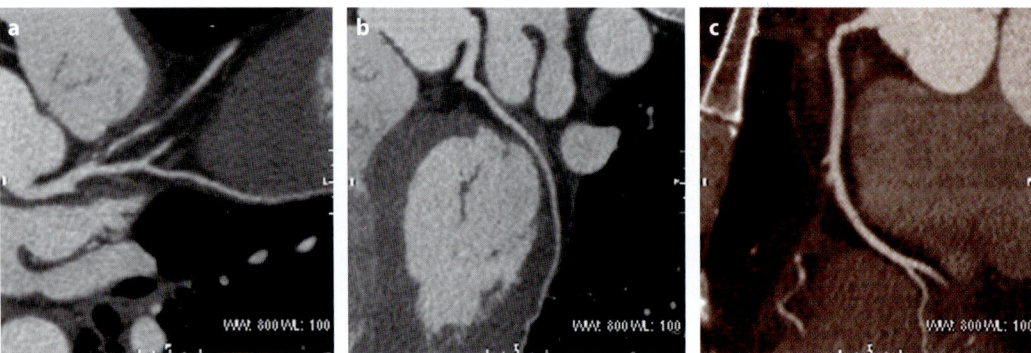

Fig. 2 a-c High-grade LAD stenosis with normal LCX and RCA

Case 53
Dangerous False Negative Stress Test Results

Patient: 45-year-old white female with chest pain. Risk factors consisted in +FHx, ex-smoker. Single-photon emission computed tomography (SPECT) stress performed five months before was negative, although pain persisted.

Case Description

Figure 1a-c shows 50-70% LAD stenosis. False negative stress tests are potentially dangerous; conversely, CCTA has a 100% negative predictive value.

Imaging shows normal RCA and a plaque at the LCX (Fig. 2a,b).

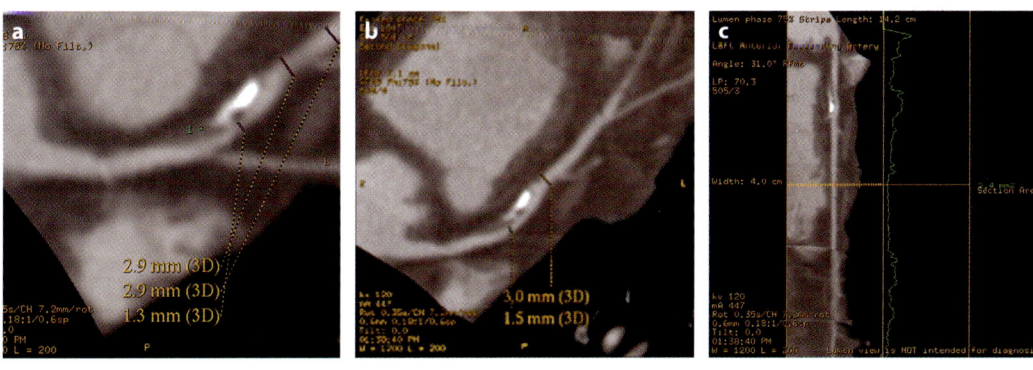

Fig. 1 a-c LAD stenosis (50-70%)

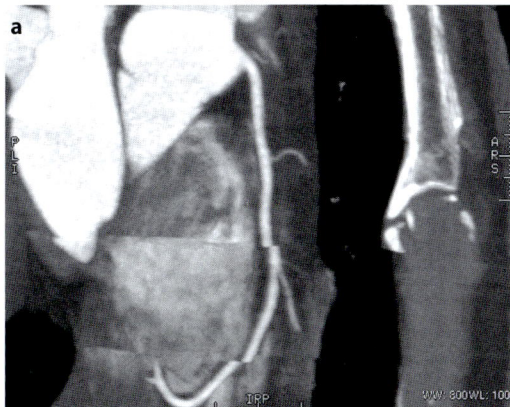

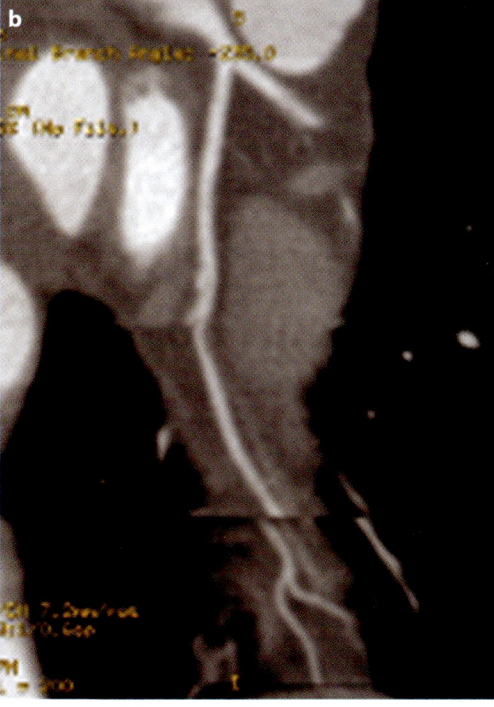

Fig. 2 a, b Normal RCA and plaque at the LCX

19.8 Valvular Disease

Case 54
Fibroelastoma of the Aortic Valve

Patient: 47-year-old white female, had suffered from cardiovascular accident (CVA) owing to an aortic valve mass. The patient could not undergo catheterization prior to valve replacement.

Case Description

Imaging shows fibroelastoma of the aortic valve (Fig. 1) and normal coronary arteries (Fig. 2a-c). CCTA can be used to rule out CAD in patients in whom coronary catheterization is contraindicated.

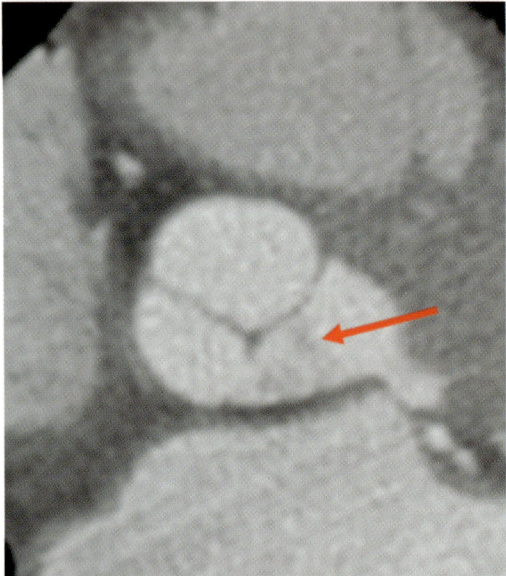

Fig. 1 Fibroelastoma of the aortic valve

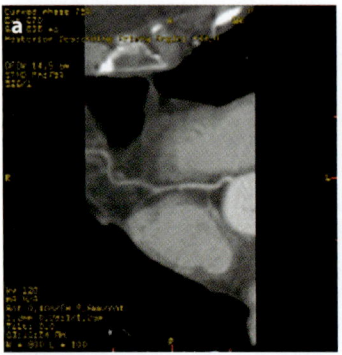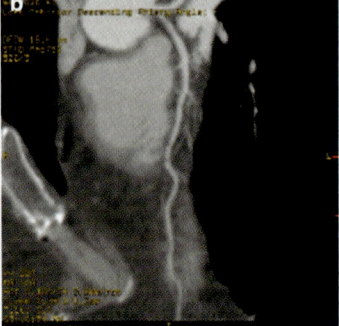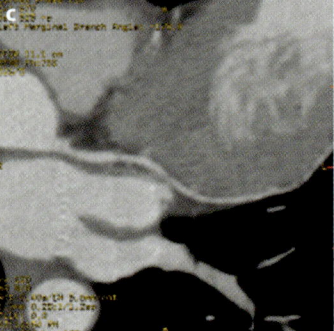

Fig. 2 a-c Normal coronary arteries

Case 55
Aortic Valvular Dehiscence in a Aortic Composite Homograft

Patient: 57-year-old white male, had undergone aortic valve composite homograft with a question of an aortic dissection.

Case Description

This patient went on to re-dissect his aorta requiring emergency surgery; imaging showed type-1 endoleak (Fig. 1a,b) and normal coronary arteries originating from the true lumen (Fig. 2a-c).

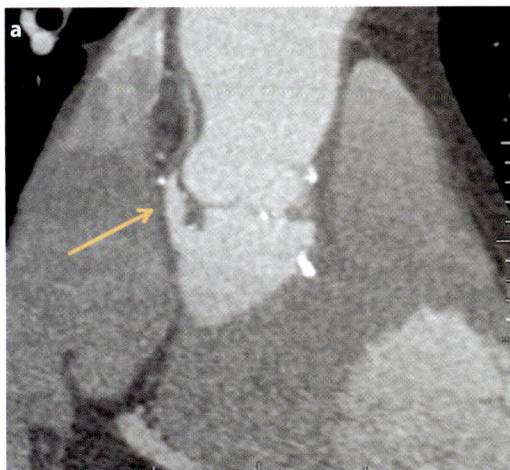
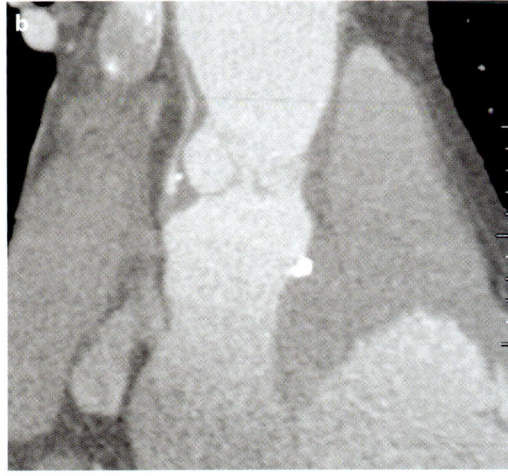

Fig. 1 a, b Type-1 endoleak

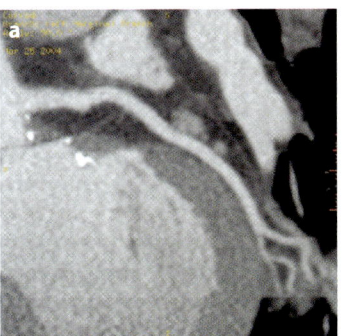
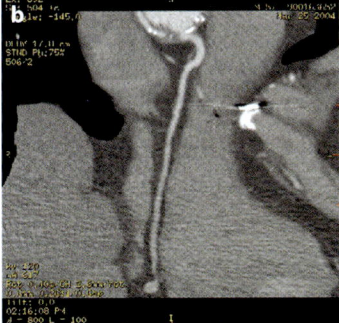
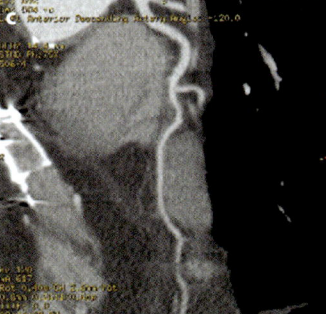

Fig. 2 a-c Normal coronary arteries originating from the true lumen

Case 56
Aortic Valvular Dehiscence in a Aortic Composite Homograft

Patient: 65-year-old white male with chest pain and history of a heart murmur.

Case Description

Bicuspid aortic valve with borderline hypertrophic cardiomyopathy (HCM) are depicted in Figure 1a-c.

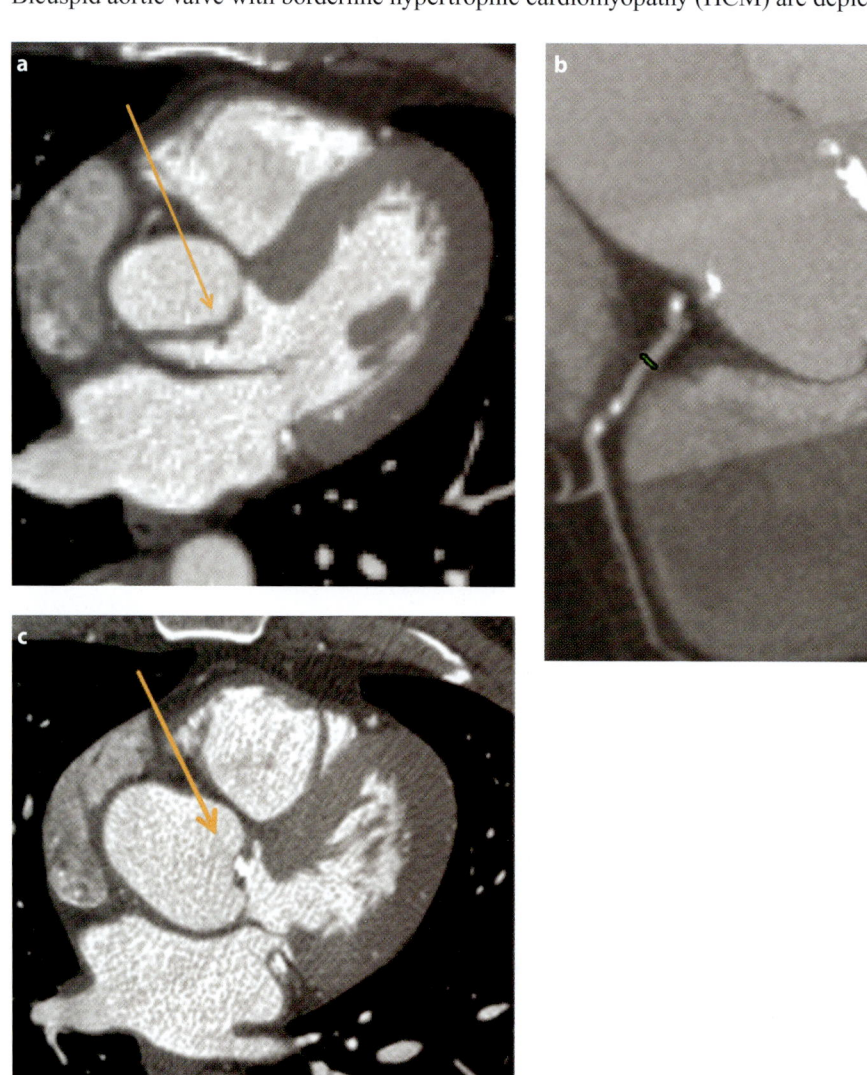

Fig. 1 a-c Bicuspid aortic valve with borderline HCM

19.9 Myocardial Infarction

Case 57
Arterial Expansion by Thrombus in an Acute, Anterior Wall Myocardial Infarction

Patient: 60-year-old white male with new EKG findings compatible with anterior wall myocardial infarction (AWMI).

Case Description

Imaging shows critical stenosis with/without thrombosis of the LAD (Figs. 1a-c, 2).

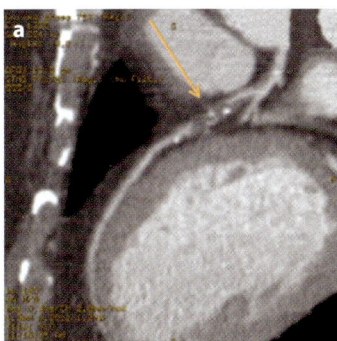
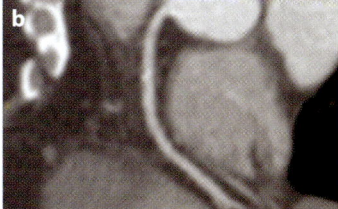
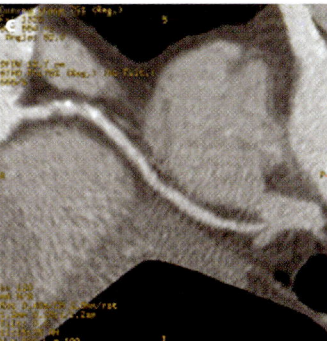

Fig. 1 a-c Critical stenosis with/without thrombosis of the LAD

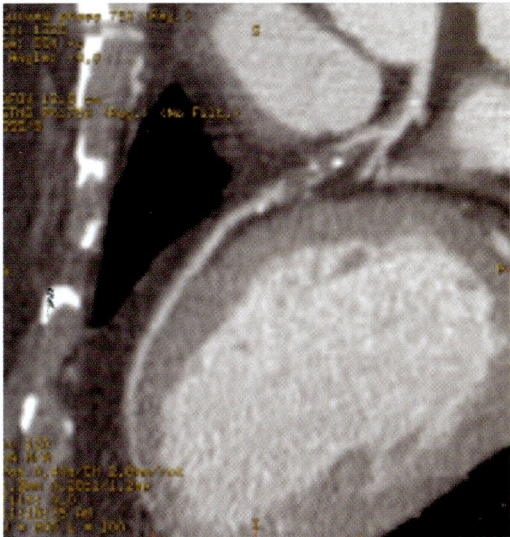

Fig. 2 Critical stenosis with/without thrombosis of the LAD

Case 58
Chronic Myocardial Infarction with Recanalization of the Left Anterior Descending Artery

Patient: 37-year-old asymptomatic Hispanic female with a history of an anterior MI in 1996. A scar was evidenced on SPECT Myoview.

Case Description

Imaging showed apical infarct (Fig. 1a,b), normal LCX, and mild RCA disease (Fig. 2a,b). Mild LAD disease is also present, which probably represents the healed remains of a ruptured vulnerable plaque (Fig. 3a,b). Recanalized vessels may lead to infarcted myocardium.

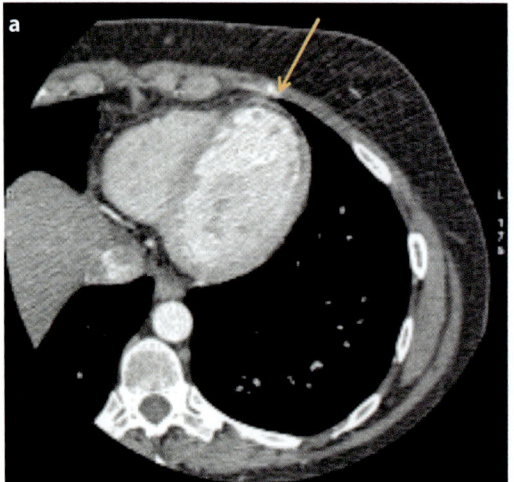 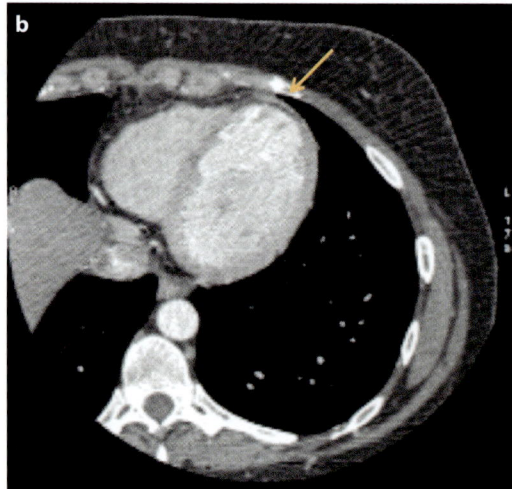

Fig. 1 a, b Apical infarct

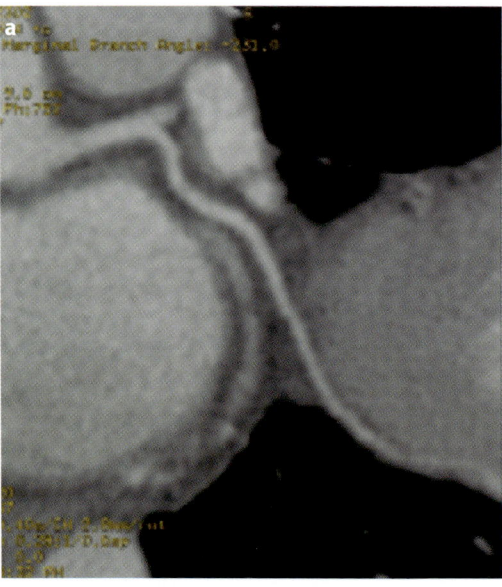 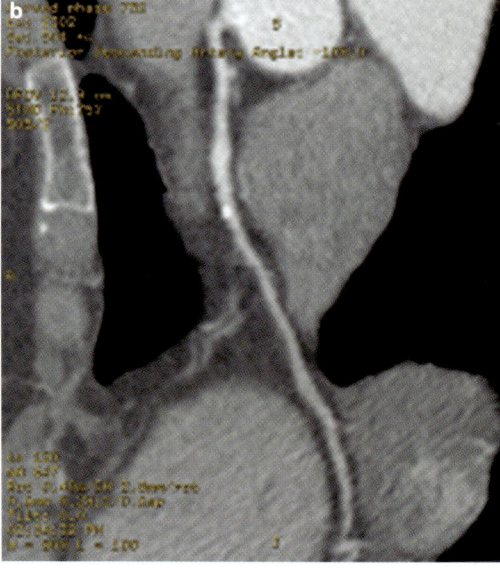

Fig. 2 a, b Normal LCX and mild RCA disease

19 Clinical Cases

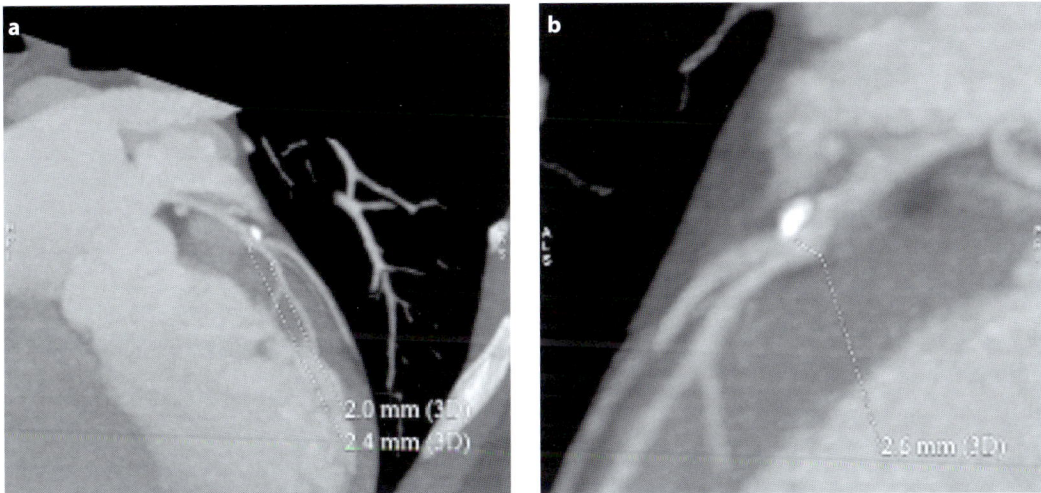

Fig. 3 a, b Mild LAD disease

Case 59
Clinical Diagnosis of Myocardial Infarction in Two Patients with Completely Normal Coronary Arteries

Patients: 55-year-old female and 65-year-old male, both diagnosed with acute myocardial infarction (clinical symptoms, positive enzymes, and EKG changes indicative of non STEMI). CTA was performed at follow-up, after 6 months, and again one year from the clinical episode.

Case Description

Figure 1a, b shows the axial slices from the coronary CTA acquisition. In Figure 1b, there is a mild subendocardial hypodensity of the myocardial tissue, indicative of previous infarction. In the VRT images of the coronary arteries shown in Figure 1c, d, the findings are completely normal: there are no stenoses nor is there parietal atheromatous involvement.

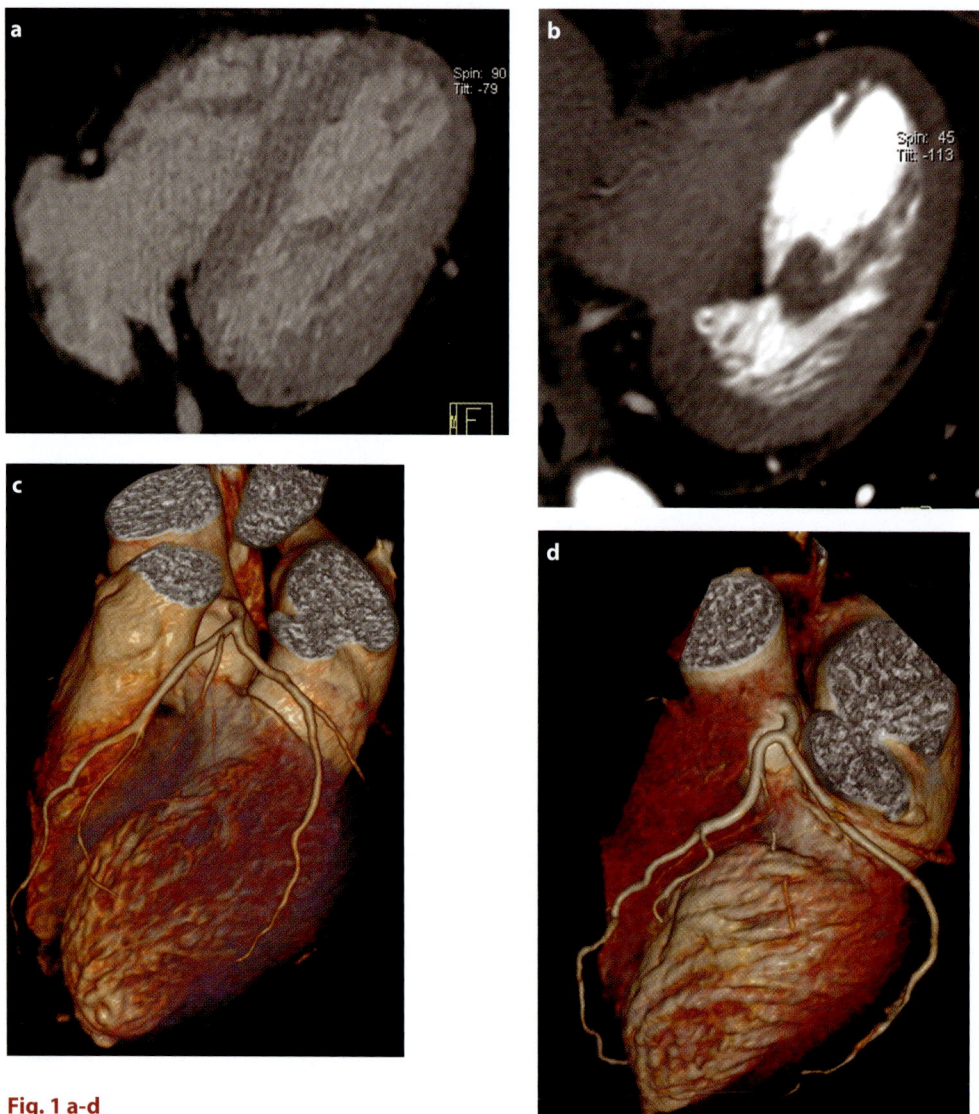

Fig. 1 a-d

19.10 Coronary and Cardiac Anatomical Defects

Case 60
Interarterial Coronary Artery Anomaly

Patient: 70-year-old white male with intermittent exertional angina.

Case Description

Interarterial anomalous left main artery (LMA) is depicted in Figure 1a,b. When coronary artery anomalies pass between the aorta and pulmonary artery they carry a 1% risk of sudden death. The risk of sudden death increases if it is the left coronary artery crossing to the right side and if the vessel has an acute angle off of the aorta. Figure 2a,b shows mild RCA and LCX disease.

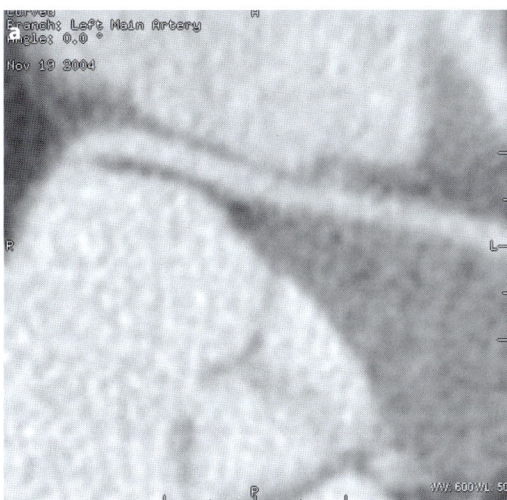 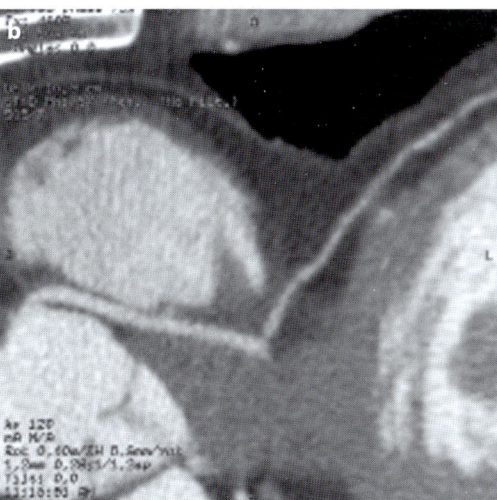

Fig. 1 a, b Interarterial anomalous LMA

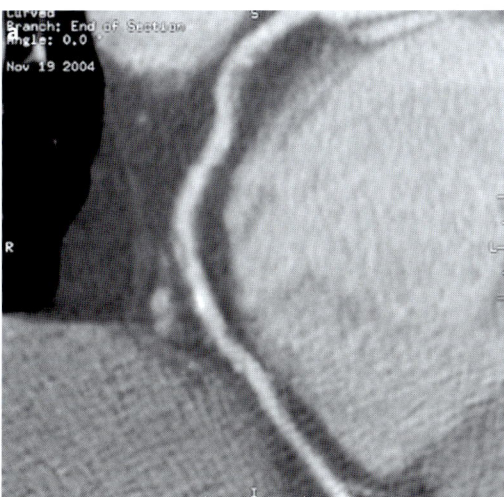 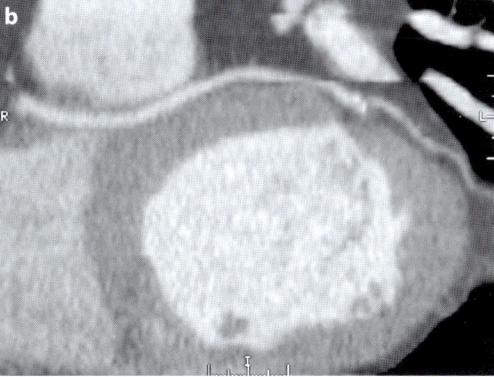

Fig. 2 a, b Mild RCA and LCX disease

Case 61
Atherosclerotic Coronary Artery Aneurysms

Patient: 50-year-old asymptomatic white male with a history of MI 16 years before. Risk factors consisted in +FHx, hypercholesterolemia, and HTN.

Case Description

RCA atherosclerotic aneurysms are depicted in Figure 1a-c. Diffuse arterial ectasia is a risk factor for myocardial ischemia secondary to slow flow.

Diffuse coronary ectasia is present (Fig. 2a-d)

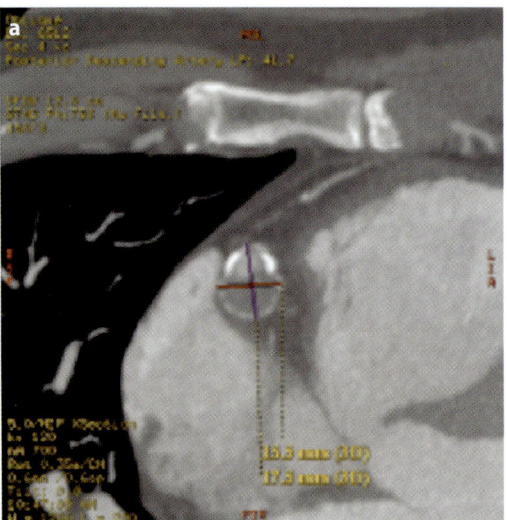
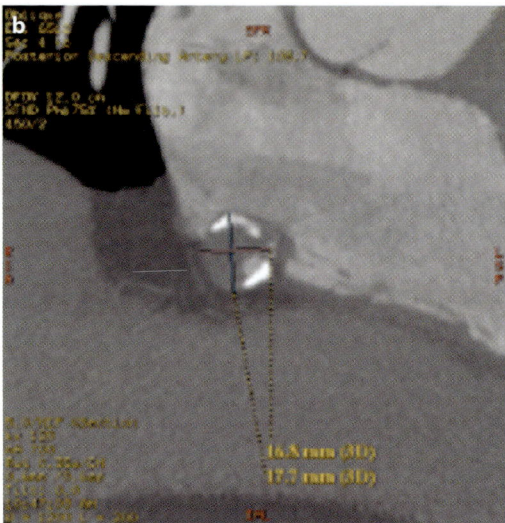
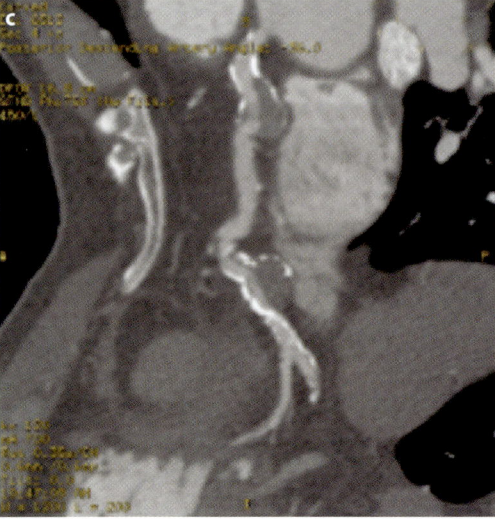

Fig. 1 a-c RCA atherosclerotic aneurysms

19 Clinical Cases

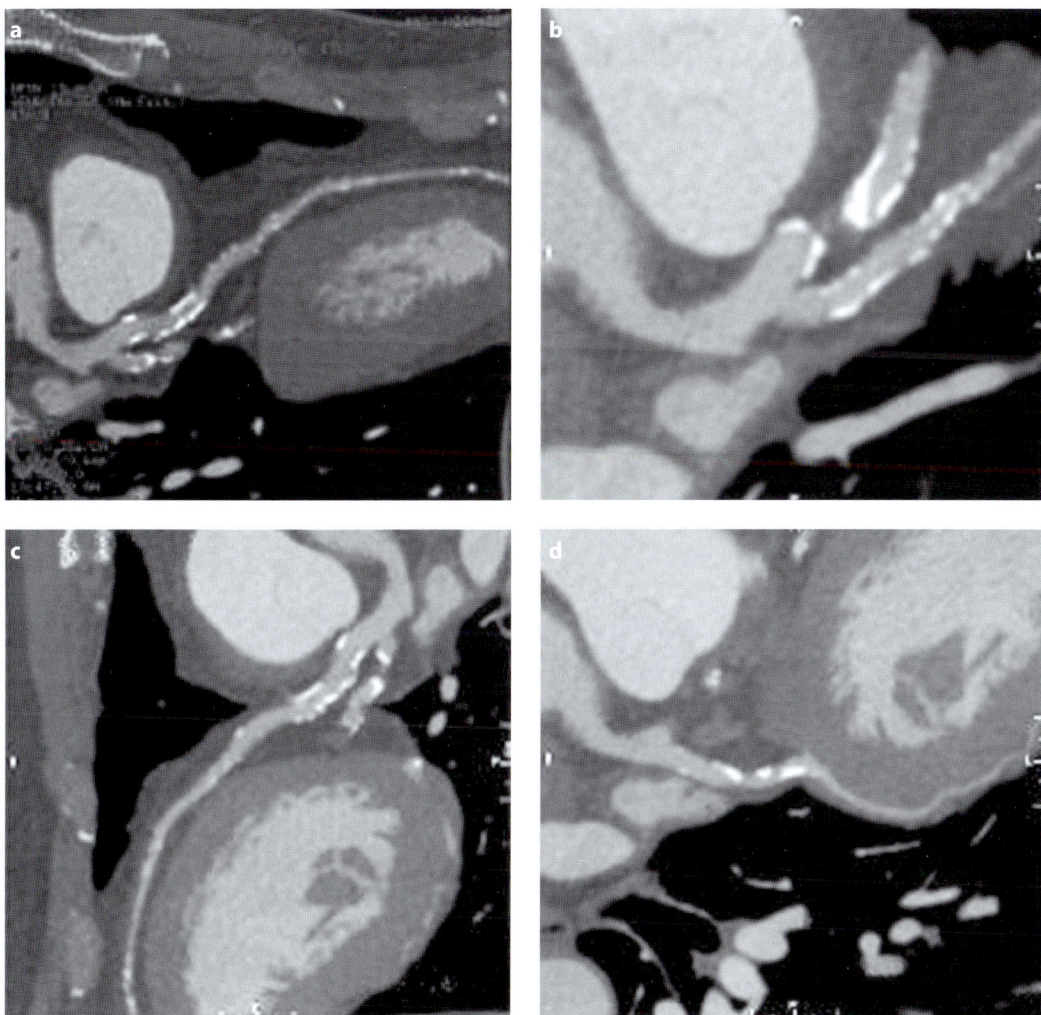

Fig. 2 a-d Diffuse coronary ectasia

Case 62
Right Coronary Artery to Pulmonary Artery Fistula with Coronary Steal from Left to Right Shunt

Patient: 62-year-old white female with chest pain.

Case Decription

Images show abrupt caliber change at the RCA (Fig. 1a,b), patent LAD and LCX. Something is highlighted in the right lower lobe (RLL) (Fig. 2a-c).

Bronchiectasis is present, with left to right systemic-pulmonary collaterals (Fig. 3). The right internal mammary artery (RIMA) and bronchial arteries to the RLL (Fig. 4a-c) and the RCA to RLL left to right shunt are also visible (Fig. 5a-c).

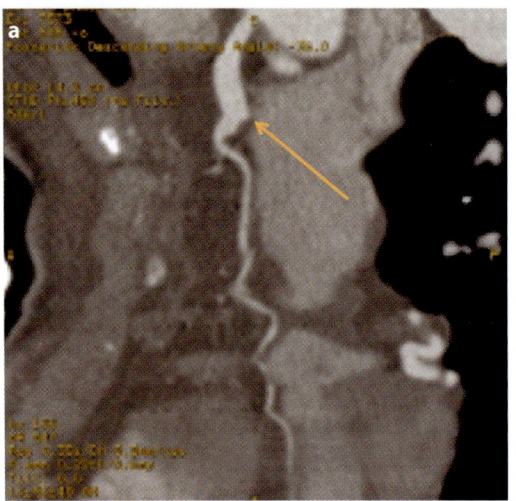
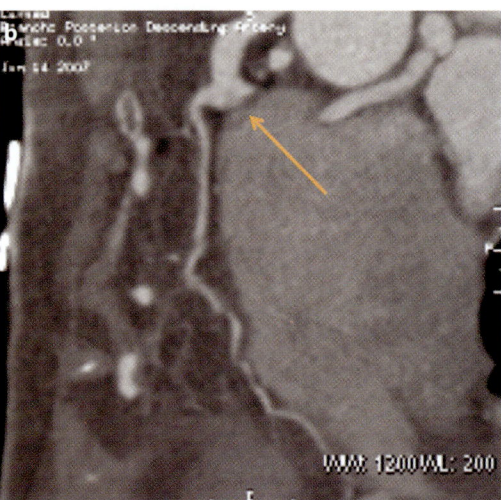

Fig. 1 a, b Abrupt caliber change at the RCA

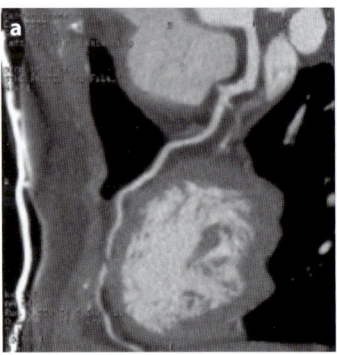
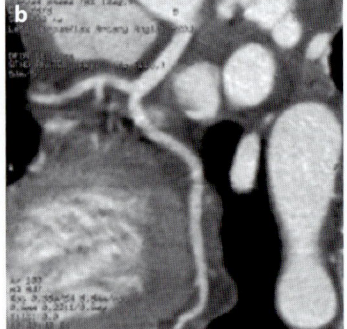
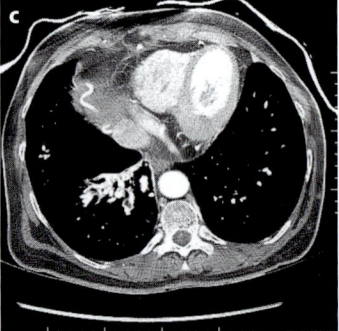

Fig. 2 a-c Right lower lobe

19 Clinical Cases

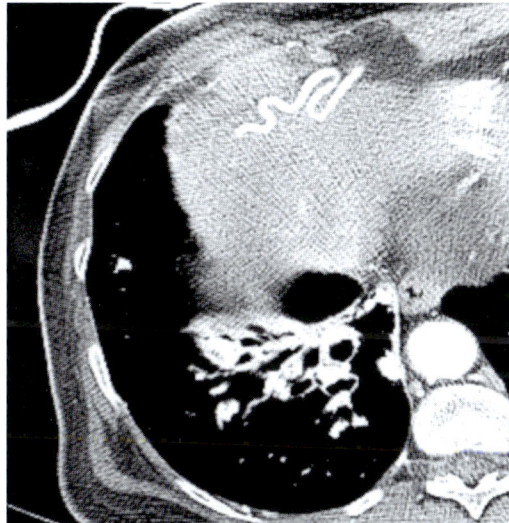

Fig. 3 Bronchiectasis with left to right systemic-pulmonary collaterals

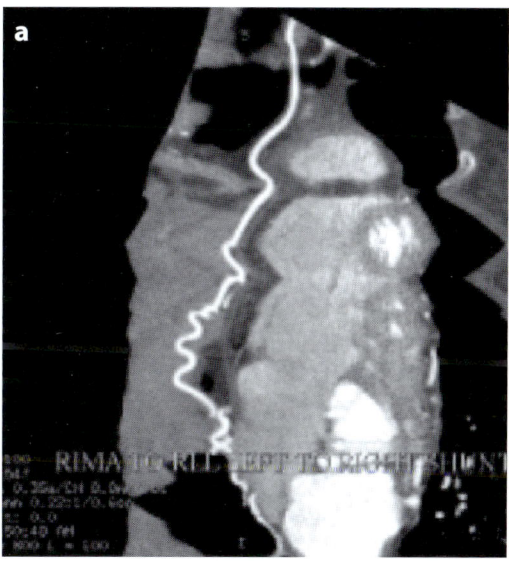

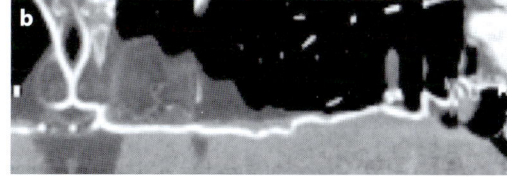

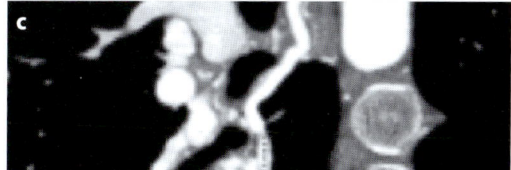

Fig. 4 a-c RIMA and bronchial arteries

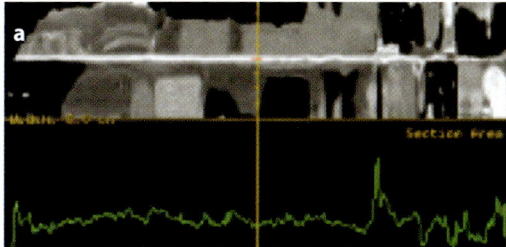

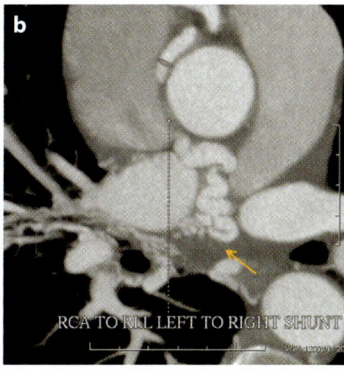

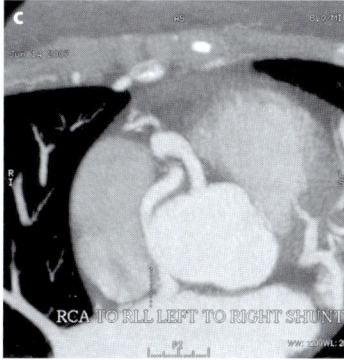

Fig. 5 a-c RCA to RLL left to right shunt

Case 63
Different Coronary Artery Anatomy in Identical Twins

Sometimes identical is not so identical: in this case the study concerned a couple of twins, whom we called "Baby A" and "Baby B".

Case Description

In Baby A, the RCA was normally positioned (Fig. 1a,b), whereas Baby B had an interarterial anomaly of the RCA (Fig. 2a,b), which proves that even identical twins can have different coronary artery anatomy.

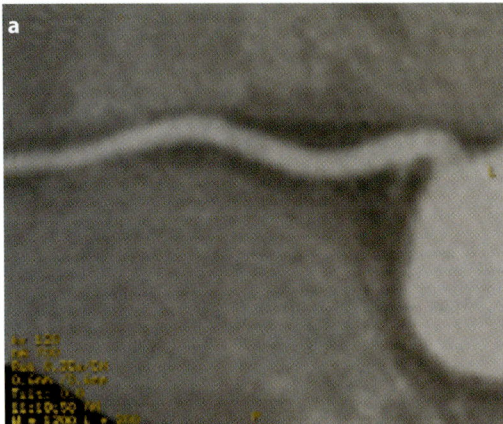
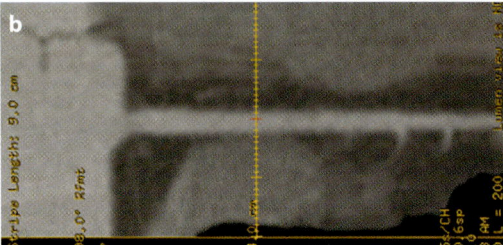

Fig. 1 a, b Baby A: normally positioned RCA

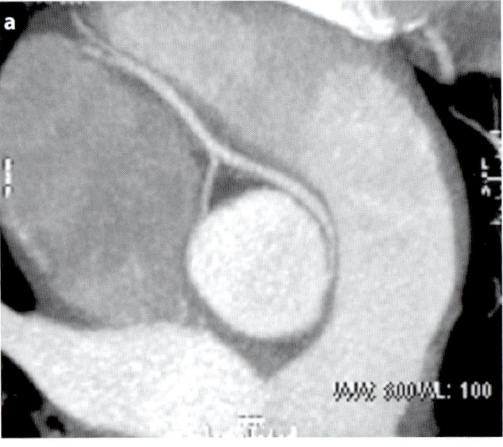
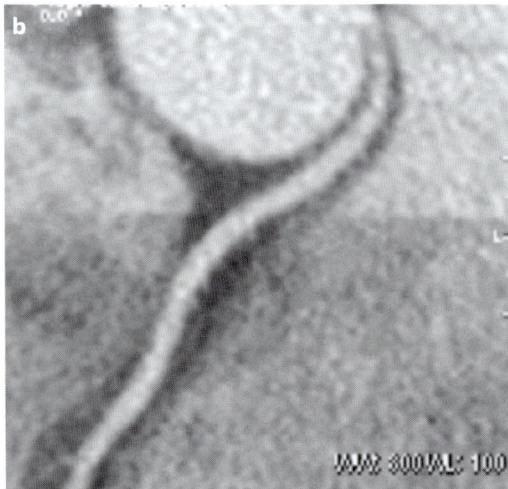

Fig. 2 a, b Baby B: interarterial anomaly of the RCA

Case 64
Intracavitary Right Coronary Artery

Patient: 60-year-old white female being worked up for pericarditis. The possible diagnosis may be of systemic lupus erythematosus (SLE) or scleroderma.

Case Description

Figure 1a-c shows pericardial effusion, and the RCA can not be identified. Further imaging shows an intracavitary RCA (Fig. 2a-d). Intracavitary coronary arteries are extremely rare. They should be pointed out prior to coronary artery dissection as part of bypass surgery.

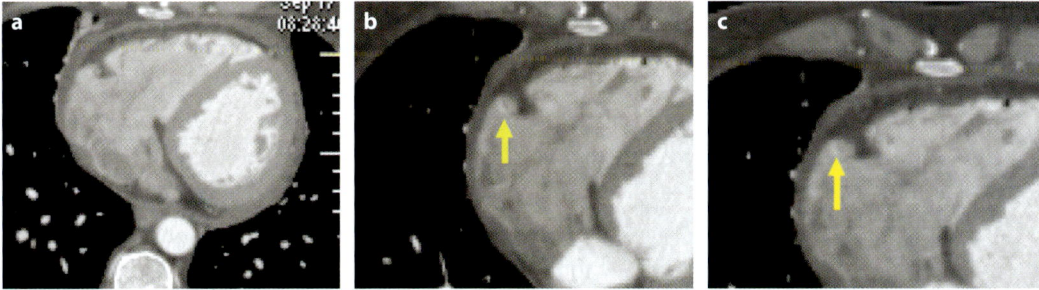

Fig. 1 a-c Pericardial effusion

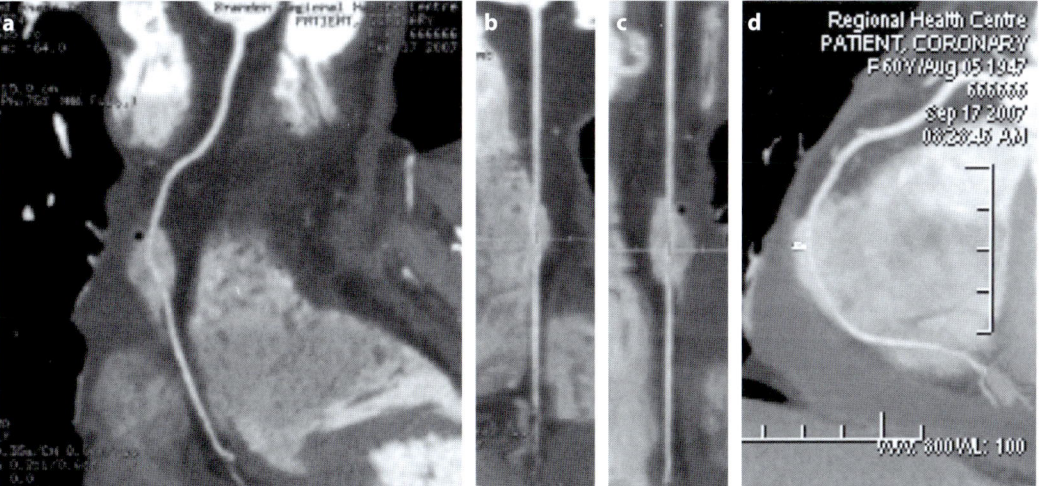

Fig. 2 a-d Intracavitary RCA

Case 65
Situs Inversus with Left Atrial Appendage Thrombus

Patient: 75-year-old white male with chest pain. The patient had undergone recent successful cardioversion for atrial fibrillation (A-fib).

Case Description

Imaging shows situs inversus and mild CAD (Fig. 1a-d) and a proven thrombus in the left atrial appendage (LAA) (Fig. 2). CCTA may yield false positive results for LAA thrombus secondary to under-filling.

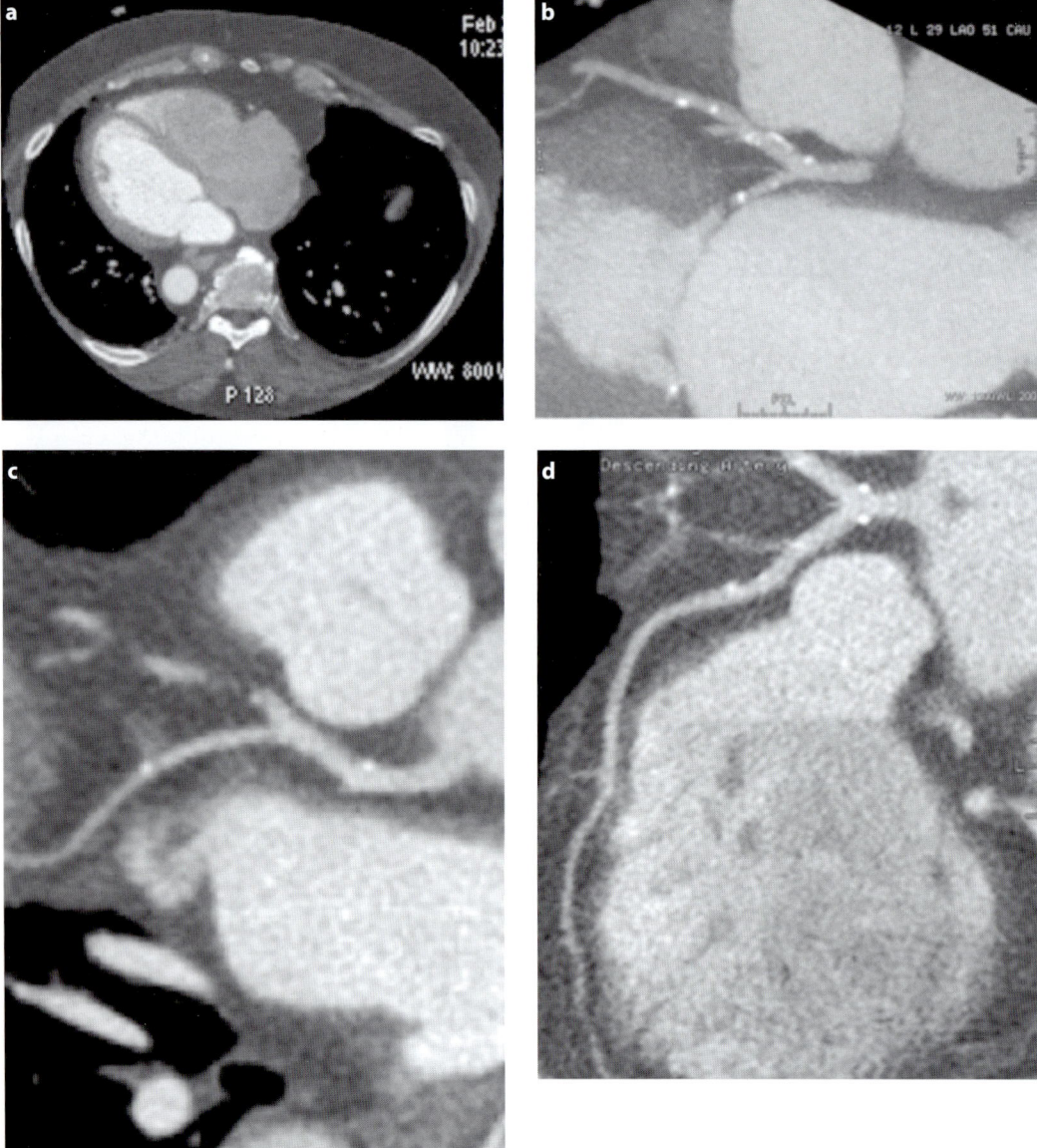

Fig. 1 a-d Situs inversus and mild CAD

19 Clinical Cases

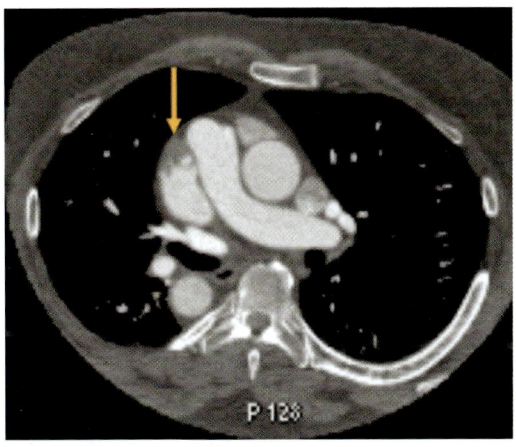

Fig. 2 LAA thrombus

Case 66
Coronary Artery Fistula with a Left to Left Shunt

Patient: 76-year-old white female with chest pain and SOB.

Case Description

Figure 1a,b shows epicardial arteriovenous malformation (AVM) supplied by LAD, PDA, LIMA and celiac arteries; epicardial AVM is also visible in Figure 2a-c.

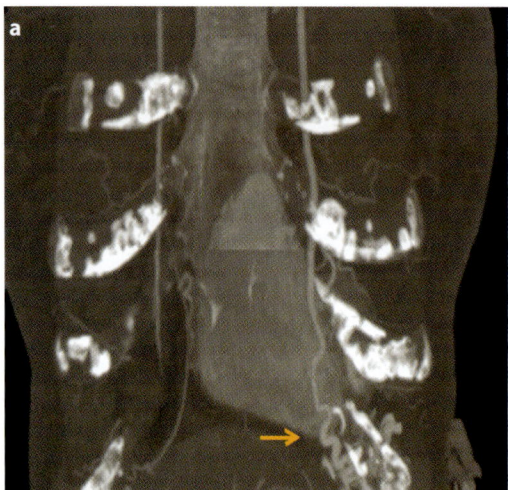
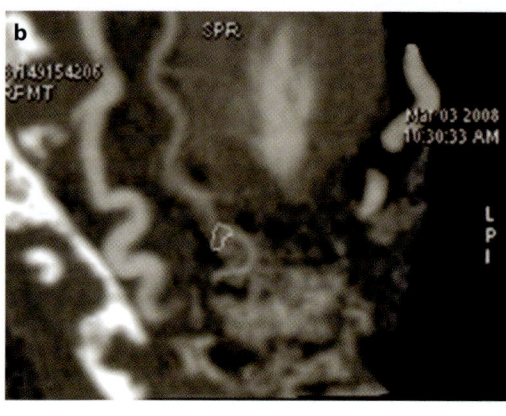

Fig. 1 a, b Epicardial AVM

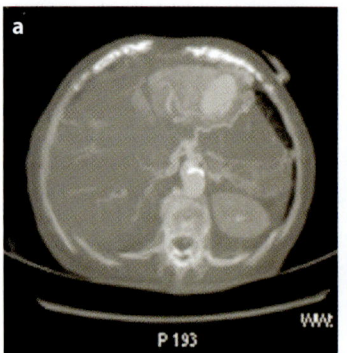
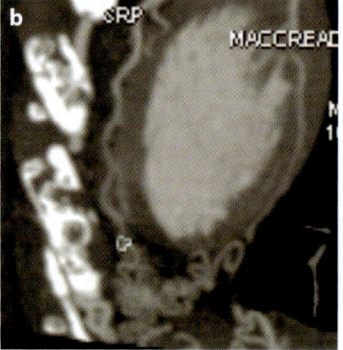
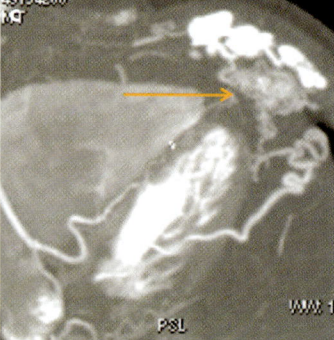

Fig. 2 a-c Epicardial AVM

Case 67
Patent Foramen Ovale

Patient: 65-year-old white female with shortness of breath (SOB) and abnormal EKG. The SPECT stress test was equivocal.

Case Description

Imaging shows a patent foramen ovale with mild CAD (Fig. 1). Careful examination of the source axial images should be performed to look for adult congenital heart disease.

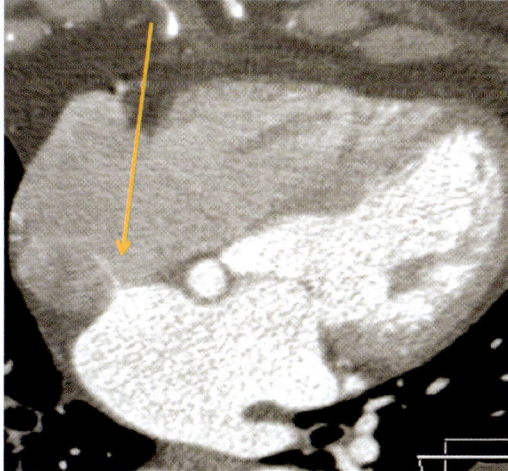

Fig. 1 Patent foramen ovale with mild CAD

Case 68
Anomaly of the Coronary Arteries

Patient: 48-year-old patient with intermediate risk factors (hypertension, smoking) who underwent coronary CTA as a screening procedure.

Case Description

An anomalous origin of the left coronary artery from the right coronary sinus is seen in Figure 1a, b.

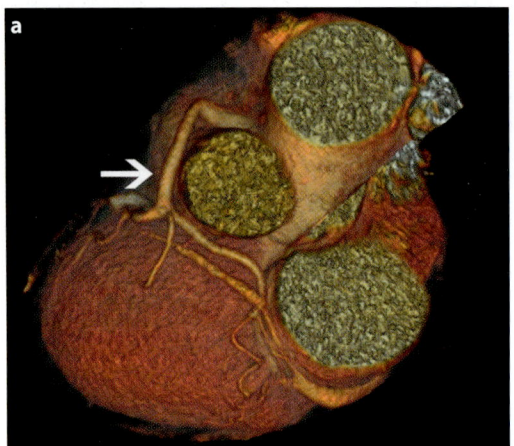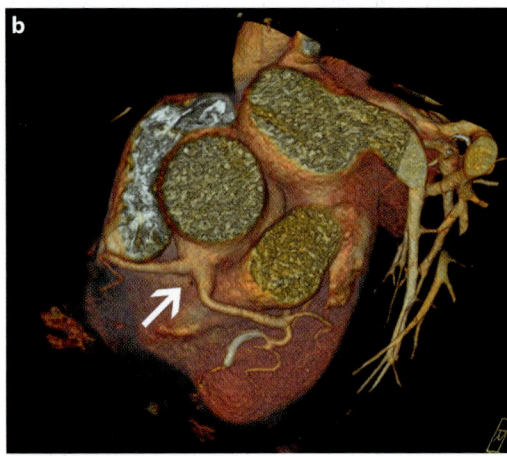

Fig. 1 a, b Anomalous origin of the left coronary artery from the right coronary sinus

Case 69
Adult Congenital Heart Disease

Patient: 60-year-old white female with chronic chest pain, presents with mild coronary artery disease (CAD) (Fig. 1a-c) with large atrial septal defect (Fig. 2).

Case Description

It is important to evaluate axial source images. In this case, we found evidence of adult congenital heart disease in the form of an atrial septal defect with aneurysmal dilatation of the interatrial septum.

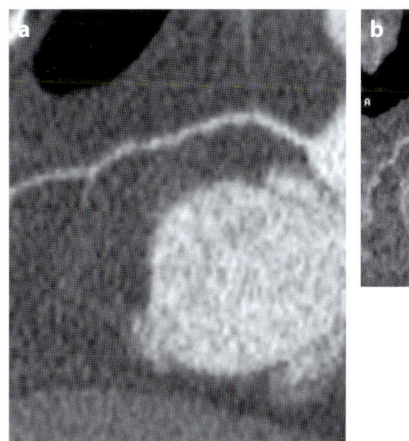
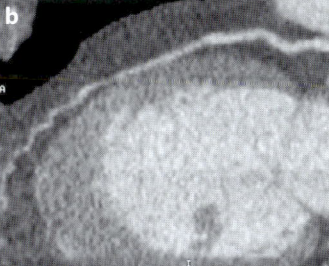
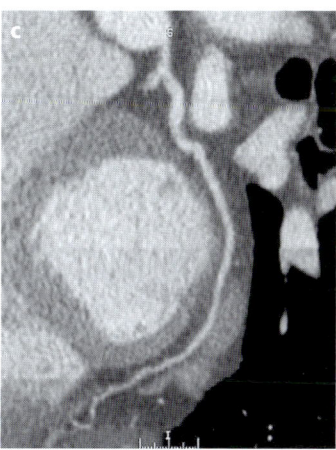

Fig. 1 a-c Mild CAD

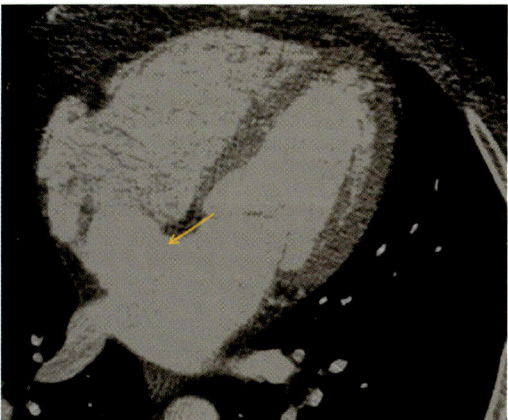

Fig. 2 Large atrial septal defect

Case 70
Congenital Coronary Artery Aneurysm

Patient: 39-year-old white female, asymptomatic, presents for evaluation of a known congenital aneurysm of the LAD.

Case Description

Imaging shows congenital LAD aneurysm (Figs. 1, 2a-d). The most common etiologies of coronary artery aneurysms are atherosclerosis, Kawasaki's Disease, congenital and post-traumatic causes.

Normal LCX and RCA are depicted in this case (Fig. 3a,b).

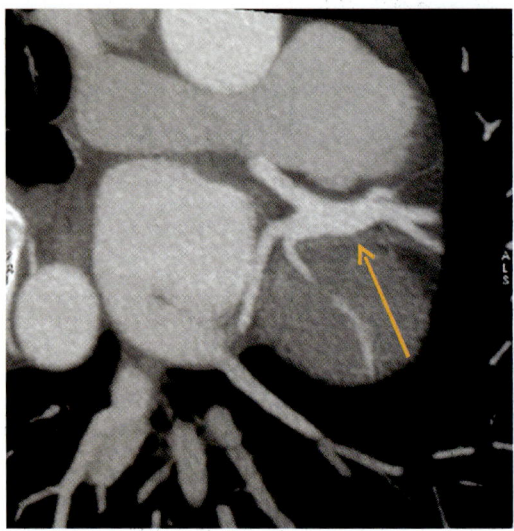

Fig. 1 Congenital LAD aneurism. Note that the first septal perforator, the LAD, the LCX and the first obtuse marginal arteries all originate off of the aneurysm

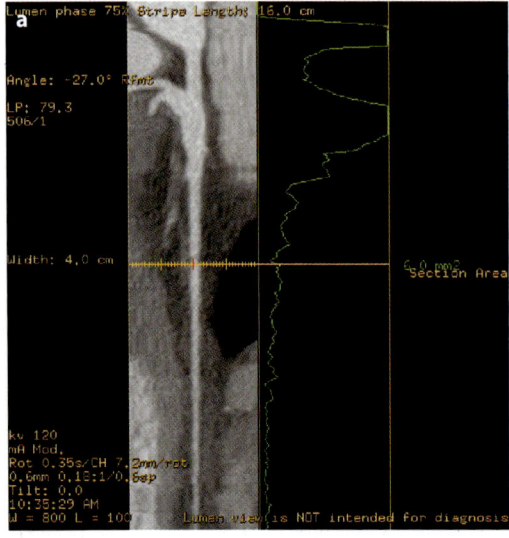
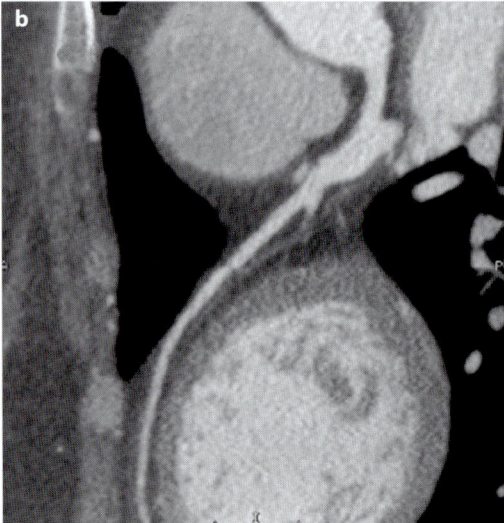

Fig. 2 a, b Congenital LAD aneurysm (*cont.* →)

19 Clinical Cases

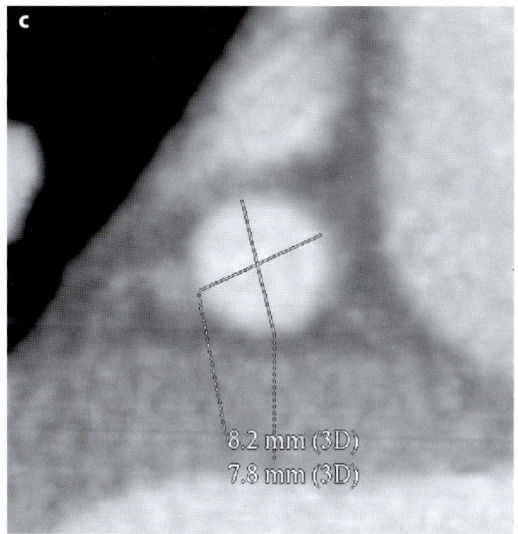
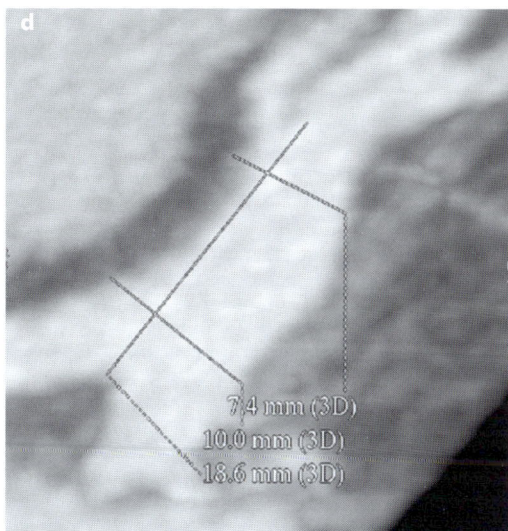

Fig. 2 c, d (continued)

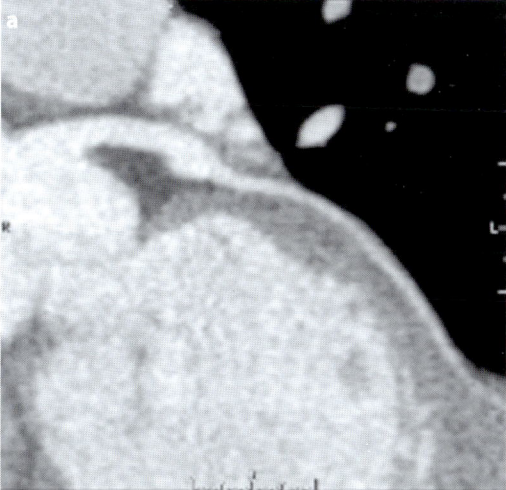
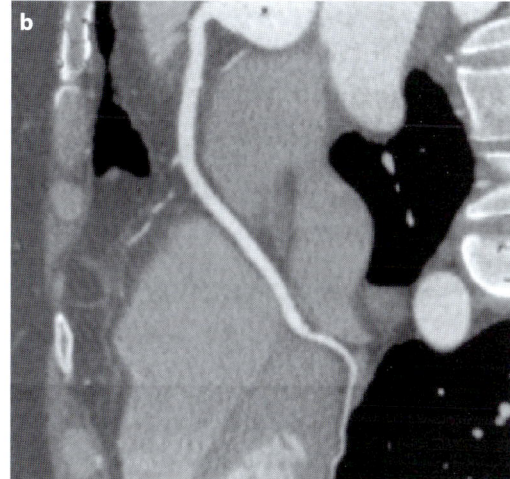

Fig. 3 a, b Normal LCX and RCA

Case 71
Myocardial Bridging

Patient: 81-year-old white male with chest pain.

Case Description

Imaging shows myocardial bridging of RCA and LAD (Fig. 1a,b). Myocardial bridging is a common variant of coronary artery course. Bridging occurs in up to 33% of patients and may be symptomatic when it involves the LAD (Fig. 2).

When myocardial bridging is combined with the idiopathic hypertrophic subaortic stenosis (IHSS) subtype of hypertrophic cardiomyopathy, there is an increased risk of sudden death (Fig. 3).

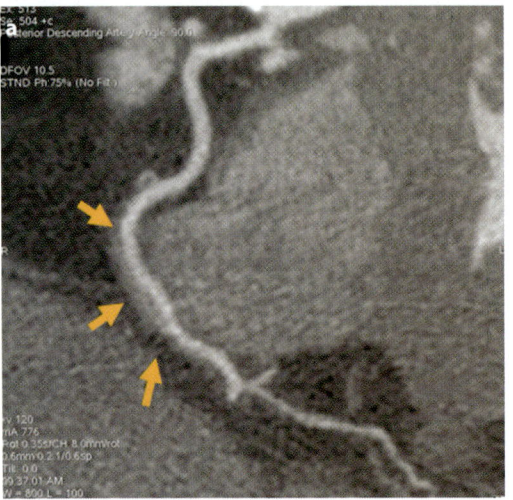

Fig. 1 a, b Myocardial bridging of RCA and LAD

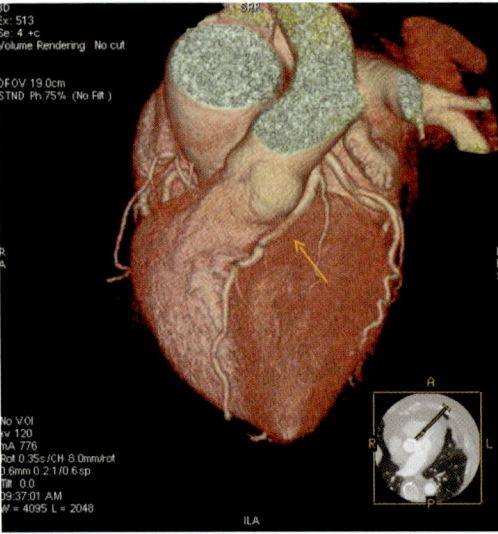

Fig. 2 Symptomatic bridging involving the LAD

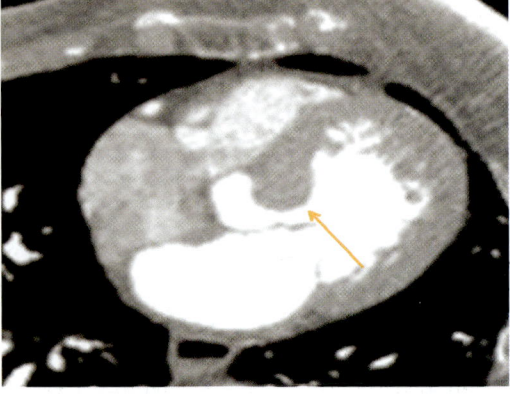

Fig. 3 Myocardial bridging combined with IHSS

Case 72
Coronary CTA Screening and an Incidental Diagnosis of Lung Cancer

Patient: 56-year-old male, non-smoker. No symptoms were present in this patient who underwent coronary CTA screening.

Case Description

The MPR (Fig. 1a) and VRT (Fig. 1b) images of the coronary arteries do not show evidence of stenosis. However, in this screening protocol, low-dose CT of the complete lung was also performed, which revealed a 3-cm lung lesion in the upper left lobe. Biopsy confirmed the diagnosis of lung cancer and the patient was submitted to surgery. We routinely complete coronary CTA with whole-lung acquisition. In fact, coronary CTA allows imaging of more than half of the lung volume. As radiologists, we feel that complete coverage of the chest should always be recommended.

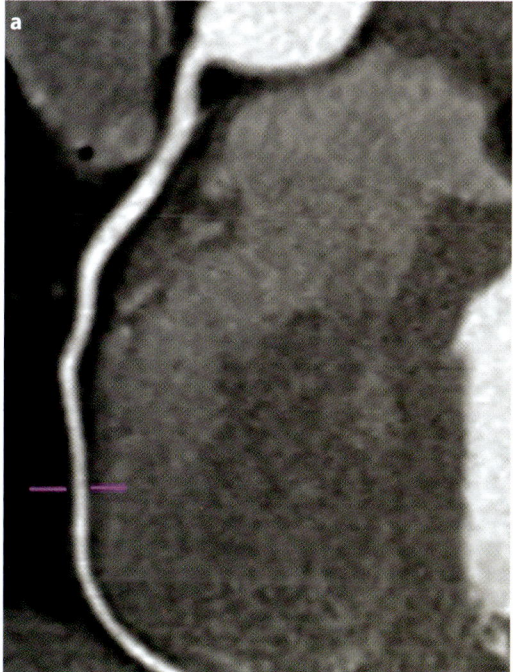 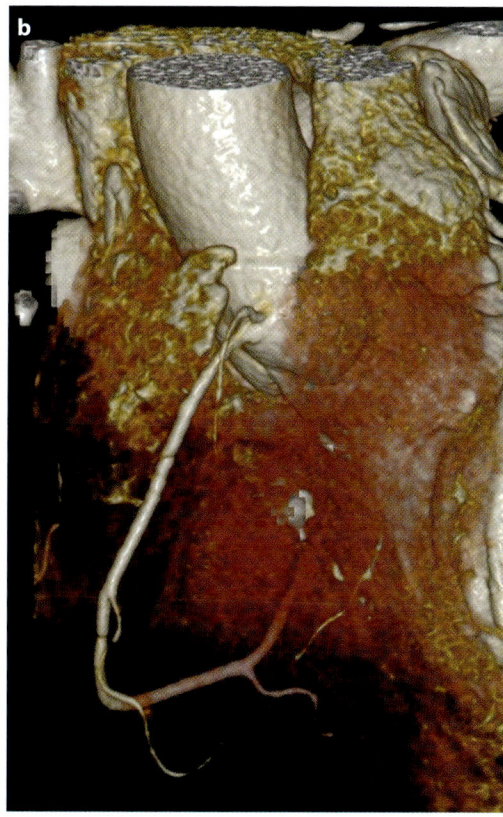

Fig. 1 a, b (*cont.* →)

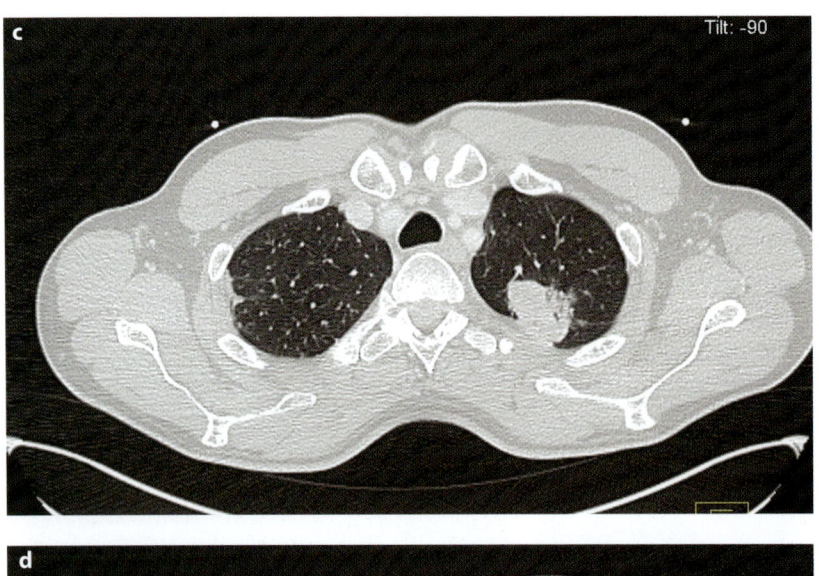

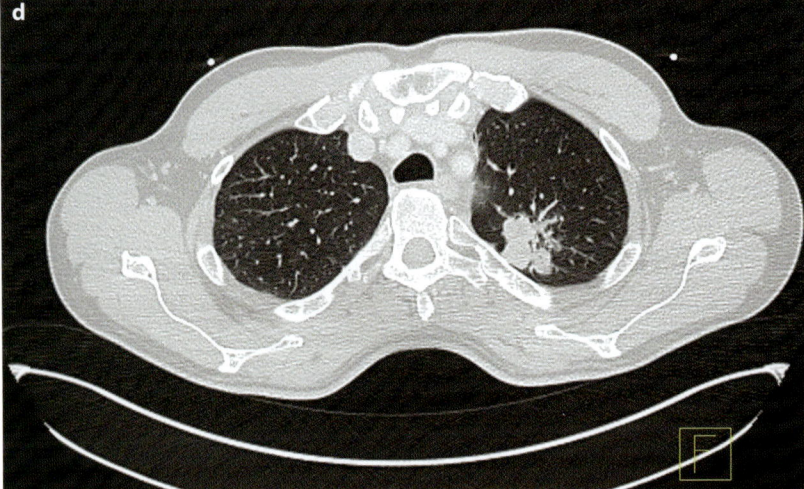

Fig. 1 c, d (continued)

Index

320-detector-row scanner 116
3D imaging 34

A

Acute coronary occlusions 78
Adenosine 41
Ambiguous lesions 142
Atherosclerotic burden 44, 70, 75
Atherosclerotic plaque 64, 71
Avantgarde 109
Axial images 29

B

Beam-hardening artifacts 118
Biodegradable polymer technologies 110
Blooming artifact 33, 117

C

Calcific plaque 66
Calcified plaque 72
Calcium 139
Cardiac energy metabolism 41
Cardiac volumes 97
Catheter angiography 80
Closed-cell 105
Coatings 105
Collateral vessels 122
Collimation 119
Convolution kernel 118
Coronary angiography 43, 44
Coronary artery bypass graft (CABG) surgery 91
Coronary artery segments 94
Coronary flow reserve 42
Coronary plaque 63
Coronary stenosis 44, 45
CRE8 108

Culprit 141
Curved reformatting 30
Curved images 33

D

Degree of stenosis 72
Density 29
Disease progression 94
Drug-eluting stent (DES) 106, 112, 115
Dual-source computed tomography (DSCT) 116

E

Endothelial cells 139
Engineering variables 102
Epicardial fat tissue 31
Everolimus 107

F

Fibrolipidic plaque 66
Fibrous cap 141
Fibrous plaque 140
Filtered back projection techniques 134
Fractional flow reserve 42

G-H

Graft kinking 91
Graft occlusion 93
Graft type 92
Hemodynamic consequences 71
High-pitch spiral acquisition mode 116
Hyperemic flux 44

I

Image editing 37
Indications for stent imaging 124

In-stent intimal hyperplasia 122
Intermediate lesions 142
Internal hemorrhage 67
Interpretation of cardiac CT 119
Intimal dissection 67
Intimal hyperplasia 118
Intravascular ultrasound (IVUS) 44
Ionizing radiation 131
Iterative reconstruction 117, 133

L

Large-diameter coronary stents 124
Lipid pool 139, 141
Lumen 64
Lumen caliber 74

M

Macrophages 141
Magnesium alloy 111
Malapposition 143
Maximum intensity projection 120
Medical therapy 70
Metallic clips 96
Minimal lumen area 142
Minimal lumen diameter 44
Mixed plaque 68
Multi-planar reformatting (MPR) 30
Myocardial capillaries 41, 42
Myocardial oxygen demand 42
Myocardial perfusion 76

N

Native arteries 97
Neointima formation 143
NEXT study 109
Non-invasive cardiac imaging, appropriateness criteria 124
Non-symptomatic individuals 125
Nuclear medicine procedures 135

O

Occlusion 78
Oncological risk 135
Open cell 104, 105
Optical coherence tomography (OCT)
    contrast medium 138
    frequency domain (FD) 137
    penetration depth 137
    pull-back starting point 138
    safety of FD-OCT 138
    stent guidance 143
    time domain (TD) 137
ORSIRO 107

P

Percutaneous coronary intervention (PCI) 115
Plaque
    burden 66
    components 64
    evolution 70
    rupture 141
    size 70
    volume 70
    vulnerable plaque 45, 67, 141
Polytetrafluoroethylene (PTFE) 106
Post-anastomotic segments 94
Post-processing techniques 120
Preoperative diagnostic tool 94
Prospective ECG-synchronization 116
Prospective gating procedure 132

R

Radiation exposure 81, 131
Radiosensitivity (of growing organs) 134
Ratio of uncovered/total stent struts 145
Redo intervention 94
Remodeling 77
Revascularization 125

S

Sequential grafts 92
Significant stenosis 76
Silent ischemia 48
Sirolimus 106
Snap and shoot approach 132
Soft claque 78
ST segment elevation myocardial infarction (STEMI) 49
    Non-STEMI 49
Stabilized atherosclerotic disease 68
Stable angina 48
Stenosis 63
Stenosis 71
Stent 101
    balloon-expandable stent 103
    fabrication method 103

follow-up 144
geometry 104
implantation 115
occlusion 121
patency
   sensitivity 123
   specificity 123
self-expanding stent 103
Subclavian arteries 96
Surgical approach 99
Syndrome X 51

T
Thrombosis 143, 144
Thrombus
   red thrombus 140
   white thrombus 140
Tissue components 139
Types of artifacts 118

U-V-X
Ulceration 67
Unstable angina pectoris 49
Vascular wall 63
Vasospastic or variant angina 51
Virtual endoscopy 39
Virtual lighting 35
Volume rendering 33
X-ray radiation exposure 135
X-ray tube 131

Printed in November 2012